A CULINARY JOURNEY

NEW COLOR EDITION REVISED AND EXPANDED

A CULINARY JOURNEY

A Personal Voyage into the World of Herbs, Spices, and Vegetarian Cuisine

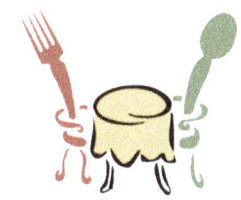

JOAN GREENBLATT

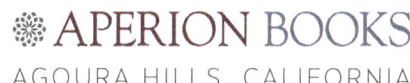

AGOURA HILLS, CALIFORNIA

APERION BOOKS™
Agoura Hills, California

Copyright © 2013-2022 by Joan Greenblatt

All rights reserved. No part of this book may be reproduced or transmitted in any form or by any means, electronic or mechanical, including photocopying, recordings, or by any information storage and retrieval system, without written permission from the author, except for the inclusion of a brief quotation in a review.

9 8 7 6 5 4 3 2
First Edition 2013
Revised and Expanded Color Edition 2022
Printed in the United States of America

ISBN: 978-0-9856039-6-0
Library of Congress Control Number: 2021924661

Book design by Joan Greenblatt
www.DynamicBookDesign.com

DEDICATION

The first edition is dedication is to my mother, Alice; my Grandma Molly; and Grandma-in-law, Pauline, whose love of cooking and feeding others seeped into my heart unknowingly. Then, one day, as I prepared my first meal in this lifelong culinary journey, the spirit of cooking rose from my soul like a released butterfly. It was always there, just waiting for the right moment to awaken.

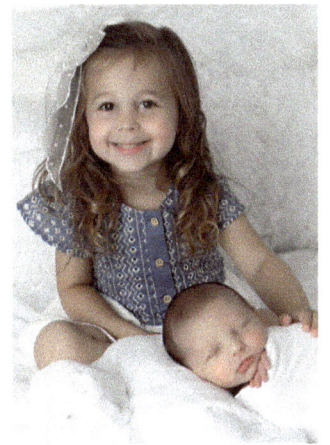

The second edition is dedicated to my grandchildren. To Ellie, who loves to bake with her Gaga, and Milo who loves to munch on "koukies" and "muffies." They bring boundless enthusiasm and joy to my life.

ACKNOWLEDGMENTS

"When eating bamboo sprouts, remember the man who planted them."
—Chinese Proverb

THIS COOKBOOK WAS COMPILED OVER A PERIOD OF OVER FORTY YEARS. There are more people who contributed to it than I can ever thank. Gratitude is sent to the many friends who joined our meals, filled with laughter and conversation, which often brought new insights long after the candles burned down.

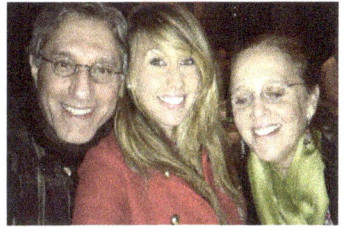

But most of all I would like to thank Matthew, my husband, who knew me well before I could prepare even the simplest of dishes. He has always supported me in the many projects I've undertaken and is the ultimate sounding board for many of these recipes.

Throughout the years of my experimentation in the kitchen, Ramani, our daughter, has learned to love tofu and discovered exotic spices that often wound up on our table. Many years ago, she gave me one of the most precious gifts I have ever received—a hand-made recipe box with the words, "Mom and Ram's Recipes," so that we could share and remember the times we created and discovered new culinary delights.

For years, my own mom was just a phone call away, offering support, love, and advice. I inherited her "Cook's Corner" box, which contains memories, recipes, and hundreds of newspaper clippings that bridged a lifetime of cooking with joy.

I also express deep gratitude to my recipe testers—those special friends who took their time and energy to test the recipes and offer invaluable advice. Without the following people this cookbook could not have been completed: Jeanne Salzman, Nancy Copen, Phyllis Kahaney, Robin Devine, Beverly LaRock, Judy Gordon, my sisters-in-law: Amy Ring, Carol Faro and Paula Faro, and especially to my sister of the heart, Chetna Bhatt.

Also, many thanks to the following contributors: Ki Holcomb, Garden Taste, Gina Bell Bragg, Nathan McMahon, and Dasaprakash. It was lovely spending time with each of these cooks and restaurateurs and gathering their special recipes and stories.

I am grateful to the two talented copy editors who helped to define the cookbook through valuable advice. Terrin Lovett not only created a style guide but also put on her apron and joined in testing several recipes. And my dear friend, Joan Loomis, who read the manuscript on several occasions, offered great editorial and style suggestions.

It was a joy to work on this unique cookbook with the support and love of such a unique team.

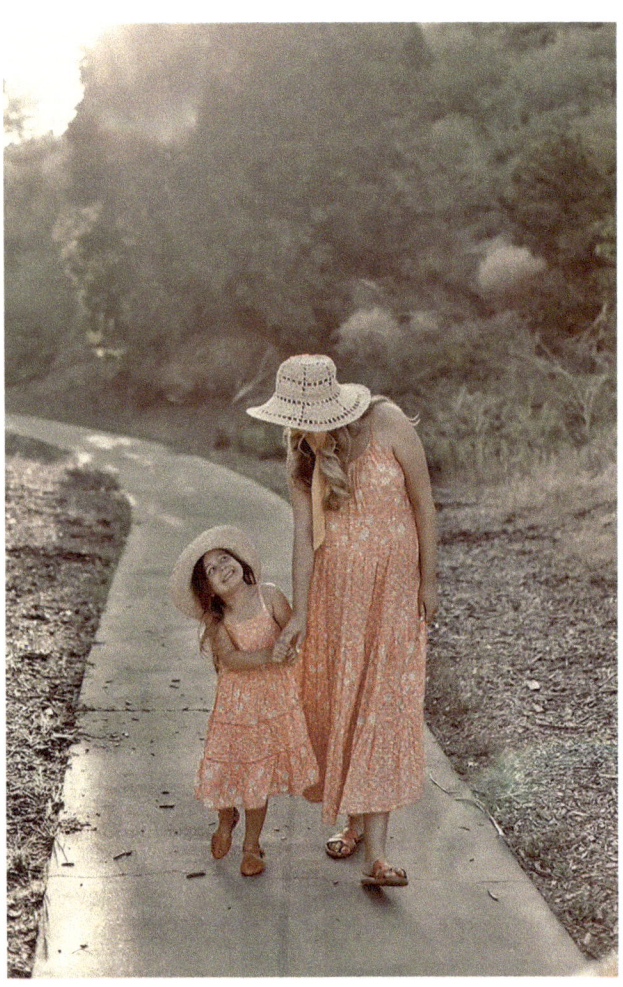

"THE MOST INDISPENSABLE INGREDIENT OF ALL GOOD HOME COOKING: LOVE FOR THOSE YOU ARE COOKING FOR."
—SOPHIA LOREN

TABLE OF CONTENTS

ACKNOWLEDGMENTS 7

INTRODUCTION
ABOUT THE SECOND EDITION 14
THE INTERDEPENDENT CIRCLE 15
EXPLORING HERBS, SPICES, AND HEALING FOODS 17
THE GENESIS OF A MANUSCRIPT 20

CHAPTER ONE: HEALING FOODS

MAGICAL GREENS 24
HEALING SOUPS 28
COOKING WITH FLOWER ESSENCES 33

CHAPTER TWO: THE BLUE ZONES

BLUE ZONE DIET 38
BLUE ZONE BREADS 46

CHAPTER THREE: VEGETABLES AND TOFU

- VEGETABLES FROM THE FARM 54
- A DAY IN THE LIFE OF TOFU 63
- VEGGIE BURGERS 67
- SATURDAY MARKET MORNING 72
- SUMMER TOMATOES 75

CHAPTER FOUR: BREAKFAST, BREAD, AND SOUP

- THE ROOSTER'S CALL 82
- BREAD OF LIFE 87
- SOUP DAZE 96

CHAPTER FIVE: QUICK & SIMPLE

- THE PASTA & SAUCE PARTY 104
- SIMPLE YET ELEGANT 109
- A MAJ JONGG AFTERNOON 112

CHAPTER SIX: SAUCES, SALADS, DRESSINGS, AND SPICES

- TOPPINGS THAT SING 118
- DRESSINGS THE SALAD 124
- SPICE MIXTURES 128
- HERBS DE PROVENCE 133

CHAPTER SEVEN: SEASONAL DISHES

SPRING LIGHTNESS..138
SPRING FARE 142
SPRING CLEANSING 146
NEW YEAR'S FEAST: 2001 151
COMING TOGETHER: 2003 156

CHAPTER EIGHT: INTERNATIONAL CUISINE

GRANDMA'S SPECIALTIES..162
STUFFING THE PITA 169
A JAPANESE MEAL 173
MISO 178

CHAPTER NINE: GUEST RECIPES

KI'S 184
GARDEN TASTE 189
KITCHEN CONSCIOUSNESS 193
BAKING AT THE EDGE OF THE UNIVERSE..201
DASAPRAKASH 207

CHAPTER TEN: COOKING FOR KIDS

FUN PROJECTS IN THE KITCHEN 212
KID'S MEALTIME 214
SNACKS AND HEALTHY DESSERTS..219

CHAPTER ELEVEN: EAST INDIAN COOKING

A DAY IN THE INDIAN KITCHEN: INDIAN VEGETABLES 226
AN INDIAN MEAL 231
SOUTH INDIAN SPECIALTIES 237
TIFFIN 241
CHUTNEY 246
RICE 250
DHAL DAY 257
MUMBAI KITCHEN 262

CHAPTER TWELVE: TIMELESS SWEETS

PIES 268
CAKES, COOKIES AND BARS 277
CREAMY CREATIONS 291
INDIAN DESSERTS 296

APPENDIX

STOCKING THE PANTRY 304
FOR EVERYTHING THERE IS A SEASONING 312
RESOURCES 317
THE ALLERGY CONNECTION 319
DEFINITION OF TERMS 325
RECIPE INDEX BY CHAPTER 331
RECIPE INDEX BY TITLE 335
GENERAL INDEX 339

ABOUT THE AUTHOR 345

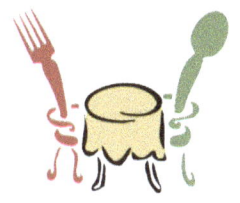

INTRODUCTION

ABOUT THE SECOND EDITION

THE INTERDEPENDENT CIRCLE

EXPLORING HERBS, SPICES, AND HEALING FOODS

THE GENESIS OF A MANUSCRIPT

ABOUT THE SECOND EDITION

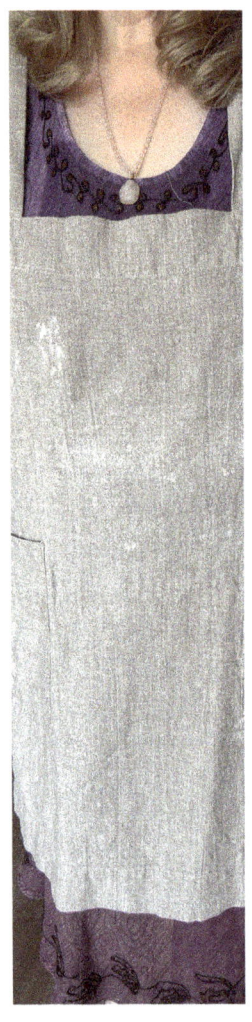

IT IS HARD FOR ME TO BELIEVE THAT IT HAS BEEN SO MANY YEARS since I published this cookbook. In the years that have passed the majority of the book stays remarkably fresh. Though I did go through and touch up recipes, a bit here and there, and added news ones. I also created two extra indexes, transformed it into this color version and added two chapters, "The Blue Zone Diet" and "Cooking for Kids." One ingredient I changed throughout most of the recipes was using avocado instead of canola oil.

In the last few years I grew fascinated with the Blue Zones around the world, where individuals eat sustainable, local food, which seem to help them often live into their 100s. The other development, a delightful new adventure, was grandchildren and discovering new recipes that include healthy foods that are yummy.

The Covid-19 pandemic actually gave me the time and space to take up the enormous project of working on the 2nd edition of this cookbook. Putting on my French linen apron that Matthew bought me for my birthday I started working on making sourdough bread, since yeast was almost impossible to get during that time. Flour was pretty scarce, too, but we found some incredible mail order organic flour companies: Azure Standard, Dufur OR and Janie's Mill, Ashkum, IL, so shipments started coming in of bread flour, whole wheat, artisan, rye, corn and oats. Soon buckets of freshly ground flour filled every corner of the house.

Love of cooking and creating recipes remains my great passion. Every day that we sustain ourselves with freshly cooked food, we bestow the gift of health and happiness to ourselves and those we feed.

THE INTERDEPENDENT CIRCLE

QUITE A FEW YEARS AGO, I spent an afternoon going through my extensive cookbook collection, trying to pare it down a bit. One particular book, *The Training of the Zen Buddhist Monk,* by Daisetz Teitaro Suzuki (originally published in 1934) caught my attention. The book opened to the section titled, *Life of Service,* and though I obviously don't live in a zendo, the following words rang especially true:

> "To serve as a cook in Zendo life means that the monk has attained some understanding about Zen, for it is one of the positions highly honored in the monastery and may be filled only by one of those who have passed a number of years here. The work is quite an irksome one, and, besides, a kind of underground service which is not very much noticed by superficial observers. Just because of this, to be the cook in the monastery affords the monk a good opportunity 'to accumulate merit,' which is turned over to their own enlightenment, as well as its universal realization."

We are all familiar with the saying, "you are what you eat," and most of us have all felt the effects of food that has not been properly prepared. Since the body and mind are interdependent it is essential to provide the body with simple, nourishing food that not only keeps us light and fit but allows the mind to remain focused and clear. What we eat and how we prepare food make all the difference. Food sustains our natural inner and outer harmony, as well as subtly affecting the people we cook for. By choosing to cook and serve food with love and zen-like attention, the spirit of both the giver and receiver is uplifted and enriched.

Most of our homes resonate with the mundane clutter of pots, pans, and dishes, yet we can feel disconnected from the daily work of cooking and cleaning. However, an ideal opportunity is available to use our hands and hearts for creating life-affirming, energy-enforcing meals. When the simplest of tasks like chopping vegetables, rubbing dried spices between our fingers to wake them up, or plucking fresh basil leaves from the window garden is undertaken with complete attention, it can transform the moment into something quite special, yet remarkably ordinary—at the same time. A delightful paradox!

My Culinary Journey

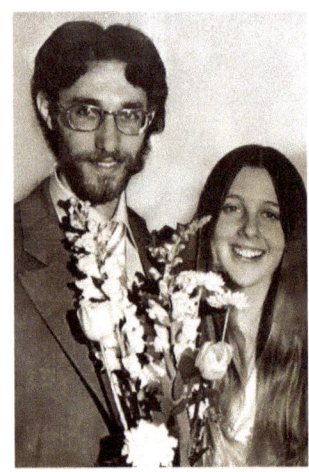

Wedding Day, March 1971

In 1971, as the world changed around us, Matthew and I were married in a simple ceremony in the backyard of my childhood home. Since neither of us had cooked a meal in our lives, we entered into a contract: Matthew would cook, and I would wash the dishes. This lasted for about a week, forcing me to face my destiny rather quickly: I would be cooking for the rest of my life. This was to be either a life sentence or a delightful adventure. It was all up to me.

Becoming both a vegetarian and cook at the same time was one of those memorable life changes. Once I adjusted to this new challenge, I found it to be a very creative and relaxing process. Yet, I doubt that over fifty years ago I could have envisioned sitting here, working on the second edition of this cookbook.

Since my first encounter in the kitchen, much has transpired in my life, and some of these events have been recorded and woven around the recipes that form the core of this book. Life has taken many paths since growing up in the small, northern New Jersey town of Glen Rock. When Matthew and I were just twenty-one, we found ourselves living in a meditation center and working farm in Nova Scotia, Canada. After about six years, life took us to a holistic community in the upstate New York countryside. Not long after, we spent three years in a hermitage in South India, in the shade of the Arunachala mountain, working on a book project. We then lived in Rochester, New York (where our daughter was born), Sarasota, Florida, and now—for over twenty-five years—in the Southern California area.

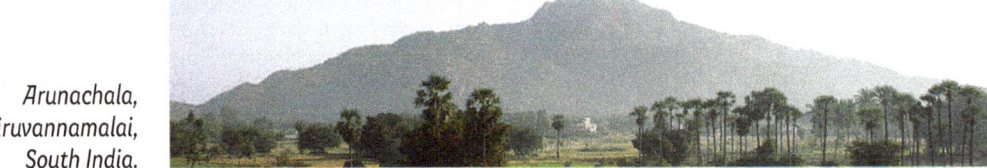

Arunachala, Tiruvannamalai, South India.

EXPLORING HERBS, SPICES, AND HEALING FOODS

MY INTEREST IN SPICES, HERBS AND HEALING FOODS BEGAN AROUND THE SAME TIME I LEARNED TO COOK. As I began to grow, store, and cook my own food, I discovered a new world—and three aspects of this world especially intrigued me. The *first* was the art of cooking; the symphony that consists of cutting vegetables, collecting spice jars, growing a thriving herb garden, preparing grains, and the simple pleasure of pouring liquid into measuring cups. I think of it as, "the elegant dance of ingredients."

The *second* aspect was the certain vibrations of specific food items, which inspired me to prepare dishes that were both delicious and energetically sustaining. I discovered this during the time we were living in Nova Scotia. At the same time, I also became fascinated with flowers and their healing properties. (Some years later, I studied both flower essence therapy and aromatherapy and have been using them in my daily life.)

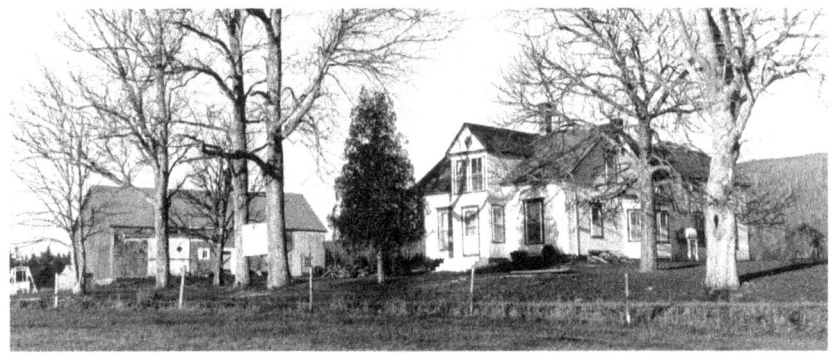

Farmhouse and barn in Nova Scotia, Canada.

Early on, I recognized how food and condiments not only support our bodies, but also affect our minds. I realized that food should give energy to the body without taxing it, and that balancing one's body chemistry also acts as the foundation for a peaceful mind.

When I ate properly, I found that I was able to move through life easier, with less resistance and more grace. At the same time, I became more aware of the parade of emotions that passed through me—often at lightning speed. During those early, exciting days of discovery while experimenting with the creativity and adventure of cooking, there awoke in me an intuitive and respectful understanding of food's potential.

Through this new realization, I began to study the properties of healing foods and how they react on the nervous and digestive systems. I began to use more healing foods in my own kitchen, including organic vegetables, legumes, amazing herbs, and a range of potent spices. I also discovered that sprouting grains and seeds were a boon to overall digestion. It was only years later that I added organic eggs to my vegetarian diet.

The *third* aspect was the manner in which food is handled and cooked. When I was a bit frazzled and cooked in a hurry or with an agitated mind, this energy was imparted into the food. Our time in India was instrumental in teaching us that food is a precious gift, and we learned to cherish even a grain of rice. In fact, in the days before refrigeration, the Indian cook was skilled in determining just the right amount of food to be cooked each day. There were rarely any leftovers, which meant that each meal was cooked fresh daily, and nothing was wasted.

Throughout the years I adjusted recipes for Matthew, who developed a number of food sensitivities (see appendix for allergy information and research). In the last few decades there are a growing number of people who are affected by these often-debilitating conditions—more than I had ever imagined. Even if one is simply sensitive to these foods, rather than allergic, avoiding the problem food may improve one's general health in a significant, sometimes dramatic way. With this in mind, I've tried to provide an alternative to almost all the recipes in this book, especially for: eggs, gluten, milk, yeast, soy, nuts, and seeds. Learning to substitute is quite a simple process once some basic rules are established and applied.

During my years of research, I found many interesting examples of the healing property of foods. One such study was done with rabbits that had high cholesterol. After they were given a regimen of eggplant juice, researchers found that cholesterol development in the main artery (that returns blood to the heart) was significantly reduced. Additionally, "green tea" seems to hold significant healing properties. In 1998, scientists at the Mayo Clinic found that the active component in green tea, called *epigallocatechin gallate*, triggered *apoptosis* (programmed cell death) in human prostate cancer cells.

The Color of Healing Foods

As a graphic designer by trade (and temperament), I have always been interested in color. I was delighted to discover a simple way of categorizing the health benefits of fruits and vegetables—by color. It made it easy for me to prepare dishes as colorfully as possible. I think of it as a healthy, "culinary rainbow." Here are just a few examples of the beneficial properties inherent in colored vegetables.

- **Blue/Purple**: contains varying amounts of properties especially beneficial for the urinary tract, memory function, and age-related issues.

- **Green**: contains lutein and indoles, helps with vision, strong bones and teeth, and lowers the risk of some cancers.

- **White**: contains allicin, found in the onion and garlic family, which benefits the heart and controls cholesterol.

- **Yellow/Orange**: contains vitamin C, carotenoids and bioflavonoids. It is beneficial to the heart, vision, and the immune system.

- **Red**: contains lycopene and anthocyanins, which benefit the heart, memory, and the urinary tract.

THE GENESIS OF A MANUSCRIPT

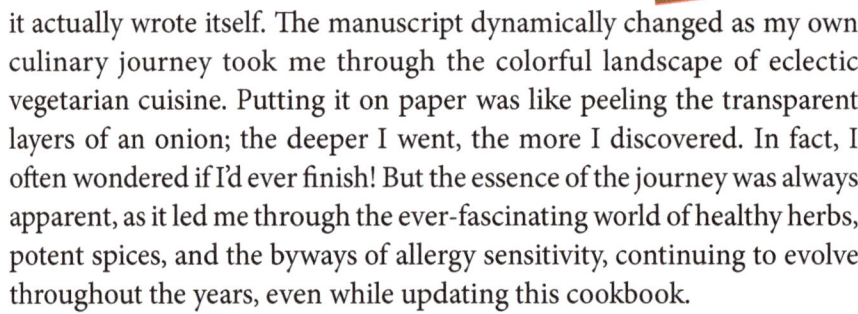

Recipe Abbreviations

Cup = C
Tablespoon = T
Teaspoon = t

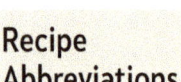 Healing Properties

 Hints & Tips

 Sidebar Information

Allergy Icons

G No Gluten
M No Milk
E No Eggs
N No Nuts/Seeds
S No Soy
Y No Yeast

I DIDN'T SET OUT TO WRITE THIS COOKBOOK; it actually wrote itself. The manuscript dynamically changed as my own culinary journey took me through the colorful landscape of eclectic vegetarian cuisine. Putting it on paper was like peeling the transparent layers of an onion; the deeper I went, the more I discovered. In fact, I often wondered if I'd ever finish! But the essence of the journey was always apparent, as it led me through the ever-fascinating world of healthy herbs, potent spices, and the byways of allergy sensitivity, continuing to evolve throughout the years, even while updating this cookbook.

Organizing the manuscript turned into an interesting biographical retrospective. Some of the recipes are from a cooking column I wrote in a small newsletter called, *Pathways,* which was started in 1987. However, the majority of the recipes are from a column I wrote in the *Inner Directions Journal,* called, "Natural Kitchen." The *Journal,* now online, is published by Inner Directions, a nonprofit organization Matthew and I founded in 1992. The *Inner Directions Journal* presents articles, dialogues, poetry, and stories that express authentic Eastern and Western spiritual teachings.

Throughout this cookbook I created highlighted areas, using call outs: *Healing Properties, Hints & Tips* and *Sidebars,* which reflect my passion to delve into the history and properties of ingredients, herbs and spices. Although some of the recipes include a lot of components, I have tried as far as possible to offer simple dishes with dietary alternatives.

CALL-OUT CATEGORIES:
- *Healing Properties* of specific ingredients.
- *Hints & Tips* about an ingredient, cooking method, or an alternative.
- *Sidebar* contains interesting tidbits and historical facts.

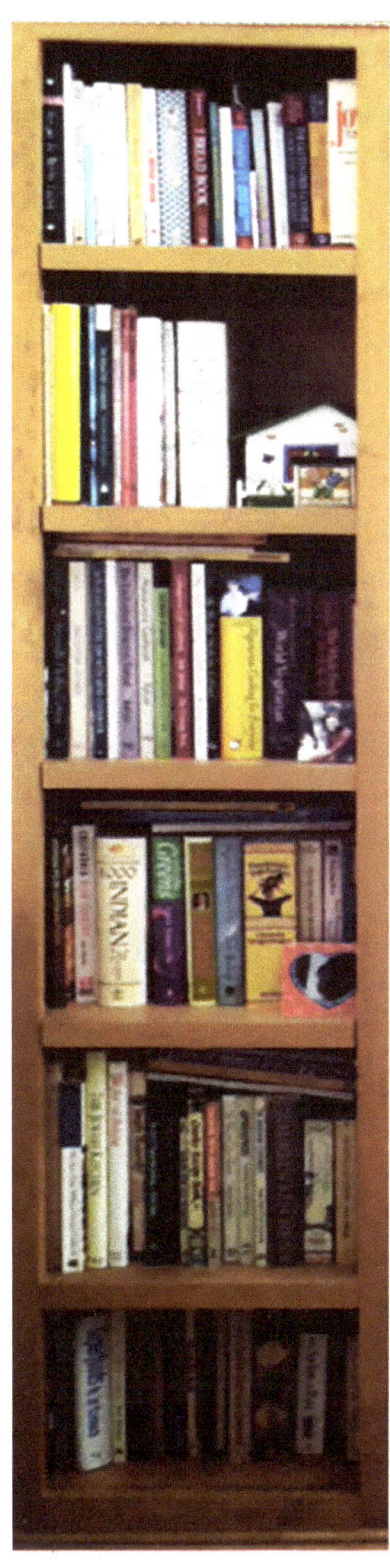

I have also included allergy icons for each recipe to help you quickly determine which recipes are free from common food allergens.

Working with allergy-free alternatives and simple cooking concepts is a dynamic and transforming process. It can be as simple as switching from peanut to olive or avocado oil, grating fresh ginger into a pot of steaming bean soup or stew, adding cumin seeds, bay leaves and a piece of kombu to beans for digestion, cooking with turmeric for neuro-antioxidents, or switching from Teflon pans to stainless-steel, cast iron, or enamel.

This cookbook is not meant to be a nutritional guide. I am not a nutritionist. I simply draw attention to scientific evidence concerning the wonderful healing properties of certain vegetables, fruits, grains, herbs, and spices. Like me, you may simply want to sit down and enjoy reading an interesting cookbook as if it were a novel. For years I collected cookbooks and especially enjoy the writing and culinary insights I cull from them.

There is no specific beginning or end to this book; the entries follow the seasons and bring back memories of events that span over fifty years. The focus of the early *Pathways* reflected experiences of living in India for three years, as a result, most of these recipes were Indian-inspired cuisine. When writing for the "Natural Kitchen" column in the *Inner Directions Journal*, the recipes became more eclectic. Since many of the entries were originally written as articles, they often followed a specific theme. Therefore, I categorized them to achieve a sense of order. Yet, they often change country and season in quite a spontaneous way.

The recipes in this book can be used by anyone interested in incorporating whole, healing foods derived from natural ingredients into their diet. My favorite meals are often unplanned. By looking inside the refrigerator and pantry and discovering what ingredients are waiting for me, I enjoy the adventure of creating on a blank canvas.

Living in Harmony

"Harmony" is one of my favorite words. Harmony is the balance between body and mind, which is vital because if either one is out of sync, it can affect the other in a fairly dramatic way. If we truly yearn to be at peace with ourselves—if we honor both a peaceful mind and energetic body—we can live in true harmony, which is our birthright.

In exploring this adventure, I leave this journey in your hands.
Make it your own.
—JG

View from my writing desk where I finished this new edition in the Conejo Valley mountains' presence.

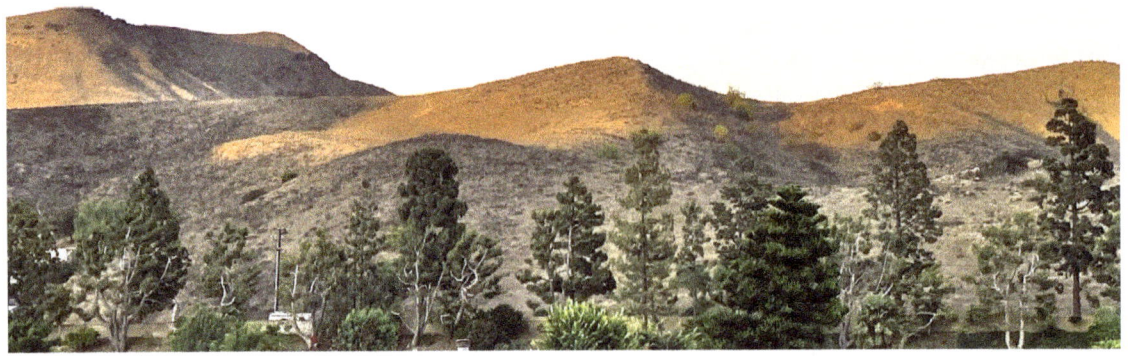

"Happiness is not a matter of intensity, but of balance, order, rhythm and harmony."
—Thomas Merton

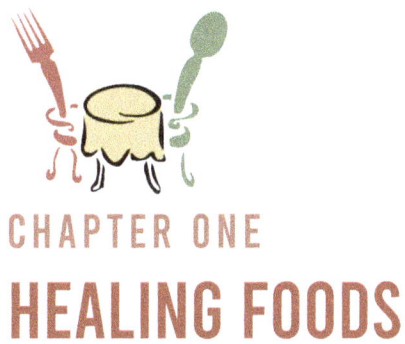

CHAPTER ONE
HEALING FOODS

MAGICAL GREENS

HEALING SOUPS

COOKING WITH FLOWER ESSENCES

MAGICAL GREENS

"I yam what I yam."
—Popeye the Sailor Man ("toot, toot")

MOM AND POPEYE WERE RIGHT ALL ALONG, they both told you that spinach was really good for you. We grew kale in Nova Scotia, and it was literally indestructible; it grew clear into November's first snow, and the more you picked, the more it grew. With a light steam and double bagging, it freezes very well.

Leafy greens are powerhouses and have extensive health benefits: they are ideal for weight management, helpful in reducing the risk of cancer and heart disease, high in dietary fiber and rich in folic acid, vitamin C, potassium, and magnesium. They also contain a host of phytochemicals such as lutein, beta-cryptoxanthin, zeaxanthin and beta-carotene. A study showed that even one daily serving of green leafy vegetables lowered the risk of cardiovascular disease by 11 percent. Due to their high magnesium content and low glycemic index, green leafy vegetables are also valuable for persons with type 2 diabetes.

The delightful kaleidoscope of colors of these leafy vegetable's range from the bluish-green of kale to the bright kelly green of leaf spinach. Greens run the gamut of flavors, too, from sweet to bitter, and from peppery to earthy. If you have a choice, always choose plants with young and tender leaves. Even if your greens are organic, make sure to wash them carefully to avoid little bugs that may have inadvertently been harvested along with the greens. I have personally met with an amazing assortment of tiny green bugs and spiders.

Hint: An item to have handy in your refrigerator is a lemon spray. Squeeze 4 to 5 lemons into fresh juice, add 1 t lemon zest and put in a small spray bottle. You can spray fresh lemon juice onto greens, rice or soup just before serving them. It will instantly wake them up.

My current favorite green right now is rainbow chard. We get fresh bunches almost year round from local organic farms in Southern California.

SAAG PANEER (OR TOFU)

Serves 2 to 4

GMENSY

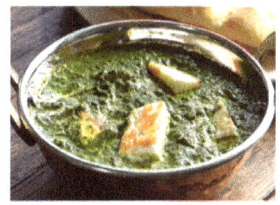

*Saag (greens) Paneer is a creamy spinach dish with paneer—a homemade Indian cottage cheese. You can, however, also substitute tofu for paneer. It's a popular dish in India where they use various types of greens as well, which include mustard and fenugreek (methi) leaves. The weed, lamb's quarters (*bathua *in Hindi), was the first plant to invade our garden in early summer and it would take over if we weren't vigilant. One day, while I was weeding the Nova Scotian garden, a friend from India who was staying with us told me not to throw the lamb's quarters away, that she would make a traditional dish out of them. A few years later while visiting a tiny village in Bihar, Northern India, this dish was given to us as a delicacy. It's prized for its many health benefits, which is the essence of greens.*

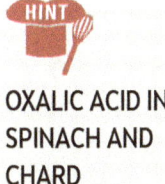

OXALIC ACID IN SPINACH AND CHARD

One warning about greens: swiss chard and spinach contain high amounts of oxalic acid. People who are pre-disposed to kidney stones from an excess of oxalic acid should not overeat spinach; kale is a great substitute.

Matthew discovered this problem when he was in the hospital painfully passing a kidney stone. The lab results came back, "oxalic!"

2 medium tomatoes, chopped
1 T fresh ginger, chopped
1 t coriander powder
½ t turmeric powder
½ t cayenne powder
2 T whole wheat flour or rice flour
½ C fat-free half-and-half, or ½ C soy or almond milk

1½ C fresh paneer or tofu (see page 227 for paneer recipe)
4 T avocado oil
½ t cumin seeds
Pinch of asafetida (hing)
4 C spinach or any greens, chopped
½ t salt, or to taste

1. BLEND tomatoes and ginger to make puree.
2. MIX coriander, turmeric, and cayenne (you can make it as mild or spicy as you like) with tomato puree and set aside.
3. MIX flour with cream (or alternative milk) and set aside.
4. CUBE the paneer or tofu in half-inch pieces. Pan fry them with 3 T oil on medium high heat, for just a few minutes, so paneer or tofu becomes very light gold in color. Drain on paper towel, so extra oil is absorbed.
5. HEAT remaining 1 T oil, add cumin seeds and *hing* (asafetida). After cumin seeds brown, add the tomato puree mixture and let it cook for a few minutes, until the tomato puree is reduced slightly by half.
6. ADD spinach and salt, cook on low-medium heat for about 10 minutes.
7. ADD pan-fried paneer or tofu and fold gently into spinach. Cook for an additional 2 to 3 minutes.
8. ADD cream or milk mixture, simmer 4 to 5 minutes, uncovered.

KALE AND WHITE BEAN SOUP

Serves 6 to 8

G M E N S Y

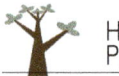

HEALING PROPERTIES

Kale
- High in fiber
- Contains antioxidants
- Anti-Inflammatory
- Cardiovascular Support
- A great detox
- Vitamins K, A, C

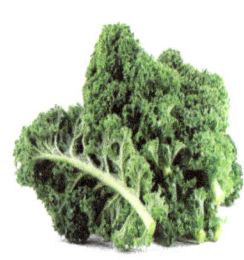

I love a hearty soup on a cold weekend. This recipe is packed with lots of veggies and creamy beans. Kale takes longer to cook than traditional greens, so make sure it's nice and tender before serving. This soup makes enough to freeze. When you defrost and reheat it, add a splash of lemon juice and more fresh herbs to wake it up.

2 T olive oil
1 onion, diced; 2 carrots, diced; 2 celery stalks, diced
2 to 4 garlic cloves, smashed and roughly chopped (optional)
5 C vegetable broth or 5 C water with vegetable broth cube
1" piece ginger, minced
1 bay leaf

1 t fresh dill or ½ t dried dill
1 t salt
4 C kale, de-veined, chopped small
1 (14 oz.) can diced fire-roasted tomatoes
2 zucchinis, diced
1 (14.5 oz.) cannelloni beans, double rinsed and drained
Splash lemon juice

1. HEAT oil over medium heat; cook onion, carrot and celery until onion is translucent.
2. ADD garlic and cook 2 additional minutes.
3. ADD broth or water (with broth cube), ginger, bay leaf, dill, salt, kale, tomatoes, and zucchini; then cover.
4. COOK 20 to 25 minutes or until kale and veggies are tender.
5. ADD beans and lemon juice and heat thoroughly, remove bay leaf.
6. SERVE hot with a drizzle of olive oil on top.

SIDEBAR   THE HISTORY OF KALE

Kale has been cultivated for over 2,000 years. In much of Europe it was the most widely eaten green vegetable until the Middle Ages when cabbage became more popular. Historically, it has been particularly important in colder regions due to its resistance to frost.

In the nineteenth century "Scotland kale" was used as a generic term for "dinner," and all kitchens featured a kale pot for cooking. Kale was given protection from the elements through what was called a "kale yard." Almost every house had a kale yard, and kale was generally preserved in barrels of salt, similar to German sauerkraut. Kale was also fed to livestock through the winter months, and it continued to be an extremely important food until potatoes came to the British Isles toward the end of the eighteenth century.

HEALING GREEN DRINKS

Serves 2 to 4

GMENSY

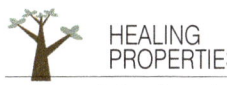

HEALING PROPERTIES

Fenugreek Seeds and Leaves
- Balance cholesterol
- Control diabetes
- Lower blood sugar
- Topical treatment for skin problems
- Helpful for fever
- Balance hormonal issues

FENUGREEK WATER

Take fenugreek seeds and grind it into a powder. Mix the ground powder with enough warm water to form a paste. It has been known to help with weight loss.

Having spent some time in a fasting clinic and drinking three cups of handmade organic wheat grass daily, I grew to respect the energy that green drinks provide. The varieties are almost endless.

VEGGIE DRINKS

Detox Green Drink
2 C spinach
2 large kale leaves
1 cucumber (approximately 1 cup)
1 celery stalk
1 t ginger juice
½ C parsley
2 T fenugreek water
1 apple
1 lemon, juiced
4 ounces spring water

Potassium Juice
3 carrots
3 celery stalks
2 beets, peeled and cubed
1 apple, cubed
1 C spinach
½ C parsley

BLENDER DRINKS

High Blood Pressure Reducer
1 garlic clove
1 handful parsley
1 cucumber
4 carrots
2 celery stalks

Yummy Green Drink
1 C spinach
2 large kale leaves
¼ C orange juice, fresh
½" fresh ginger, chopped
1 small banana
1 kiwi

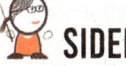 **SIDEBAR**   **BENEFITS OF GREEN DRINKS**

Green drinks have a great impact on the immune system. Since they are highly alkaline, they encourage new cell growth and ward off any toxins that may have entered the body. The alkaline, along with protein that may be in a green drink, also helps to increase energy. Green drinks are also helpful when trying to lose weight.

HEALING SOUPS

EVERY SUMMER MY FRIEND CHETNA DREAMS UP great, innovative, cold soups, which are not only delicious but have many health benefits as well. I am delighted when she shares her new creations with me. She often tells me delightful stories about her childhood in Ahmedabad, India, and the many healing spices and remedies her grandmother used for both daily cooking and medicinal purposes. Once, when I had a recurrence of an ankle sprain Chetna told me that her grandmother would apply a poultice of turmeric and warm oil to heal a sprain. Although I walked around with a bright yellow ankle for weeks, it really did help.

From ginger to fenugreek, each spice holds the seed of ancient healing. Most families in India are aware of the healing effects of herbs and spices through generations of life experience, incorporate them into their food every day. Now science is confirming what the Indian grandmas always knew. The incidence of Alzheimer's disease in India is uncommonly low, and this phenomenon is generally attributed to the widespread daily use of turmeric, the primary ingredient used in curry powder.

"Cookery means the knowledge of all herbs, fruits, balms, and spices,

and all that is healing and sweet in the fields and groves.

It means carefulness, inventiveness, willingness, and readiness of appliances.

It means the economy of your grandmothers and

the science of the modern chemist; it means much testing and no wasting."

—JOHN RUSKIN *(Quoted in the first edition of the Boston Cooking-School Cook Book, 1896)*

CHETNA'S CHILLED SUMMER SOUPS

Serves 4 to 6

GMENSY

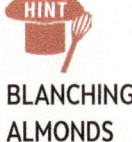

BLANCHING ALMONDS

1. Place almonds in a bowl. Pour boiling water to barely cover them.
2. Let the almonds sit for 1 to 2 minutes.
3. Drain twice, rinsing under cold water.
4. Pat dry and slip the skins off.

Tip

If you let almonds sit in hot water too long they will lose their crispness.

CANTALOUPE SOUP

This is a simple and refreshing soup. The fennel garnish adds depth and a unique overall flavor.

1 cantaloupe, chopped
2 C orange juice
½ t ginger powder
¼ t nutmeg, freshly grated
½ t salt
Pinch of cayenne powder

Garnish
1 T fennel fronds (top of fennel bulb), chopped

1. BLEND six ingredients together until well-combined.
2. TOP with fennel fronds.

GMESY

GRAPE SOUP

This is one of Chetna's original creations. At first I was a bit skeptical about putting scallions in this soup, but it works in ways I didn't expect.

2½ C green grapes
1 C low-fat milk or soy, rice or almond milk
½ C blanched almonds (see hint)
3 scallions, chopped
1 lime, zest and juice
½ t salt

1. BLEND all ingredients well.
2. CHILL before serving.

FIRE ROASTED GAZPACHO

Serves 4 to 6

GMENSY

CILANTRO OR CORIANDER LEAVES

Gazpacho is a healthy, cold tomato-based soup. I can't eat raw onions but discovered that sautéing the onions for this soup is an easy fix. If you use raw onions, the gazpacho is more authentic. If your blender is not large enough to make this recipe in one batch, you can easily split the ingredients into two batches.

What's in a name? The Latin name for this herb is *Coriandrum sativum*, from which the word "coriander" is derived.

In England, its leaves and stalks are known as "coriander leaves," in Mexico, and Spain as "cilantro" and in India as *dania* leaves.

1 (28 oz.) can fire-roasted tomatoes, whole
1 C salsa, fresh or prepared
½ C green pepper, rough chopped
½ C cucumber, chopped (reserve 2 T finely chopped for serving)
¼ C cilantro (reserve 2 T for serving)
½ C croutons, from whole grain bread or gluten-free bread
¼ C onion, diced (option: sauté in ½ t oil until translucent)
2 T red wine vinegar
2 T olive oil
1 to 2 garlic cloves, rough chop
1 jalapeño pepper, de-vein, de-seed, chop small
1 T cumin powder
½ to 1 t salt, to taste
½ t black pepper, freshly ground

1. PLACE all ingredients (not reserved items) into the blender. Cover, pulse on medium, don't over blend.
2. COVER and refrigerate for at least 1 hour (longer is better).
3. TOP with reserved cucumber and cilantro.

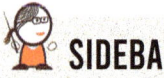 **SIDEBAR**   **GAZPACHO: STUDY ON STRESS**

A study was conducted by Antonio Martin, a physician specializing in nutrition and inflammatory responses at Tufts University in Boston, Massachusetts. The researchers fed twelve healthy volunteers—six men and six women—two bowls (17 ounces, total) of gazpacho every day for two weeks. Stress molecules, which are secreted by the body as a normal response to stress, was measured, and they were found to significantly decrease after the soups' consumption.

CHILLED MANGO SOUP—TWO WAYS

Serves 2 to 4 G M E N S Y

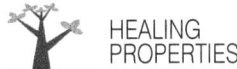

Mango
- An excellent source of copper and potassium
- Contains traces of magnesium, manganese, selenium, calcium, iron and phosphorus
- Rich in vitamin C and vitamin A
- High in fiber

SMOKY MANGO CHIPOTLE SOUP

In Mexico, the traditional way of eating mangoes is by sprinkling them with a bit of chili, salt and lime. This chilled soup takes those Mexican flavors and turns it into a cold, perky, fruit soup, which is perfect for a hot summer day.

2 mangoes (reserve 4 T for garnish)
1 lime, juiced and ½ t lime zest
½ t ginger powder
Dash salt and pepper, to taste
½ to ¾ t chipotle powder
2 C water
¼ C cilantro (reserve a few leaves for garnish)

1. PUREE all ingredients together in a blender or food processor, until smooth and creamy.
2. ADD more chipotle and salt to taste, chill and serve cold.
3. SERVE with 1 T chopped mango and a few pieces of cilantro on top.

Serves 3 to 4

INDIAN MANGO DESSERT SOUP (LASSI)

One year we found ourselves in North India during mango season. The implications of this are enormous because every day, sometimes a few times a day, a mango preparation is served. This mango dessert was often served along with a dollop of homemade vanilla ice cream, an Indian creamsicle.

3 mangoes pitted and skinned, chopped, or 1 (24 oz.) can mango pulp
1 C low or non-fat milk or almond milk
½ C yogurt (you can substitute with dairy-free yogurt)
¼ C agave syrup (omit if mango pulp has sugar in it)
½ t cardamom powder and a few strands of saffron

1. PUREE all ingredients together in a blender or food processor until smooth and creamy. Chill.

GRANDMA'S HUNGARIAN CABBAGE SOUP

Serves 6 to 8

GMENSY

In the wintertime Grandma Pauline would venture out into her local Brooklyn neighborhood vegetable stand to get the ingredients for her famous cabbage soup. It was loaded with lots of vegetables and plenty of garlic. I added the ginger as a digestive element.

3 T olive oil (grandma used chicken fat!)
1 onion, diced
3 carrots, chopped
2 celery stalks, chopped
½ C green pepper, chopped
2 garlic cloves, roughly chopped
½ green cabbage, sliced and chopped
1 (14.5 oz.) can crushed tomatoes
8 C vegetable broth or water with a bouillon cube
¼ C parsley, freshly chopped
1 t fresh ginger, minced
1 T kosher salt, without bouillon cube (1 t with bouillon cube)
½ t black pepper, freshly ground
1 t Hungarian paprika

This is an old-world Hungarian recipe.

Cabbage was a stable, since it lasts far into the winter months.

1. SAUTÉ onion, carrots, celery and pepper in oil in a heavy-duty soup pot.
2. ADD garlic and stir fry for a few moments.
3. ADD the rest of the ingredients.
4. BRING to a boil then lower heat, cook with lid ajar for 1 to 1½ hours, until cabbage is well cooked.
5. DRIZZLE with olive oil and eat with a crusty loaf of fresh bread.

 SIDEBAR WHY GRANDMA USED KOSHER SALT

Grandma Pauline liked to feel the large grains of kosher salt. It was how she determined how much to use in each dish as she never used a recipe. The size and shape of the salt allows it to absorb more moisture than finer grains of salt. She was convinced it simply made the dish taste better.

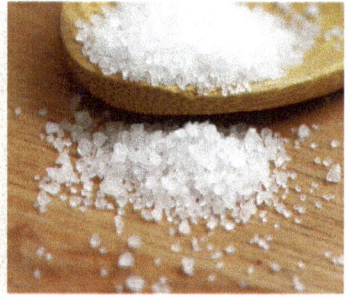

A Culinary Journey

> "The most beautiful plants and herbs to be found in the pharmacy of nature are divinely enriched with healing powers for the mind and body."
>
> —Dr. Edward Bach

COOKING WITH FLOWER ESSENCES

The recipes in this chapter are inspired from my book, *Healing with Flower Essences*

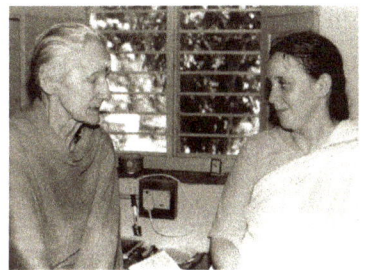

Lucy Cornelssen

Flower essences ideally lend themselves to be incorporated into recipes. t's a new twist on the "Alice B. Toklas" brownie. The challenge in creating these recipes was to eliminate any heat, that would change the flower essence's molecular structure.

I HAVE WORKED WITH FLOWER ESSENCES for almost Four decades. Their energetic healing properties were re-discovered in the 1930s by the pioneering work of Dr. Edward Bach. Flower essences bring relief from the many emotional challenges and physiological stresses that arise in our lives.

I discovered my passion for flowers one spring day when I walked to a meadow in the back of the Nova Scotia farm. When I reached the open space, a blanket of wildflowers took my breath away. I felt their healing power and heard their gentle voices. My heart re-awoke to the wonder and delight of flowers amidst the silence and harmony of nature. During that brief morning of "flower meditation," I knew that I had touched upon the mystery and majesty of an ancient world, and it opened me up to its limitless possibilities.

Years later, my husband Matthew and I found ourselves in South India working on a special publication, It was where I first discovered the healing aspects Flower Essences. Lucy Cornelssen, was a dear friend and teacher who I often spent time with. One day, I saw her take a vial from an end-table drawer and put two drops onto her tongue. When I asked about it she handed me an Indian edition of a book on Bach Flower Essences. I devoured the book; it was a revelation to me, and a clear understanding of something I intuitively knew to be true.

An example of the power of flower essences is the story of Beth Beasley, a dedicated mother of Jarrett, an autistic child. He was on 22 medicines a day, including antidepressants. She decided to incorporate flower essences into her son's daily routine and change them according to his changing needs. Jarrett began to show empathy and affection, and a new inclination to listen and follow directions. Jarrett's doctors were amazed, and he told his therapist, "Mommy made me better with the flowers from God."

Healing Foods

TRANQUILITY POTATO SALAD

Serves 5 to 6

G M E N Y

BACH FLOWER ESSENCE:
2 Drops Gentian

This salad will help make your day carefree and tranquil.

This is a great potato salad recipe with a twist. It balances the carbohydrates of potatoes with the protein of edamame, and a little wasabi to kick it up a notch.

8 unpeeled red potatoes; bake until soft, then cube.
½ C edamame, steamed
1 C corn kernels, cut from roasted cob or canned or frozen
½ C carrots, shredded
½ t ginger, freshly grated
1 t yellow, whole grain mustard
1 t salt
¼ to ½ C mayonnaise or vegenaise, add ½ t wasabi paste (optional)
½ t smoky paprika
¼ C fresh parsley, chopped fine plus 2 T fresh chives, chopped fine

1. MIX ingredients together while potatoes are still warm.
2. DROP flower essence on top and mix in.
3. CHILL at least one hour before serving.

 SIDEBAR   **HEALING POWER OF FLOWER ESSENCES**

In the early 1900s, Dr. Edward Bach trained at University College Hospital in England and held diplomas in public health, homeopathy, and bacteriology. During his work at the Royal London Homeopathic Hospital, Dr. Bach made an important discovery: those patients with the same emotional difficulties needed the same homeopathic treatment, irrespective of their physical illness. For Dr. Bach, these homeopathic treatments became the vehicle to rediscover the healing power of flower essences.

As a result of his newfound passion for energetic healing, Dr. Bach decided to leave his comfortable medical practice and move deep into the English countryside. It is here that he observed and intuited the flowers around him, discovering that each plant held an imprint that corresponded to a specific emotional state. Like healers before him, Dr. Bach noted that the dew on the flowers became impregnated with the plant's healing properties. To re-establish what nature had shown him, he created a way to reproduce this dew, which resulted in the Bach Flower Essence family—seven groups of remedies that correspond to 38 different challenging states of mind. They are "complementary" remedies that can restore each condition to a positive, natural state of harmony and well-being.

CONTENTED HUMMUS LAVASH ROLL

Serves 6 to 8 | Preheat Oven to 350 Degrees   GMENY

BACH FLOWER ESSENCE:
2 Drops Impatiens

This roll will help you slow down and smell the tahini.

This is a great party roll. I make it ahead of time and cut it into pieces just before serving. Adding fresh ginger makes the beans easier to digest. Be sure to double rinse and drain the beans very well.

2 roasted garlic cloves; cover with aluminum foil and roast in an oven for 20 to 30 minutes until soft.
2 C chickpeas or cannelloni beans, canned
¼ C sesame paste (tahini)
2 T olive oil
3 T lemon juice, fresh
1 T lemon zest
1 t soy sauce or Braggs Liquid Aminos
½ t salt
1" fresh ginger, minced
½ t ground cumin
¼ t ground coriander
¼ t smoky paprika and ¼ t cayenne pepper

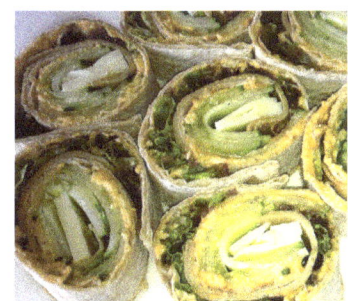

2 cucumbers, sliced paper thin, using a mandolin
8 pieces, thin sliced tofu
1 C arugula
1 large whole wheat or gluten-free lavash style flat bread

1. PROCESS the roasted garlic and rinsed beans in a food processor. Pulse the machine only a few times.
2. ADD tahini, olive oil, lemon juice, zest, soy sauce and salt. Stop the processor occasionally to scrape down the sides of the bowl.
3. OPEN the lid and add the salt, ginger, cumin, coriander, paprika, cayenne, parsley, and flower essence. Process until thoroughly blended. If the puree seems too thick for spreading, use up to ¼ cup of water for consistency, adjust salt.
4. TRANSFER the puree to a bowl. Cover with cling wrap and refrigerate to chill well.
5. SPREAD hummus over entire bread. Top with one layer of sliced cucumber, tofu and arugula, then roll up tightly on short side.
6. WRAP roll with cling wrap and refrigerate for at least 1 hour.
7. CUT into 2" to 3" pieces just before serving.

CONFIDENT LASSI DRINK

Serves 4

GMENSY

BACH FLOWER ESSENCE:
2 Drops Larch

This is a great drink when you need a boost of confidence.

My first rose milk experience was in the 1970s, in South India, on a dusty, blistering hot bus ride to Chennai (Madras). We stopped on the way and took shelter in a tiny yogurt drink shop where we were transported to rosewater heaven the moment we tasted the smooth, frothy, icy cold, rose-flavored yogurt beverage.

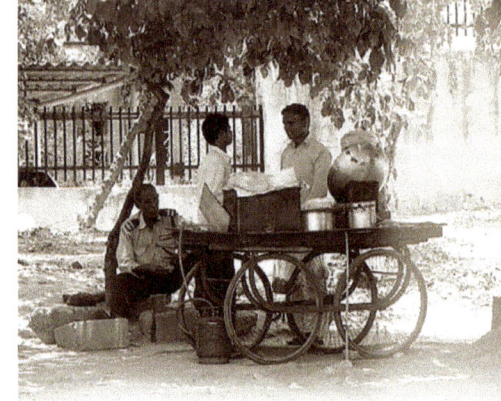

4 C low or nonfat plain yogurt or yogurt alternative
5 T lavender, or any mild honey or agave syrup
2 drops pure rosewater (available in an Indian grocery store)
½ t cardamom powder, freshly ground
2 C ice, roughly chopped

1. WHIP first four ingredients together in a blender with flower essence, blend until well-mixed.
2. ADD ½ C ice to glass, fill with yogurt mixture.

Serves 4 to 6

BACH FLOWER ESSENCE:
2 Drops Olive

This is a pick-me-up boost; great for a late afternoon slump.

ORANGE MANGO ENERGY PUNCH

4 C orange juice
1 C mango pulp
1 C raspberry spritzer
½ orange, cut into thin slices, remove seeds
¼ C raspberries, fresh
8 mint leaves

1. BLEND juice, pulp, spritzer, and flower essence together.
2. ADD 1 C of punch to glass.
3. TOP with orange slice, a few raspberries, and mint leaves.

36 | A Culinary Journey

CHAPTER TWO
THE WORLDWIDE BLUE ZONES

BLUE ZONE DIET
BLUE ZONE BREADS

2

BLUE ZONE DIET

There are a few variations in how many blue zones there are around the world. Here are the most mentioned zones: Okinawa (Japan); Sardinia (Italy); Nicoya (Costa Rica); Icaria (Greece); and among the Seventh-day Adventists in Loma Linda (California).

> "Before each meal she takes a moment to say *hara hachi bu*, and that keeps her from eating too much."
>
> "Hara hachi bu?" I repeated.
>
> "It's a Confucian-inspired adage," Craig chimed in. "All of the old folks say it before they eat. It means 'Eat until you are 80 percent full.'"
> —Dan Buettner, *The Blue Zones*

WHEN WORKING ON THE REVISION FOR THIS COOKBOOK I accumulated a number of recipes and information about the Blue Zones around the world and their healing recipes, related to people who seem to live the longest. Obviously, no one knows when one's life will be over, but adding a few elements from the blue zone diet research can go a long way in making whatever time we have here healthier and happier. Adding this new chapter was the perfect opportunity to address this very fascinating aspect of food and longevity.

In the new world in which we live, where cancer, autism and now covid's viral reality touch so many households throughout the world, the blue zones give us a window into the world of eating simply and locally. If you have never heard of the blue zones, let me give you a brief history of them and the studies that have risen out of observing the lifestyle and eating habits of people who seem to outpace our normal lifespan, often into their 100s.

The main researched findings include a few common traits about the people living in these areas: eat as much food that is local, seasonal, and ingredients that are common to the region you live; exercise regularly, walking is the most common form of exercise; have a positive attitude to one's purpose in life; relax more, be accepting and present; eat smaller portions at each meal; limit red meat; drink more good quality water, reverse osmosis with added minerals is great alternative; and be aware of the abundant power of love and gratitude.

These concepts might sound very logical but put together it is a simple and organic way to live. With our lifestyle choices of grabbing a muffin "to go" at Starbucks and skipping breakfast, if we are running late, it is not always easy to incorporate these simple solutions. We may need to make an effort to work them into our day life.

During the time we lived in Nova Scotia, we actually followed this routine. We ate our main meal at lunchtime, grew most of our own vegetables, and canned, froze, or stored some of them on basement shelving and the root vegetables in hay. With daily milk from our cows, we made our own yogurt, butter, bread, and cheese and stored big bags of rice and lentils in the pantry.

Of course, once we left the farm, we left this diet there too. But, even today we still try and keep up these habits, as best we can, in the fast pace that life finds us. So, if we simple slow down, just a little bit, and integrate a few of these traits into our lives, it can be a game changer.

THE BLUE ZONES

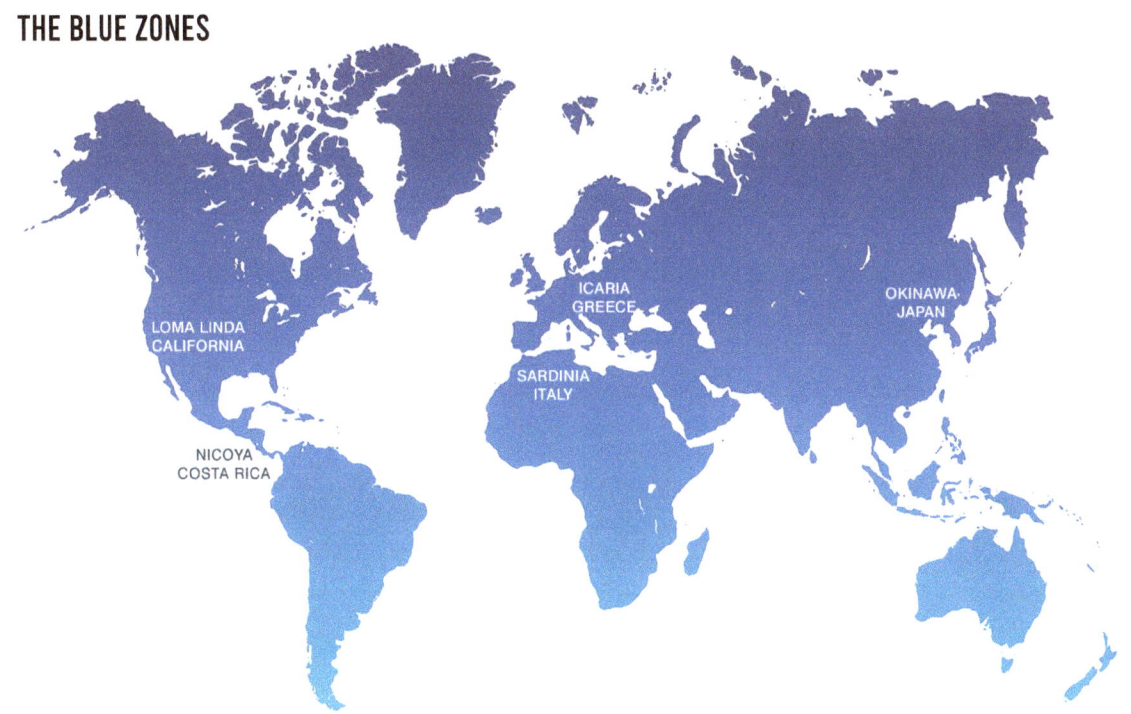

The Worldwide Blue Zones

LEMONY RED LENTIL STEW

Serves 6 to 8   GMENSY

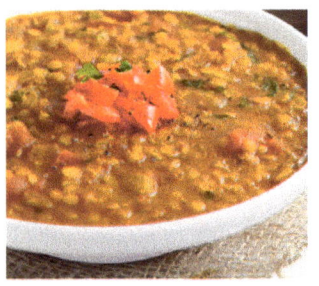

Lentils are used widely throughout Italy, India, and Greece. This is a great powerhouse staple recipe to cook and also freeze.

Boil
2 cups red lentils
8 cups water or vegetable broth or combination of both
1 large carrot, diced
½ t turmeric and 1 t ginger powder
1 T salt

HEALING PROPERTIES

Lentils essential nutrients:
 folate
 iron
 manganese
 phosphorus
 thiamin
 potassium
 vitamin B6

Lentils also contain:
 riboflavin
 niacin
 pantothenic acid
 magnesium
 zinc
 copper
 selenium

Sauté
1 T avocado or olive oil
1 t cumin
½ t paprika, smoked
1 t oregano
2 T tomato paste

Add
1 large onion, diced
2 zucchinis, diced
½ C parsley, chopped
2 T lemon zest and ¼ C lemon juice
1 tomato, chopped

1. BOIL red lentils (wash in a strainer first), water or broth, carrots, turmeric, ginger and salt and place on medium heat to boil, lower heat and simmer until very tender, about 15 minutes.
2. SAUTÉ spices in avocado oil for a few moments, add tomato paste. Then add onions, fry until translucent. Add zucchini and parsley, cook until zucchini is soft.
3. MIX cooked vegetables in pot with soft lentils.
4. ADD lemon zest and juice and adjust salt and water to make the consistency you wish, thicker or thinner.
5. REDUCE heat to medium, cover pot, cook for an additional ten minutes, serve with 1 T chopped tomatoes for each bowl.

SIDEBAR   THE COLOR OF LENTILS

Brown Lentils: Ranging in color from light to dark, the varieties are: Spanish, German, or Indian. The blackest and tiniest ones are Beluga, with a rich and earthy flavor.
Green Lentils: The green-brown color has a glossy exterior are more peppery than their earthy brown cousins, they are firmer, so they work well in salads.
Red Lentils: The range in colors from golden, vibrant orange and red. These hulled lentils are sweet, nutty, quick cooking and are the easiest to digest for delicate stomachs.

SIMPLE EVERYDAY SOUP

Serves 4 to 6

GMENY

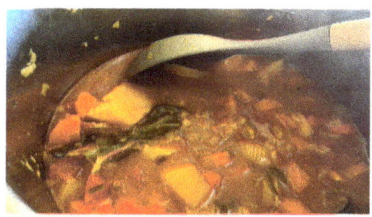

Blue Zone cooking utilizes food that is local, in season and easily available. My go-to soup is simply seeing what I have on hand. It can be any number of vegetables, sauces, and spices. Here is a simple recipe to start you on your own soup adventure.

1 T avocado oil
3 scallions, chopped
½ inch fresh ginger, grated or 1 t ginger powder
½ t turmeric
½ t cumin
½ t Aleppo chili pepper
½ C tomato sauce
1 red pepper, I also use jarred red peppers, chopped
2 carrots, chopped large
2 celery sticks, chopped (I peel them if the outside is a bit tough)
1 potato, chopped big
2 zucchini, chopped
3 C vegetable peel stock* or water
2 T red miso, dissolve in a cup of hot broth before adding to pot

Also known as a Halaby chili, the smoky **Aleppo Pepper** is named for the Syrian city in which it originated. It was grown by Christian and Muslim farmers and migrated through Sephardic Jewish spice merchants, who traded along the Silk Road.

1. HEAT oil and add scallions, and spices. Fry until soft.
2. ADD tomato sauce, heat until bubbling.
3. ADD the rest of the ingredients and bring to a boil.
4. COOK until vegetables are tender.

 SIDEBAR HERBY VEGETABLE PEEL STOCK*

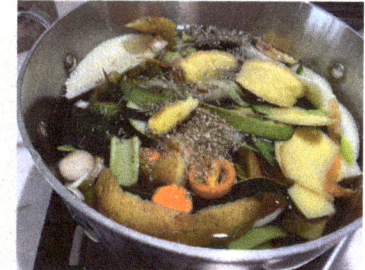

Whenever you wash and peel your veggies, you have an opportunity to make soup stock. I use carrots, celery, mushrooms, zucchini, potato, and I usually have fresh ginger and add that, as well. If you eat garlic, you can add 2 to 3 cloves.

1. PUT all the vegetable peels in the pot, fill with water to the cover the veggies.
2. ADD 1 T salt, pinch cayenne pepper, pinch turmeric powder, 1 t dried oregano, 1 t dried thyme and 1 t dried rosemary.
3. BRING to a boil and simmer for 1 to 2 hours.
4. STRAIN and put the liquid in the fridge, it lasts for 1 week, or you can freeze it.

SIMPLE SPICY TOFU STIR FRY

Serves 3 to 4

G M E Y

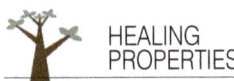

Health Benefits and Warning of Sprouts

Lower Cholesterol
Sprouts contain high levels of phytonutrients, and have antioxidant properties, which can help to lower cholesterol.

Manage Blood Sugar
Antioxidants in sprouts help to decrease insulin resistance and improve vascular health.

Anti Inflammatory
Antioxidants in sprouts may have several powerful anti-inflammatory effects.

Adverse Effects
Since bacteria thrives in warm, humid environments, the exact conditions in which they are grown, there is a possibility of food bourne illness associated with raw sprouts. Making your own is the best way to assure they are clean and safe. Also, they are best used fully cooked.

Soy products are a protein powerhouse. In the Blue Zone of Okinawa this simply tofu dish blends wonderful flavor and texture with the digestive and health benefits of ginger and bean sprouts.

2 T sesame oil
12 oz. firm tofu, cut into chunks
½ C red onion, diced
½ C mung bean sprouts
1 garlic clove, minced
2 C spinach or kale, chopped
1 t chili powder
1 T tamari

1. SAUTÉ tofu on both sides in 1 T sesame oil, about 3 to 4 minutes. Set aside, in a bowl.
2. STIR FRY onions 1 T sesame oil, over medium-high heat, so they brown for 2 to 3 minutes, add sprouts, garlic and fry for an additional minute. Remove from pan and add to bowl with fried tofu.
3. ADD greens, chili powder and tamari to the pan and cook until greens are wilted, about 2 minutes, depending on greens used.
4. TOSS all ingredients together, cook another 2 to 3 minutes. Serve with rice.

 SIDEBAR   MAKING YOUR OWN SPROUTS

1. RINSE and pick over beans. Mung beans and lentils are easy and fast to sprout. Make sure to use the best quality beans.
2. PLACE beans in jar with water. Use 2 T of beans to 3 C water. Fill with cool, clean filtered water.
3. SOAK. Cover with a cap with holes or put cheesecloth on top and secure with a rubber band, soak for 8 to 12 hours.
4. RINSE and drain completely, place in a sunny area, continue to rinse a few times a day.
5. STORE. When sprouts are fully formed, rinse and drain really well and place in refrigerator. They will last for about a week.

GREEN PESTO

Serves 6 to 8

GMESY

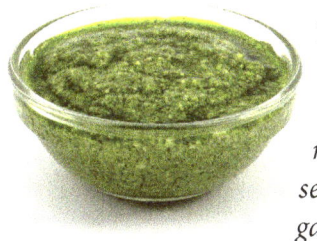

This is a healthy low-fat and delicious pesto alternative, and the green variations are limitless: spinach, chard, or beet greens are just a few suggestions. You can also change the nuts: walnuts, almonds or macadamia work well. In the Blue Zone tradition use what is local and seasonal and try different combinations. I omit the garlic or use roasted garlic, as I am sensitive to it raw. It all depends on your own taste and sensitivity.

 HEALING PROPERTIES

Combining ingredients like kale and basil is a superfood offering.

Pesto contains disease-preventing antioxidants such as vitamins A and C, plus it's rich in heart friendly mono and polyunsaturated fats.

2 C chopped kale or any greens you have on hand
½ C basil leaves
2 T Italian parsley
1 clove garlic (optional)
1 T lemon juice
1 t lemon zest
¼ t Aleppo chili pepper
¾ t salt
½ C pine nuts
2 to 3 T olive or avocado oil
2 T water
¼ C Parmesan cheese or vegan alternative

1. BLEND all ingredients together.
2. ADJUST seasoning, add more water, salt or chili, as needed.
3. OMIT cheese or use a Parmesan cheese alternative, if you prefer to make it vegan.

 SIDEBAR THE MORTAR AND PESTLE OF PESTO

"If you are in Pra and you don't grow basil, you are nobody."
—Roggerio Rossi, basil farmer

Pesto is simply a generic word for anything that is made by pounding, blending or crushing, leaves making it endlessly flexible. The word for "pesto" in Italian means, to pound, or crush and in the traditional Italian home is often prepared with a marble mortar and wooden pestle, crushed with a circular motion. You can interchangeably use different nuts and greens, depending on your taste. You can also make it a vegan option, or simply omit cheese.

The Worldwide Blue Zones

BLACK BEAN CORNBREAD CASSEROLE

Serves 6 to 8 | Preheat Oven to 350 Degrees | Bake: 35 to 40 Minutes   M N S Y

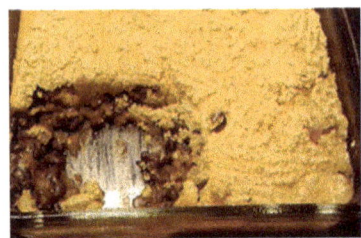

Black beans and corn masa are a staple of the Blue Zone South American diet. The secret is soaking the dried beans overnight, draining the soaking water and rinsing them very well the next morning before cooking. Adding bay leaves also aids in digestion. I add ginger, as well and include greens. This is an innovative way to add black beans and corn into your diet.

1 C dried black beans, soaked overnight (for cooking in Instant Pot, see Hint)
¼ C olive oil
1 onion, chopped small
½ t ginger powder
2 C spinach or local greens, chopped
3 bay leaves and 1 garlic clove, roasted
1 T lemon juice and ½ t lemon zest
1 t salt
4 C water or broth

HINT

INSTANT POT BEAN COOKING

Rinse and sort dried beans. For each cup of beans add 3 cups of water and the rest of the ingredients to the pot.

Cook on high pressure for the directed time.

When done, let the pressure release naturally.

Minutes to Cook
Black Beans: 30
Chickpeas: 40
Kidney Beans: 35
Pinto Beans: 25
Navy Beans: 30
Great Northern: 35

1. STIR FRY onion in oil until transparent.
2. ADD all the rest of ingredients.
3. TOP with water or broth.
4. BOIL for about 10 minutes and lower heat to medium, cook until beans are tender, removed bay leaves and drain extra water. You can use an Instant Pot, as well, see Hint.
5. ADD cooked beans to on oiled casserole dish. Follow cornbread topping recipe below, and baking instructions.

MASA CORNBREAD TOPPING

Dry Ingredients
1½ C masa harina
½ C whole wheat pastry flour
1 t salt
2 t baking powder

Wet Ingredients
2 eggs
¼ C agave
1¼ C almond or rice milk
4 T avocado oil

1. COMBINE dry and wet ingredients in separate bowls.
2. WHISK together, until just blended
3. SPOON on top of the black bean casserole
4. BAKE until cornbread in done and golden on top.

A Culinary Journey

SARDINIAN MINESTRONE STEW AND LEMON COUSCOUS

Serves 6 to 8

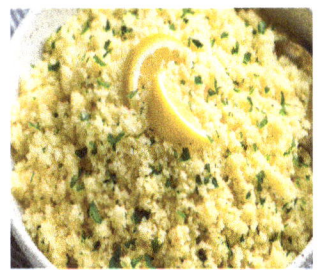

Inspired by the long-living residents of Sardinia, Italy, this thick stew is easy to prepare and perfect to make in large batches and freeze for another time. Serve over a warm bed of luscious lemon couscous.

3 T olive oil
½ t oregano, dried
2 T tomato paste
1 onion, chopped
1 carrot, peeled and chopped
1 celery stalk, chopped
1 broccoli stalk, peeled and chopped
1 sweet potato, peeled and diced (about 1 cup)
1 garlic clove, minced or roasted
2 cans Northern white beans, double rinse, drain well
1 (28 oz.) can crushed fire roasted tomatoes
½ C parsley leaves (save 2 T for garnish on the top)
2 T basil leaves, chopped
Kosher salt and freshly ground black pepper (to taste)
3¼ C vegetable broth

Lemon Couscous
1 T olive oil
¼ C pine nuts
½ C lemon juice, ¾ C water and ½ t salt
1 C couscous

Garnish
¼ C Romano Cheese or vegan alternative, grated (optional)
Extra virgin olive oil

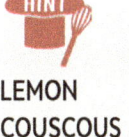

LEMON COUSCOUS

Roast pine nuts in 1 T olive oil, until light brown. Add lemon, water, and salt to pot and bring to a boil.

Add couscous to the boiling liquid and stir in well. Cover and remove from the heat. Let it stand covered for 10 minutes and then fluff with a fork.

1. HEAT the oil in a large soup pot, add the oregano and tomato paste, sauté. Then add the onions, carrots, celery, broccoli, and sweet potatoes, stirring frequently, until all the vegetables are softened.
2. ADD the garlic, sauté a few minutes. Mix in the remaining ingredients.
3. ADD broth and bring to a boil, then lower the heat and simmer for about 20 to 30 minutes.
4. ADJUST the salt and pepper as needed.
5. SERVE on top of couscous.

The Worldwide Blue Zones

BLUE ZONE BREADS

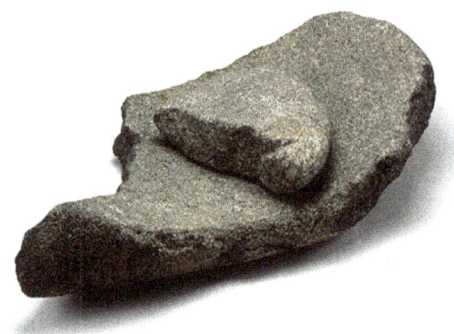

An ancient quern stone.

THE HISTORY OF BREAD IS THE HISTORY OF MANKIND. The earliest evidence of using flour and water to make flatbreads are 8,000 B.C. in the Middle East and South America. A quern stone is the first known grinding tool for ancient grains. The surface of the stone is dotted with tiny crevices that make it into a more efficient grinder. These stones are found all over the world and is the centuries-old living voice and proof of people making bread for their families.

The first breads were baked on fire-heated rocks and became a staple in early man's diet. The grains they used were wild barley, einkorn wheat, oats and tubers. Yet, no one knows exactly when grains were mixed with water, left to ferment and rise, and then baked as flatbreads and sourdough loafs.

In the Blue Zones, each zone has a unique bread: Japan: sweet potato cake; Italy: sourdough; Costa Rica: corn tortillas; Greece: flatbread; and Loma Linda, California: unleavened communion bread. The basic characteristic of Blue Zone breads is that the majority of the ingredients rely on a variety of organic whole grains.

Sourdough leavening is used in many Blue Zone bread recipes, where natural fermentation lowers the glycemic load of an entire meal by 25%. Simple flatbreads, such as tortillas and pitas are another local staple.

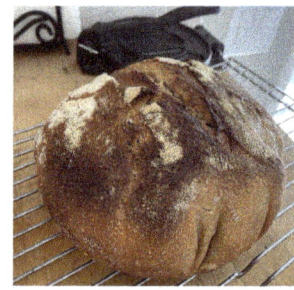

A Culinary Journey

LIMEY SWEET POTATO CAKE

Serves 4 GMENY

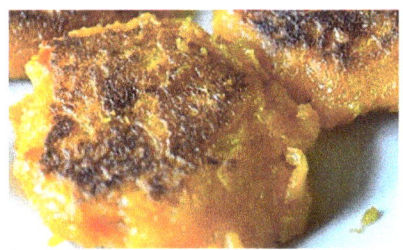

In honoring the Japanese Blue Zone for its use of Sweet Potatoes, this is a lovely pan-fried cake you can use as a base for many types of toppings. They can be made into patties or into one big cake, for whatever base you are using it for.

3 sweet potatoes, grated
4 T avocado oil
2 shallots, finely chopped
1 garlic clove, roasted
1 t ginger powder
2 T brown rice flour
2 T potato starch
½ t wasabi paste
1 T tamari
2 T parsley, finely chopped
1 lime, juiced and zested

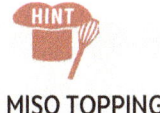

MISO TOPPING

1 T white miso
2 T rice wine vinegar,
½ t grated fresh ginger
Pinch of cayenne
1 T dark sesame oil
1 T avocado oil
2 T mayonnaise

Blend all together until smooth.

1. RINSE the grated sweet potatoes and squeeze into a towel to remove the excess water.
2. SAUTÉ shallots in 2 T oil, until translucent.
3. MIX cooked shallots with the sweet potatoes, garlic, ginger, flour, starch, wasabi, tamari, parsley, lime juice and zest.
4. ADD 2 T oil to a fry pan, heat the oil.
5. MAKE into small patties or use all of it for one large cake.
6. COOK on medium heat. Fry first side about 4 minutes, a bit longer if it is one large cake. Turn and cook another 3 minutes until brown.
7. SERVE with sour cream, miso topping (see Hint), salsa or guacamole on top.

SIMPLE SOURDOUGH

1 Loaf | Preheat Oven to 450 Degrees | Bake: 40 to 45 Minutes   MENS

SOURDOUGH STARTER

First day. Mix ½ C warm water, ¾ C bread flour and 1 T of rye flour. **Next day.** Remove some of the previous day's starter, add water/flour mixture (after two days omit rye flour) In about 5 to 6 days starter should begin to double, have bubbles and a yeasty, sourdough smell. Refrigerate, and replenish water/flour mixture every week.
To Use: The morning you're baking, feed the starter. Between 7 to 8 hours starter may begin to sink, use at its peak, it is ready when you put a spoonful in water, and it floats.

Sourdough is a very satisfying experiment. Though it took a while to get used to the feel of this dough, since it is much different than yeasted dough; it is more hydrated (this recipe is 75% hydration) and sticky. My inclination, at first, was to add more flour. I implore you NOT to do this. Stickiness (hydration) is essential. I found the secret is letting the dough rest and absorb the water throughout the process; this overnight version finally did the trick. The other trick is to heat a cast iron skillet, pot or pan in a very hot oven and bake the bread with the top on to create steam. The challenge for me was we had just moved into a new house, which we renovated, but hadn't replaced the original wall oven, so I was forced to bake in a toaster oven. After quite a few tries, I finally figured it out!

½ C very bubbly, active sourdough starter (see Hint)
1½ C plus 1 T warm water
3¾ to 4 C bread flour
2 t fine sea salt

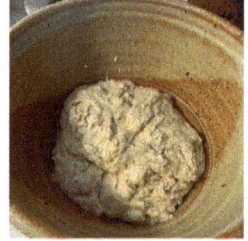

Shaggy dough

1. START the dough around 4 p.m. Whisk starter and water together vigorously in a large bowl. Add just enough flour (I use 3¼ C to start, you will be adding more flour, as needed) to make a very wet shaggy dough. Cover with a damp tea towel and initially rest for 30 minutes, to let the flour absorb the water.
2. SPRINKLE salt on top and mix into the dough. Add just a little more flour, to be able to handle the dough. Then begin the "Stretch and Fold" intervals (see Sidebar below).

 SIDEBAR   STRETCH AND FOLD SOURDOUGH METHOD

This is where you give the dough a chance to create the traditional holes that develop a light, springy sourdough loaf. With lightly floured hands grab a corner of the dough and pull it up and into the center. Rotate the bowl and repeat this a few times, letting the covered dough rest for 30 minutes in between the stretching and folding action. Continue two more 30-minute intervals. If you have the time, you can do it 2 more times.

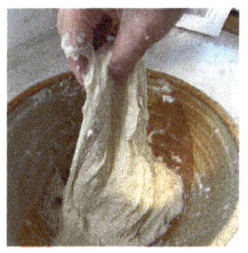
Stretch and Fold

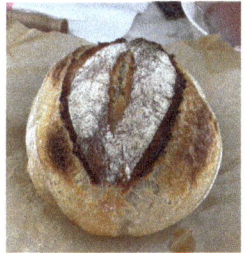
Finished Loaf

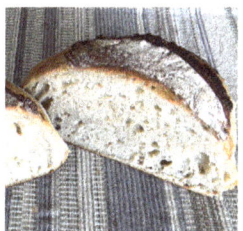
Inside the Loaf

Sourdough Bread Tools: *Bannaton proofing basket, scoring razor, bread whisk, and brush.*

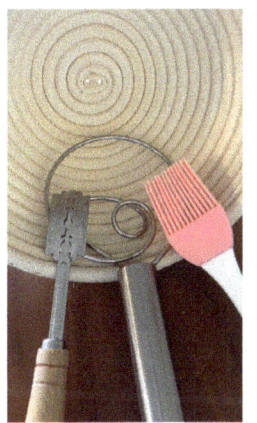

3. RISING the dough. The bulk rise is overnight. Put it in the refrigerator with cling wrap on top of the bowl and a tea towel on top of that. Let it sit anywhere from 8-18 hours. The dough should rise, even in the cool refrigerator and have some bubbles on top.
4. PREPARING the dough. In the morning place the dough onto a lightly floured surface (I use a Silpat, so it doesn't need too much flour). With floured hands shape it into a rough circle, folding the top into the center, rotate the dough and repeat until it is a nice circle. Add just enough flour to be able to work with it to create tension. Let the dough come to room temperature in a covered bowl for about 60 minutes.
5. LINE an 8-inch bowl with a tea towel or use a traditional proofing basket with a tea towel or proofing cloth insert. Dust generously with coarse flour (rice flour, semolina, or cornmeal work well). Using a bench scraper or your floured hands, shape it once again, see step 4. Place the rounded dough into your lined bowl, seam side up.
6. PROOF. Cover the dough and let rise for 60 minutes or return to the refrigerator for up to 24 hours. The dough should rise a bit, not too much, since the bulk of the final rise will be in the oven. At this stage you can put the bread vessel in the oven to preheat for 30 minutes.
7. REMOVE the cast iron, Dutch oven pot or loaf pan carefully from the oven where it has been heating.
8. CUT a piece of parchment to fit the size of your baking pot. Place the parchment over the dough and release the dough from the final rising bowl. Add a sprinkle of flour to the top of the dough and with the tip of a small knife or a razor blade, score the dough. There are endless ways to score the top of the dough. In the beginning a simple "X" is fine. Remove excess flour with a brush and transfer the final dough, on the parchment, into the heated baking pot.
9. BAKE, covering the pot or pan, for 30 minutes. Then remove the lid and lower the temperature to 400 degrees and continue to bake for an additional 10–15 minutes. Check the loaf by lifting it out of the pot and if necessary place directly onto the oven rack for the last 5 minutes.
10. COOL on a wire rack for 1 hour before slicing.

 SIDEBAR   **USING EXTRA SOURDOUGH STARTER**

Rather than simply throwing out the excess starter each day, use it in other recipes. If you add 1 cup of starter to a recipe, reduce the flour and liquid in the recipe by ½ cup.

CORN TORTILLAS

Makes 16 to 18 Tortillas

GMENSY

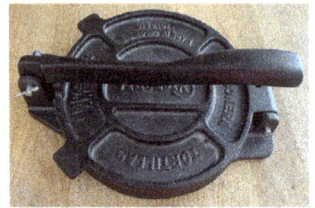

KNEADING THE TORTILLA DOUGH

In the beginning the dough will be a little rough but becomes more pliable as you knead it.

Continue to knead it, as you would any bread, but a little gentler, until it is pliable and smooth ball and feels like Playdough.

You can always adjust the dough by adding more water or masa. It takes a little practice to know the right consistency, not too dry or too wet.

Corn Tortillas are made with Corn Masa. Masa is corn flour that has been treated with calcium hydroxide or "lime," which releases the niacin in the corn, making it easier to digest. You can buy masa flour at Mexican markets or online. When looking to buy masa harina, make sure it only has two ingredients corn and lime and it says it is for tortillas. There is no reason why you can't make the tortillas by hand: form into a small ball between your hands, but it takes an experienced hand to do so. The easier method is using a tortilla press, which is available at most Mexican markets or online, they can be wood or cast iron.

2 cups masa harina
½ t salt
1½ to 2 C very warm water

1. MIX flour and salt, then begin adding 1½ C of warm water or follow the directions on the masa package, some brands may call for different amounts of water. It will be a slightly wet dough, which is fine. Let sit for at least 15 to 30 minutes, covered, to help it absorb the dough, don't omit this resting and absorbing step.
2. KNEAD the dough, see hint on left. Keep a damp cloth on top, so it doesn't dry out, while forming the balls.
3. FORM balls of dough by pinching off a piece and rubbing it between your lightly wet hands to shape into a ball, the size of a plum, or a slightly large golf ball. Shape all the balls and cover with a damp cloth.
4. PREPARE the tortilla press with two sheets of wax paper or a large Ziplock plastic bag, cut into two pieces. Place the ball of dough between the sheets and press gently to make a tortilla 4" to 5" wide.
5. HEAT a griddle or a cast iron skillet on high heat. Remove the tortilla from the press carefully and working, one at a time, transfer the tortilla to the hot pan by: allowing the tortilla to rest half on your hand, and half hanging down, and gently lay the tortilla down on to the skillet. Then, start working on pressing the next tortilla.
6. COOK the tortilla on the hot pan for 30 to 60 seconds on each side. The tortilla should be lightly toasted with little air pockets forming. If you have a gas stove, you can put them directly on the burner for a few seconds and let it pop up even further. Serve warm.

WHOLE GRAIN PITA BREAD

Makes 7 to 8 Pitas | Preheat Oven to 475 Degrees | Bake: 3 to 4 Minutes   M E N S

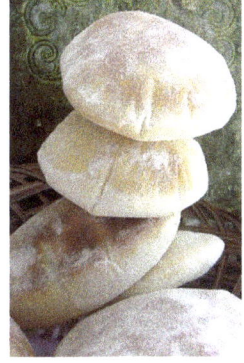

The first pita breads seem to have been made in the area West of the Mediterranean, and eventually flourished in the Greece Islands. Though there is no direct evidence, it's believed that the Amorites or the Bedouins were the people to discover them, and they soon found their way to those travelling across the desert lands. Originally, it was a simple sourdough that was left to ferment and help the bread rise and then it was discovered that yeast was a quicker and easier way to make them, and traditional bread recipes were born.

STORING PITAS

I like to freeze my pitas and take them out, a few at a time, to keep them super fresh.

- MAKE sure the pitas are completely cooled.
- STORE in doubled bagged Ziplock plastics bags.
- Freeze the pitas for up to 3 months
- To use: wrap the frozen pitas in tin foil and heat in a low-heat oven.

1 C warm water
2¼ t dried active yeast
1 t honey
1½ cup whole wheat pastry flour

½ C cornmeal
1 C unbleached white flour
1 t fine sea salt
2 T avocado oil

1. MIX water, yeast and honey in a large bowl. Add ½ cup whole wheat flour and whisk briskly for about 1 minute. Let the sponge mixture rest for at least 15 minutes, until bubbly.
2. ADD the rest of the ingredients, holding back ½ C white flour to form a rough dough. Dust a surface with a little flour and knead the dough for about 5 to 7 minutes, until smooth, adding just enough flour as you knead, since the dough should be slightly moist.
3. COAT another bowl with some oil and place the kneaded dough inside with cling wrap on top. Leave in a warm place for at least 1 hour, until the dough has doubled.
4. MAKE the pita balls, by dividing and rolling them into 7 to 8 pieces. Let them rest for a few minutes with a moist towel on top.
5. SHAPE the pitas by rolling out the balls into a circle, until they are a quarter of an inch thick. Use as little flour as necessary, so the pitas do not stick, but are pliable.
6. BAKE them in a very hot oven. Heat a flat iron pan or cookie sheet and add a few pitas at a time. Bake on the first side for 2 to 3 minutes and carefully turn and bake them for an additional minute, they should pop by then. Continue baking the rest of the pitas. Keep each batch of baked pitas covered with a clean towel while you work on the rest.

ADVENTIST UNLEAVENED COMMUNION BREAD

Makes 25 Pieces | Preheat Oven to 425 Degrees | Bake: 8 to 12 Minutes   M E N S Y

In Loma Linda, California, where a lot of Seventh-day Adventist live, they use grape juice in place of wine and this unleavened bread for their communion service. This yeast-free bread dates back to the Exodus of the Hebrews fleeing Egypt. They didn't have enough time to let the bread rise, and this flatbread was the solution. It most resembles a cracker. They have a very unique way of making this traditional bread.

½ C olive oil
3 C warm water
1½ t fine pink sea salt
2 cups whole wheat pastry flour

1. ADD oil, water, and salt into a gallon Ziplock bag. Shake the bag very well, until the mixture is frothy.
2. ADD the flour, remove air from bag and mix together and then gently knead the dough in the bag, do not over knead.
3. FORM dough into a circle, inside of the bag.
4. REST the dough for 15 to 30 minutes.
5. ROLL out the dough, inside of the bag, until it fills the entire bag.
6. CUT the top off the bag and along the sides. Remove one side of the plastic bag and put a piece of oiled parchment paper on top.
7. REMOVE from the bag and place, parchment side down and score, not slice, into even squares (see picture above) with a knife or pizza cutter. Then, "tine" each square with a fork.
8. FLIP dough onto a cookie sheet and remove parchment paper.
9. BAKE until the edges are golden, do not overbake.
10. COOL completely on a rack and break apart, into single crackers.

 SIDEBAR   ADVENTIST COMMUNITY DIET

The Seventh-day Adventist diet combines a wide variety of plant foods, fruits, vegetables, legumes, nuts, seeds, and whole grains. They eat meat and eggs in moderation, but it doesn't include pork, rabbit, or shellfish. About 50 percent are lacto-ovo (milk-and-egg-using) vegetarians and they abstain from smoking and drinking alcoholic beverages.

CHAPTER THREE
VEGETABLES AND TOFU

VEGETABLES FROM THE FARM
A DAY IN THE LIFE OF TOFU
VEGGIE BURGERS
SATURDAY MARKET MORNING
SUMMER TOMATOES

VEGETABLES FROM THE FARM

IN 1972 WE FOUND OURSELVES LIVING ON A 130 ACRE FARM IN THE CANADIAN PROVINCE OF NOVA SCOTIA. The challenge for me at the time was my introduction to a turn-of-the-century wood-burning cook stove. I remember my first meal was to attempt to cook macaroni. My inexperience with the stove and actually making wood burn produced a sticky, uncooked meal. Soon, with the challenge behind me, the aroma of freshly baked bread and three-hour bean soup was wafting its way through the country kitchen. In those quiet, snowbound winters, my lifelong appreciation of cooking and feeding others began. It was there I learned by doing and doing over again. And perhaps the biggest revelation, one that even now stays with me, was that the way one cooks is as important as using the purest ingredients.

An interesting experience for us was raising cows. Each morning and evening two huge pails of milk were brought into the kitchen. It was a challenge to find ways to use all this milk without wasting it. The cows tolerated us city slickers. There were times when the cow let us finish milking only to calmly put her hind leg into the bucket. This brought a bit of relief on my part since I was given a break from some milk preparation that day. As soon as the steaming bucket of milk came in from the barn, we separated it with an old-fashioned milk separator and made wonderful butter and ghee for frying. In summer we made homemade ice cream, along with fresh yogurt and cottage cheese. The best part was when we brought the separated fat-free milk to our neighbor's pig. In one

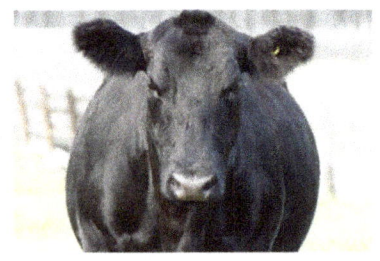

A Culinary Journey

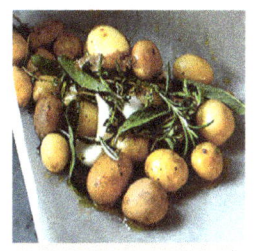

Potato Package Surprise

For this herb-infused delight, cook new potatoes and peas in parchment.

- PILE tiny new potatoes and fresh podded peas onto a large piece of parchment paper, along with 1 garlic clove.
- ADD herbs like rosemary and lemon thyme, sprinkle with salt and a drizzle olive oil.
- FOLD the parchments into individual parcels and bake in a 350-degree oven for 30 to 40 minutes.
- OPEN the packages for a dramatic presentation.

stream the entire bucket was poured into the pig's mouth. We were sure we saw a smile on his face when we left. All breads, casseroles, and desserts contained the fresh milk from those dear cows. Years later, my husband, Matthew, developed an extreme allergy to milk. I'm sure our cows would have had a hearty laugh over that.

As soon as the first sign of buds came bursting out of the ground from the potato plants, we knew a few tiny potatoes waited to be picked for a special recipe—new potato stew. I even made a little jingle of it as we picked these little gems. "New potato stew . . . is waiting just for you." Simmering away with just picked tiny carrots we gathered from thinning out the rows, and the early batch of freshly podded peas, all it needed was a little churned butter, fragrant rosemary and thyme and we experienced the essence of goodness and simplicity only vegetables one hour old can bring.

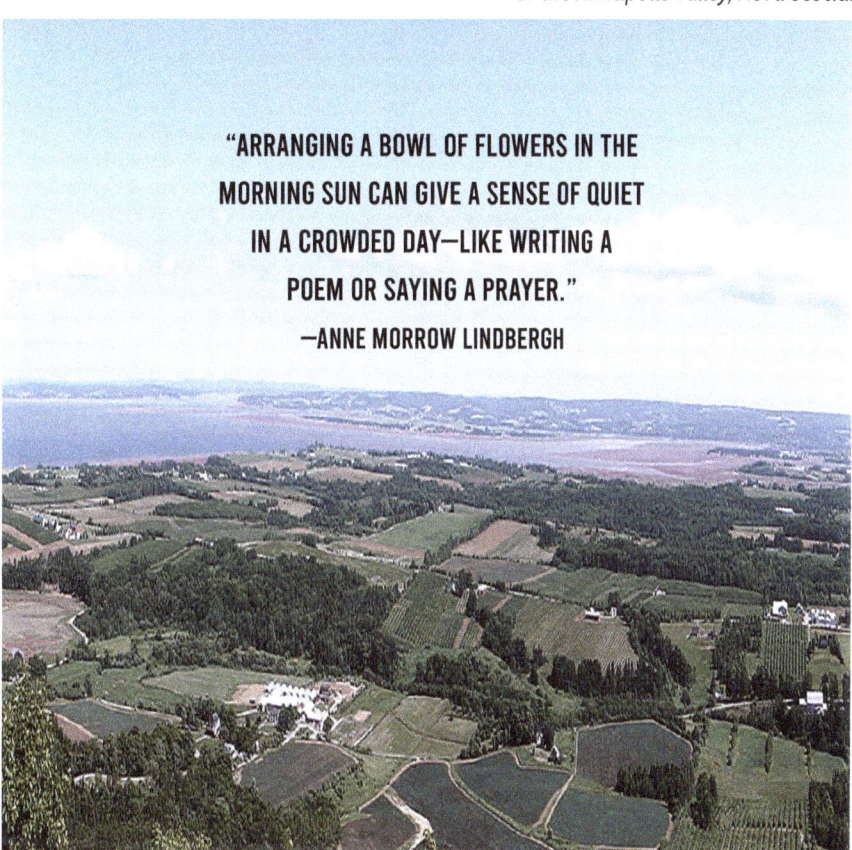

"The Lookoff," from the North Mountain, in the Annapolis Valley, Nova Scotia.

"ARRANGING A BOWL OF FLOWERS IN THE MORNING SUN CAN GIVE A SENSE OF QUIET IN A CROWDED DAY—LIKE WRITING A POEM OR SAYING A PRAYER."
—ANNE MORROW LINDBERGH

CARROT/SWEET POTATO CUSTARD BAKE

Serves 4 | Preheat Oven to 350 Degrees | Bake: 30 Minutes   G M N S Y

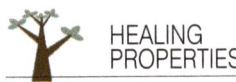 **HEALING PROPERTIES**

Carrots & Sweet Potato/Yams
- Antioxidant, helps to eliminate free radicals
- Anti-inflammatory
- Anti-diabetic, healing properties in blood sugar control

The fun of growing your own carrots is pulling them out of the ground with little bits of earth stuck to their tender roots. A small amount of carrot seed goes a long way. When you thin the rows, you also get a wonderful collection of sweet baby carrots of various sizes to use in dishes. This is a simple, fragrant, sweet, and comforting side dish for fresh summer carrots or when using them from the root cellar on a cold winter night. The protein from the eggs helps to balance the extra carbs of the carrots and sweet potatoes.

2 to 3 C large carrots, or 5 to 6 small carrots, diced small
1 sweet potato, peeled and cubed
2 T maple, brown rice, or agave syrup
2 T margarine, butter, or ghee, melted
½ C milk (low or nonfat) or soy, rice, or almond milk
½ t salt
2 eggs or 3 egg whites, beaten
¼ t cardamom powder and ¼ t cinnamon
Nutmeg, grated fresh

1. STEAM carrots and sweet potatoes together until very tender.
2. PULSE all the ingredients (including warm, not hot, carrots and sweet potatoes) in a food processor until almost smooth.
3. PLACE in a 9" x 9" square casserole dish.
4. TOP with nutmeg and bake until custard is set.

SIDEBAR   THE HISTORY OF THE SWEET POTATO AND THE YAM

Sweet Potatoes (*Ipomoea batatas*) are the root of a vine in the morning glory family, native to the New World tropics and date back to 750 B.C. in Peruvian records. Columbus brought the sweet potato to the New World from the island of Saint Thomas. At that time, potato referred to the sweet potato, and not the generic white potato as it does today. In fact, the white potato did not arrive in the northern regions from South America until 1676. The original yam is the tuber of a tropical vine (*Dioscorea batatas*) and is not even distantly related to the sweet potato. Rarely found in US markets, this yam is still a popular vegetable in Latin America and the Caribbean with over 150 varieties available worldwide. Generally sweeter than the sweet potato, this tuber can grow over seven feet in length. The word yam comes from the African words *njam*, *nyami*, or *djambi*, meaning "to eat," as it was a dietary staple.

HOMEMADE RAINBOW COLESLAW

Serves 4 to 6

GMENSY

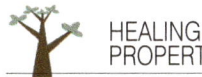 **HEALING PROPERTIES**

Cabbage
- Speeds up estrogen metabolism
- May help block breast cancer and suppress growth of polyps
- Contains anti-ulcer compounds
- Includes anti-viral powers, especially in raw cabbage
- Encourages new cell growth

This is a favorite coleslaw recipe—smoky, crispy, refreshing, a rainbow of colors, incorporating green, orange, and red vegetables, great for picnics.

¼ of a whole medium red cabbage
½ of a whole medium green cabbage
1 beet, peeled
2 carrots
½ lemon, juiced
Splash of apple cider or balsamic vinegar
1 t salt
Fresh pepper
½ C olive oil mayonnaise (or vegan mayonnaise); blend with ¼ to 1 chipotle pepper (canned) or a small amount of the adobo sauce, depending on how spicy you want it.

1. GRATE cabbages, carrots, and beet.
2. COMBINE lemon juice, vinegar, salt, pepper, and chipotle mayonnaise until well blended. Add to shredded veggies, blend well and let marinade at least ½ hour before serving.

 SIDEBAR   THE EVOLUTION OF CABBAGE

The history of cabbage is quite fascinating in its transformations throughout the centuries. Although they appear very different, kale, cabbage, kohlrabi, cauliflower, broccoli, and brussels sprouts are all the same species. Known botanically as members of *Brassica oleracea*, the only difference between these plants are the different methods used over thousands of years of human cultivation and selective propagating. In the wild, the original *Brassica oleracea* plant is native to the Mediterranean region of Europe. Soon after the domestication of plants began, people in the Mediterranean region began growing this first ancient "cabbage" plant as a leafy vegetable. By the fifth century B.C., they preferred a larger leaf, which led to the development of the vegetable we now know as kale, which translates to mean, "cabbage of the vegetable garden without a head." As time passed, however, some people began to express a preference for plants with a tight cluster of tender leaves in the center of the plant, at the top of the stem. Eventually, the cluster of leaves became so large, it dominates the whole plant, and the cabbage "head" we know today was born.

CRUSTY HOMEFRIED POTATOES & PEAS WITH SPICY DILL SAUCE

Serves 4 GMENSY

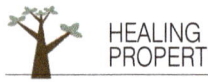

HEALING PROPERTIES

Dill
- Dill tea can be used to control flatulence
- Chewing a few dill seeds freshens your breath
- Calcium, helps prevent bone loss

Dilly Sauce

1 C low fat yogurt
½ C ricotta cheese or alternative (see Hint)
1 t avocado oil
2 t dill, fresh
1 t fresh dill
¼ t salt
¼ to ½ t chipotle powder
½ t cumin powder

BLEND until smooth creamy.

Our first experience planting potatoes occurred during our first summer in Nova Scotia and it was quite an event. Using a planting book as a guide, we meticulously cut out the eyes of the potatoes and began planting the tiny sprouts one by one. Our neighbor Mr. Connell drove by and found us on hands and knees, digging up little mounts of dirt. He looked at us gravely, cocked his head, and immediately brought over his horse and plow. Motioning us to leave the field, he began to plow up six long rows. Coarsely chopping the remaining potatoes into large pieces, he carelessly chucked them into the deep brown loosened soil and then proceeded to plow the dirt over the rows. As the sun set beyond the mountain, he quietly rode home, tipping his hat. Not a word had been spoken.

4 to 6 medium/large, red potatoes (new ones with thin skins are best), baked until almost tender, about 45 minutes to an hour.
2 T olive oil
1 red pepper, julienne, sliced thin
2 garlic cloves, crushed slightly and sliced thin
1 t kosher salt
¼ t smoky paprika
1 C fresh or frozen peas

1. CUT baked potatoes (leave skin on) into medium cubes.
2. HEAT a heavy-duty skillet and add oil, red peppers, and stir fry for five minutes, then add garlic and stir fry for another minute.
3. ADD potatoes, salt, and paprika, fry on medium heat until crusty.
4. ADD peas and fry until about 2 minutes.
5. TOP with dilly sauce just before serving.

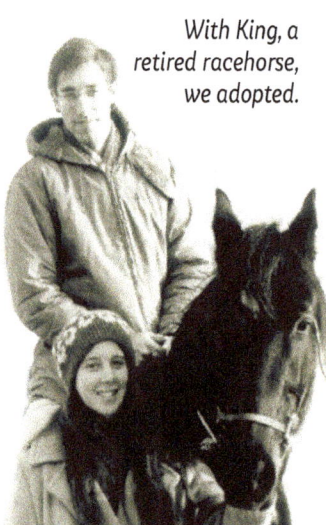

With King, a retired racehorse, we adopted.

VEGAN RICOTTA CHEESE

1½ C raw cashews, soaked overnight in bowl of water.
½ C water, 1 T apple wine vinegar,
2 T nutritional yeast, ½ t onion powder, ½ t salt.

Drain cashews and process all ingredients into a blender or food processor, until creamy. Store in an airtight container in the refrigerator.

GARDEN FRESH-BAKED HERBED TOMATOES

Serves 4 | Preheat Oven to 350 Degrees | Bake: 30 Minutes

GMENSY

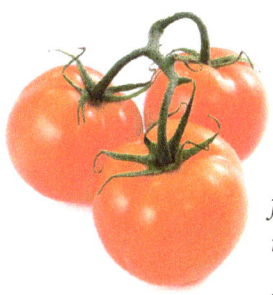

These tomatoes are truly heavenly. They not only utilize the tomatoes that are available in abundance from a summer garden or farmers market but can be cooked and frozen to bring sunshine to the cold winter days ahead when summer is a faint memory. It combines the olive oil flavor, a bevy of fresh herbs, garlic, and lemon. The dish can be used as a side vegetable or mixed with pasta as a fresh tomato sauce.

¼ C fresh parsley, chopped
3 rosemary sprigs
1 T lemon thyme, chopped
4 fresh mint leaves, chopped
3 T olive oil

2 t lemon rind, grated
1 t salt
Freshly ground pepper
5 pounds, plum tomatoes, chopped
2 to 3 garlic cloves, minced

1. MIX all the ingredients in a large bowl, toss well to combine.
2. PLACE the tomato mixture in a 13" x 9" baking dish and bake for 30 minutes. Stir a few times.
3. REMOVE from the oven and turn on the broiler. Broil for 10 minutes until they begin to brown, and peels begin to loosen.
4. REMOVE peels from blistered tomatoes and rosemary sprigs, mash slightly, drizzle 1 T olive oil at the end.

 SIDEBAR   **THE HISTORY OF OLIVE OIL**

Olives have ancient roots; their cultivation probably occurred, beginning in 5,000 B.C. and until 1,400 B.C., olive cultivation spread from Crete to Syria, Palestine, and Israel. Commercial networking and cultivation advances brought the olive tree to southern Turkey, Cyprus, and Egypt. King Solomon and King David placed great importance on olive trees. King David even had guards watching over the olive groves and warehouses, ensuring the safety of the trees and their precious oil.

The belief that olive oil conferred strength and youth was widespread. In ancient Egypt, Greece, and Rome, it was infused with flowers and grasses to be used in both medicine and cosmetics. Despite harsh winters, burning summers, and truncations, olive trees continue to grow, proud and strong, reaching towards the sky. There are about thirty varieties of olives growing in Italy today, and each yields a specific oil with its own unique characteristics.

Vegetables and Tofu | 59

CARAMELIZED DOUBLE-BAKED SQUASH

Serves 4 to 6 | Preheat Oven to 350 Degrees | Bake: 10 Minutes   GMENSY

PANKO BREADCRUMBS

Using Panko makes any recipe which calls for breadcrumbs much lighter and crunchier. These bread flakes are made in Japan from traditional Japanese bread. The loaves are slowly dried and then shredded into crispy flakes. Panko is basic to Japanese cuisine, but its texture and flavor can be added to any type of cooking. This is now readily available in most markets or online.

Personally, I love butternut squash. By now you should have figured out if you like squash and which one you like the best. Any winter squash will work in this recipe—acorn is good too. This is a great dish with a summer salad or winter soup.

2 medium butternut squashes
½ C low-fat sharp cheddar cheese or cashew cheese (see page 291)
2 T butter, ghee or olive oil
1 t salt
Pinch of cayenne or chipotle pepper powder
½ C maple, agave syrup or brown sugar
¼ C Parmesan cheese or alternative (optional)
½ C Japanese Panko breadcrumbs, traditional breadcrumbs, almond meal or gluten-free breadcrumbs.

1. CUT squashes in half and de-seed.
2. PLACE on a greased baking sheet, cut side down.
3. BAKE until tender, about one hour.
4. SCOOP out squash gently trying not to disturb the shell, mash well.
5. HEAT butter, ghee, or olive oil; add syrup or sugar and cook for a few moments to caramelize.
6. ADD crumbled cheddar or cashew cheese, salt and pepper to butter/syrup mixture then add mashed squash; mix well.
7. RETURN to shells and mix Parmesan cheese with breadcrumbs or almond meal and sprinkle on top.
8. BAKE until top is brown and bubbly.

 SIDEBAR   USING AND STORING WINTER SQUASH

As winter squash easily decays, carefully inspect it before purchasing. You should choose ones that are firm, a bit heavy for their size and have hard and dull, not glossy skin. Depending on the variety, winter squash can be kept up to six months. To extend its life it should be kept away from direct exposure to light, as well as extreme heat or cold. The best way to freeze winter squash is to first cut it into the particular size you may need for an individual recipe and parboil.

EVERYDAY GARLIC BROCCOLI STIR FRY

Serves 4   GMENSY

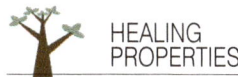 HEALING PROPERTIES

Broccoli
- Promotes gastro tract healing
- Strengthens the immune system
- Contains indole carbinol, which breaks down estrogen
- Contains antioxidant, beta carotene

This is such a simple and healthy way to stir fry any vegetables; you could easily substitute broccoli for string beans, zucchini, or cabbage.

2 to 3 T olive oil
1 red pepper, julienne cut
1 onion, sliced thin
3 to 4 garlic cloves, crushed slightly (you can pierce with toothpicks for easy removal after the dish is cooked)
1 T ginger, freshly grated
1 T thyme, fresh, or ½ t dried
¼ t turmeric
1 t paprika or smoky paprika
½ t salt or low sodium soy sauce
Fresh pepper
1 large head of broccoli, chopped into florets (save broccoli stems for coleslaw, see page 57)
Splash of lemon juice

1. SAUTÉ peppers and onions in oil until translucent.
2. ADD garlic and ginger and stir fry for 30 seconds.
3. ADD thyme, turmeric, paprika, salt, pepper, and broccoli.
4. COVER and turn heat to low-medium, cook for 15 minutes.
5. UNCOVER and cook an additional five minutes until all liquid is absorbed and broccoli is fork tender; remove garlic cloves.
6. SPLASH with lemon juice.

 LEMON JUICE EXTRACTION

Here are a few hints to extract the most amount of juice from a lemon:

1. Roll a lemon on a hard surface applying pressure with the palm of your hand.
2. Boil a lemon for 3 minutes.
3. Microwave a lemon for 30 seconds.
4. Bake a lemon in the oven for 4 minutes at 325 degrees.
5. If you don't have enough lemon juice for a recipe you can replace a small quantity of lemon juice with a mild vinegar for the same quantity of lemon juice. (If you need just drops or a splash of lemon juice, pierce a lemon with a fork, turn and squeeze.)

Vegetables and Tofu

CARROTS AND PINE NUT MEDLEY

Serves 4 to 5

GMESY

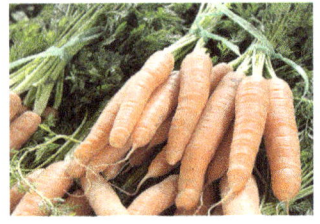

Carrots are a staple in most homes, though they can be forgotten in the back of the bin and left to sprout whiskers. They are, of course, great just eaten fresh, but the hidden secret about carrots is that they grow nutritionally as they are cooked, because the cellulose breaks down and becomes more digestible. Also, the healthy beta carotene in carrots needs fat in order to be absorbed properly. Roasting baby carrots with their furry tops on, in a simple blend of oil, spices and the contrast of some acid is one way to enjoy the humble carrot.

When we grew carrots in our large Nova Scotia garden we always had a bevy of carrots to deal with during harvest time. I would often feel challenged to create a new and interesting carrot dish. This one, a bit Middle Eastern in flavor, perfectly matches with fluffy couscous, or, if you are wheat sensitive, you can use steamed buckwheat (kasha) or protein rich quinoa.

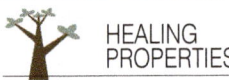

Carrots
- Rich in beta carotene
- Powerful antioxidant
- Believed to be effective against breast, ovarian, and lung cancer

Cooking Quinoa

1 C quinoa, rinsed and 1¾ C water. Combine quinoa and water, bring to a boil, then cover, reduce heat and simmer 15 minutes. Let it sit covered for 10 minutes. Fluff with a fork.

2 T olive oil
1 medium onion, diced very small
3 T pine nuts
1 t paprika
1 inch piece of ginger, freshly grated
1 T basil, fresh, or ½ t dried

3 C carrots, sliced diagonally
½ C water
2 T agave or maple syrup
1 T capers
1 T balsamic vinegar
Salt and fresh pepper to taste

1. SAUTÉ onions in oil until translucent.
2. ADD pine nuts, paprika, ginger, and basil, fry until nuts are golden.
3. ADD carrots, water, and syrup, cook on low-to-medium heat with the lid on until the carrots are fork-tender.
4. ADD capers, vinegar, salt, and pepper.
5. COOK uncovered about 7 minutes until all the liquid is evaporated and carrots are nicely caramelized.

WHAT ARE CAPERS?

Capers are the immature flower bud from the caper bush which grows in hot and arid climates, primarily southern European and on the North African coast. These buds are hand harvested and pickled in vinegar or salt cured. They add a unique and distinctive acidic and salty flavor. A simple way to retrieve them from the jar is to use a vertical potato peeler and scoop out the capers, draining the water at the same time.

A DAY IN THE LIFE OF TOFU

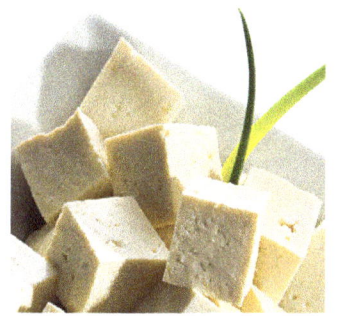

I HAVE A REAL FASCINATION FOR TOFU. For brief (and I stress brief) moments, I thought about preparing it from scratch, so it would be on hand whenever I needed it. Tofu is one of the great versatile foods.

I don't know when I first discovered tofu. It was probably many years ago, floating free in a humble bowl of miso soup. But since our first acquaintance, we have been growing together, year by year.

Tofu is definitely a daily staple in our home. Even my daughter, Ramani, when she was young, could literally eat bean and cheese burritos for all three meals, tolerated tofu in its simplest form, pan-fried with a little olive oil and soy sauce. Now as a grown woman, Ramani considers tofu one of her main proteins. It has a wonderful and almost perfect combination of protein, carbohydrate, and fat. There has been research done that Japanese women, who regularly consume soy products, reported markedly fewer menopausal symptoms than American women. It has also been noted that Japanese women have 75% less breast cancer. Yet its effectiveness in both menopausal symptoms and breast cancer is still not conclusively proven.

The recipes included in this chapter come from years of experimentation and are open to full creative expression on your part. Tofu is the canvas, so to speak, and you are the artist. The possibilities are endless.

During my daughter's kindergarten days, I prepared chili for a chili contest held yearly at her school Halloween carnival. When the contest was over (the chili was sold to raise money for the school), I went to pick up my dish, and the chili was all gone. I often wondered if people knew they were eating tofu!

> I sometimes wonder if we cannot live our life like tofu, a neutral observer, having the capacity to take on what is given to us at the moment—absorbing the texture and flavor of life without interfering.

SMOKIN' VEGGIE TOFU CHILI

Serves 6 to 8

G M E N Y

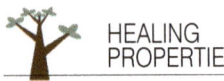

HEALING PROPERTIES

Oregano
- Anti-bacterial, inhibits growth of bacteria
- Antioxidant, helps prevent oxygen-based damage to cell structures throughout the body

2 T olive oil
2 onions, slivered
1 green pepper, slivered
1 red pepper, slivered
3 garlic cloves, minced
¼ C T fresh cilantro, reserve 1 T for top
2 T fresh parsley
¼ t turmeric
½ t cayenne pepper
½ t Hungarian smoky paprika
½ t cumin powder
½ t coriander powder
1 to 2 T ginger, freshly grated
1 T salt
1 t oregano, dried

2 carrots, shredded
2 zucchini, chopped very small
1½ C firm tofu, mashed
2 cups tomatoes, chopped or canned
½ C water with bouillon cube or veggie soup base
½ C black beans, dried and soaked overnight and cooked until tender (about 1½ hours). You could also use 1 can of cooked black beans, drained well
2 T lemon juice
2 drops liquid smoke flavor
Mild fat-free or low-fat cheddar cheese or alternative cheese for sprinkling on top.

1. SAUTÉ onion, green and red peppers in olive oil.
2. ADD garlic, herbs, and spices; cook for a few seconds.
3. COMBINE vegetables, stir fry for about 7 minutes; add tofu and fry until brownish.
4. ADD tomatoes, soup base, salt, and cooked beans. Cover and let it cook together on a slow heat for about 30 to 45 minutes.
5. ADD lemon juice and liquid smoke at the end.
6. TOP with cheese and coriander.

SIDEBAR   SMOKY PAPRIKA

We first discovered smoky paprika (*Pimenton Ahumado* in Spanish) on the village square in Sonoma, California. It was in a specialty store where they made olive oil soap right in front of you. It was the soap that drew us into the store but on the shelf the paprika was a great discovery. I took some home and found it to be a wonderful way to perk up many dishes. Paprika is made from a variety of sweet, bright red powders that are dried and ground from whole peppers. Peppers vary in size, color, and shape and all have their own distinct flavor and aroma, and Spanish paprika has a distinctive smoky flavor. You can now find this paprika in most specialty stores.

OLIVE TOFU-HERB SALAD

Serves 4   G M E N Y

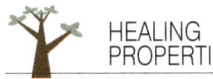 **HEALING PROPERTIES**

Tofu
- Helps to lower cholesterol levels
- Helpful with menopause symptoms
- Rich in minerals for energy and antioxidant protection
- Offers cardiovascular protection from omega-3 fatty acids

This is a simple staple; use it for a variety of sandwiches or topped on a salad. It is especially great for people who do not eat eggs. Olives give it a unique flavor (if you do not care for olives, simply omit them). This salad keeps well in the refrigerator for about three to four days and pairs well with roasted red peppers.

1 T olive oil
2 T red miso
2 T mayonnaise, or vegenaise
1 t mustard, prepared
2 T fresh parsley, chopped very fine
½ t thyme, dried
½ t grated ginger, fresh or ¼ t ginger powder

½ t turmeric powder
Generous pinch cayenne pepper
Black pepper, freshly ground
½ C black olives, chopped small
1½ C extra firm tofu, mashed

1. BLEND everything together, except tofu and olives.
2. ADD tofu and olives at the end, pulse until well combined but still a bit chunky.

 SIDEBAR   THE TOFU STORY

No one is quite sure when the Chinese began making tofu or who figured out the rather complicated process, but historic tomb markings date back to 220 A.D. There are a few varieties: silken or soft is ideal for custard-like desserts, soups and drinks; and firm and extra firm are used for stir frying, grilling and baking. Chinese tofu comes in various textures but tends to be softer than regular tofu; you may need to drain and extract the excess water by pressing it down with a heavy can. You can also squeeze, press, and freeze tofu to enhance its texture. Tofu has an astounding 20 grams of protein in each 1 cup serving.

Quick Tofu Ideas:
- Mash firm tofu with cottage cheese and seasonings for a sandwich spread.
- Stir dried onion soup mix or gomasio into soft or silken tofu for a veggie or chip dip.
- Add chunks of firm tofu to soups, stews, salads, and stir-fried vegetables.
- Blend silken tofu with melted chocolate or carob chips, sugar, or sweetener for an easy chocolate cream pie filling.

MARINADED & GRILLED TOFU WITH THAI SAUCE

Serves 4 to 6

GMEY

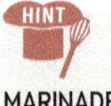

MARINADE

When marinating anything, use as little or no oil as it seals the outer layer of the protein, preventing the marinade flavor from penetrating.

1 lb. tofu, drained and blocked, cut into 1" squares

Tofu Marinade
1½ C coconut milk
1 onion, coarsely chopped
1 T garlic, minced
¾ t turmeric
1 t red pepper flakes
½ t fresh ginger, grated
¾ T kosher salt

1. PROCESS the marinade ingredients into a paste, the consistency of thin yogurt. (Reserve a small amount for basting)
2. ADD the tofu pieces to the marinade and toss, cover with cling wrap, and marinate at least six hours or even better, refrigerate overnight.
3. GRILL tofu in a lightly oiled grill pan (first remove excess marinade), grill over medium heat for approximately 5 minutes per side, or until lightly crisp.
4. BRUSH with the reserved marinade.

Serve with Thai Peanut Sauce: Makes 1 Cup
½ C roasted peanuts or 2 T peanut butter and 1 T avocado oil
1 to 2 fresh Thai chilis or any small green chilis, de-seeded and chopped
1½" ginger, minced
1 garlic clove, minced (optional)
⅓ C light coconut milk
1 t Braggs Liquid Aminos or light soy sauce
1 t honey or agave syrup
1 T lemon juice and 1 t lemon zest
1 t yellow miso
1 t cilantro and stems, very finely minced

How to Serve Grilled Tofu

Place tofu on top of rice and pour ⅛ C of sauce. Sprinkle cilantro on top.

1. ADD peanuts along with the oil to a food processor.
2. BLEND at high speed until the peanuts form a rough paste or use peanut butter.
3. ADD the rest of the ingredients except for the cilantro; blend until very smooth.

VEGGIE BURGERS

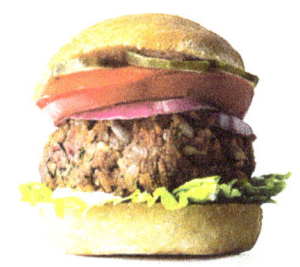

"Good painting is like good cooking; it can be tasted, but not explained."
—Maurice de Vlaminck

IN ART AND WRITING, THE WHITE SPACES SOMETIMES SPEAK LOUDER THAN THE WORDS; and when cooking, rather than following a recipe to the letter, let it guide and speak to you. It will often create itself in its own unique way. I love to simply read cookbooks. Often, I never get around to making a recipe, but something—a fragrance or subtle touch of spice—bookmarks itself and is recalled at the most unexpected moments. Because cooking and life are inextricably intertwined, it is fascinating to observe the play of life in action as we stir the dancing rice grains before turning down the heat or cut through a fresh basil leaf only to be blasted into the awareness of its unique fragrance.

Veggie burgers are so varied that you can really have fun with the ingredients. The nice thing about them is they can be made ahead of time, wrapped separately and frozen. While I was writing this column, a friend called and reminded me of his favorite almost-burger, a Jewish standard: the potato knish. When he was a child, his mother once found him crying and when she asked why, he said he wanted a potato knish. How simple life can be when all we want is a potato knish!

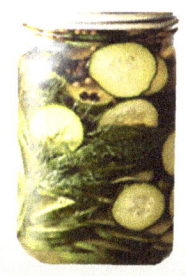

Spicy-Sweet Dill Pickles (Makes 1 (12 oz.) or 2 (6 oz.) Mason jars of pickles)

2 large or 4 small pickling cucumbers
½ C + 2 T rice wine vinegar
½ C water
2 T sugar, blended until fine
1 T kosher salt

¼ t yellow mustard seeds
¼ t red chili flakes
Dash celery seed
½ t pickling spice
1 t fresh dill
½ t ginger, minced
¼ t ground turmeric

1. SPRINKLE 1 T salt on sliced cucumbers and let sit in a sieve for at least one hour to draw out excess water; rinse.
2. COMBINE rest of the ingredients and bring to a boil. Add cucumbers and return to a boil.
3. PLACE cucumbers into jars, ladle hot pickle liquid on top. Refrigerate; jar lasts 2 to 3 weeks.

Vegetables and Tofu

SPICY JAPANESE TOFU-EGGPLANT BURGER

Serves 6

GMEY

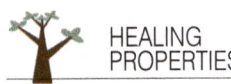 HEALING PROPERTIES

Sesame Seeds
- High blood pressure prevention
- Source of copper, known for its relief of rheumatoid arthritis
- Rich in magnesium, which supports vascular and respiratory health
- Rich in calcium and zinc for bone health

This is an elegant and simple patty that can be made ahead of time and frozen in large batches for those times when you need something prepared quickly. You can spice it up or down with extra dried red chilis.

1 medium eggplant
2 T olive oil
1 to 2 dried red chilis, crushed or ½ t cayenne pepper
1 onion, chopped small
1 red pepper, sliced thin
1 garlic clove, minced
1 lb. firm tofu, drained and slightly mashed
3 T teriyaki sauce, prepared
½ C walnuts, chopped very small
1¾ C Panko breadcrumbs or gluten-free crumbs (reserve ½ C for dredging)
2 T sesame seeds

1. BROIL eggplant on a cookie sheet until soft and the skin is charred. Scoop pulp out of skin, mash slightly.
2. HEAT olive oil and brown dried red chilis or add cayenne pepper.
3. SAUTÉ onion and red pepper until soft; add garlic for an additional minute at the end.
4. ADD eggplant pulp, tofu, and teriyaki sauce and cook slowly with the cover off for about 10 minutes to incorporate all the ingredients.
5. COMBINE tofu/eggplant mixture with remaining ingredients and mix well to form patties.
6. COAT with reserved crumbs and a thin layer of sesame seeds.
7. FRY patties in a little oil, until they are brown or bake in an oiled casserole dish until golden.

 **HINT — STORING NUTS**

We generally don't use nuts every day and because they contain so much natural oil, they tend to spoil easily. Nuts keep best in their shells in dark, cool, dry places. Store shelled nuts in the refrigerator or freezer in moisture-proof containers. Allow newly shelled nuts to dry for 2 to 3 days before refrigerating to prevent mold growth. Freeze, double bagged, for longer storage. Whole nut meats keep better than chopped or ground; unsalted, blanched nuts keep longer than salted.

PORTOBELLO LENTIL BURGER

Serves 6 to 8   G M N S Y

 HEALING PROPERTIES

Onion
- Helps to lower blood sugar
- Helps to lower cholesterol and blood pressure
- Anti-inflammatory and anti-bacterial
- Cornell University food scientists found that the more pungent the onion, the more potent

SRIRACHA MAYO

Blend well together:
1 C mayonnaise or vegan mayo
3 T Sriracha chili sauce
Juice from ½ a lemon, about 2 T
Pinch of salt

My mom and I experimented with lentil burgers for many years. After plenty of batches we compared notes and came up with this version. The addition of pomegranate juice makes it unique and adds antioxidants to the burger.

1 C lentils, brown
4 to 4½ C water and 1 C pomegranate juice
1½ t salt
½ t Aleppo chili and 1 t smoky paprika
Fresh ground black pepper
2 onions, chopped small
1 medium-sized portobello mushroom, chop very small
1 T ginger, freshly minced
2 eggs
½ to ¾ C whole wheat or gluten-free Panko breadcrumbs
2 to 3 T olive oil, for frying

1. COVER lentils with boiling water and pomegranate juice (make sure it covers the top of the lentils); add salt, Aleppo chili powder, paprika, and black pepper. Bring to a boil and lower heat. Simmer for 45 minutes, until cooked. Add water if it needs it, so it doesn't burn. Lentils should be fully cooked, but not watery. Continue to cook on a low heat, with the lid off, until all the water is evaporated, then mash.
2. HEAT olive oil, sauté onions and ginger for about five minutes; add chopped mushrooms and sauté another five minutes. Cool veggies. Add eggs and Panko breadcrumbs and form into paddies.
3. FRY in a few small batches, until golden brown and crisp.
4. DRAIN on paper towels.
5. SERVE with Sriracha Chili Mayo (see Hint)

 SIDEBAR   **HOW TO MAKE YOUR OWN POMEGRANATE JUICE**

2 C pomegranate seeds, 1 C filtered water, pinch of salt, 1 t sugar

1. ADD pomegranate seeds to the blender. Pulse for 5 to 10 seconds, just until the juice separates from the seed, don't over blend.
2. POUR the juice through a strainer and using the back of a spoon gently press the seeds down, so all the juice is released. Add water, salt and sugar.

Vegetables and Tofu

MADRAS RED PEPPER-PEANUT BURGER

Serves 4 to 5

GMESY

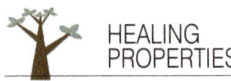

Curry Leaves
- Rich in iron
- Good for digestion and promoting a hearty appetite
- Good for diabetes, and kidney disorders

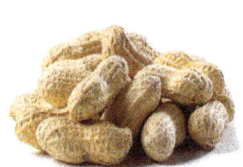

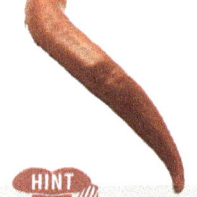

This is a quirky burger with a spicy attitude! A personal favorite of mine.

1 T avocado oil
1 t black mustard seeds and 5 curry leaves (optional)
1 onion, diced small
2 T fresh ginger, minced
1 red pepper and 1 Indian or jalapeño chili, de-seed (roast in oven with 1 T olive oil for 15 minutes, peel pepper and chili and dice)
1 T sambar powder or paste (curry powder or paste could also be used)
1 to 1½ t salt
½ C oatmeal, cooked with ¾ C water and ½ t salt (it should be thick), cool
½ C peanut butter
1 egg, 2 egg whites, beaten well, or ¼ C coconut milk
1 to 1½ C Panko breadcrumbs or gluten-free breadcrumbs

1. HEAT oil, add mustard seeds until they pop, then add curry leaves.
2. ADD onion and ginger, fry until translucent. Add roasted chili and red pepper; fry for another five minutes.
3. COMBINE sambar or curry powder and salt with approximately ⅛ C water, just enough to form a thick paste, or use a prepared paste. Add to vegetables and cook until all liquid is evaporated.
4. BLEND cooked oatmeal, peanut butter, and egg or egg substitute until well mixed; add to cooked vegetables.
5. ADD crumbs a little at a time to final mixture, just enough to be able to shape them into balls.
6. ROLL into balls, then flatten. Either pan fry or bake on a lightly greased cookie pan for 15 minutes in a 350-degree oven until golden brown.

HINT — RED HOT CHILI PEPPERS

What makes hot peppers hot? It's a chemical compound called capsaicin, which is found in the inside wall of the pepper, the seeds and in its white lining. The degree of hotness in a pepper varies between pepper types and is measured in Scoville heat units. Wilbur Scoville was a pharmacist who studied the pungency of peppers and developed the rating system in use today. Scoville units range from 0 for the common bell pepper to 350,000 for the Mexican habanero. The Anaheim chili pepper ranges between 500 to 1000 units, and the popular cayenne is 20,000 units. You may want to wear disposable gloves in the kitchen when handling and cutting hot peppers and keep your hands away from your eyes.

ZUCCHINI-BLACK BEAN-CHIPOTLE BURGERS

Serves 6 to 8

GMENSY

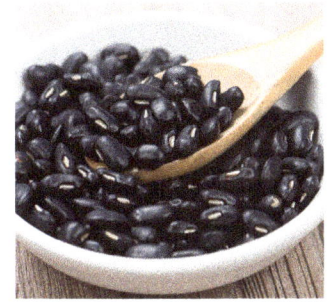

This quick, spicy, dense burger has a Latin flair.

2 T olive oil
1 C red onion, diced small
1 garlic clove, minced
2 T ginger, freshly minced
1 T cumin seeds, pan roasted and ground fresh
1 t salt
1½ C zucchini, chopped small
1 can black beans, rinsed and drained
¾ C rice, cooked, brown or white (a great way to use up leftover rice)
1 canned chipotle pepper in adobo sauce, remove seeds
1 egg or 2 egg whites (beaten well) or ¼ C coconut cream
¾ to 1 C breadcrumbs or ¼ to ½ C corn meal and ¼ to ½ C potato flour
Extra corn meal
½ C cilantro, chopped small

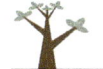

HEALING PROPERTIES

Zucchini
- Helpful for prostate health
- Helpful for cardiovascular protection and diabetic heart disease
- Rich in fiber

1. SAUTÉ onion until tender; add garlic, ginger, salt, and cumin powder.
2. ADD zucchini and sauté until tender and liquid is absorbed.
3. MASH beans very well and add to onion/zucchini mixture; fry about five minutes.
4. ADD the rest of the ingredients to the veggies and beans, with breadcrumbs or flour mixture to form a somewhat firm patty.
5. COAT patty very lightly in corn meal and pan fry until golden brown.

 SIDEBAR   THE HUMBLE CUMIN SEED

This is one of my all-time go-to spices and it seems to be a worldwide favorite too. The earliest recorded use comes from ancient Greece, but the cumin seed features prominently in Indian, Mexican, and North African cuisine. It is often used in its powdered form, but toasted whole seeds have a distinctive smoky flavor in certain dishes. I like to make my own cumin powder. It's really easy. Simply pan fry dry until brown and fragrant. You can then use either a spice grinder or the preferred method, mortar and pestle, to grind it into a powder. Make a few teaspoons at a time, so the powder is always fresh.

Vegetables and Tofu

SATURDAY MARKET MORNING

ONE WINTER MORNING IN NORTH SAN DIEGO COUNTY, while the temperature still lingered in the high 60s and the sun was strong and bright, my mom and I visited the Vista Farmers Market. There, we found an organic lettuce and cucumber farmer and vendor along with an elderly husband and wife cactus team who have been at this market since it began years ago, the crusty bread and organic egg family, the lemon and lime lady with an infectious smile, a homemade tamale team (spicy mushroom is our favorite), and an ever-energetic olive guy (you can't pass by without tasting at least one variety of spreads and, of course, some olives). There is also a Chinese wonder woman who sells seedlings of all varieties of herbs and plants—some extremely rare. She'll tell you every little detail about each seedling you glance at and offers invaluable planting and cultivating advice when you actually buy something. In other words, this sprawling outdoor market is a veritable kaleidoscope of ethnicity, color, flavor, and scent. Besides being a wonderful way to support community producers and organic farmers, it's really fun to discover what is in season at the moment, then spend the rest of the week figuring out recipes to go with whatever ends up in your cloth bags each Saturday morning.

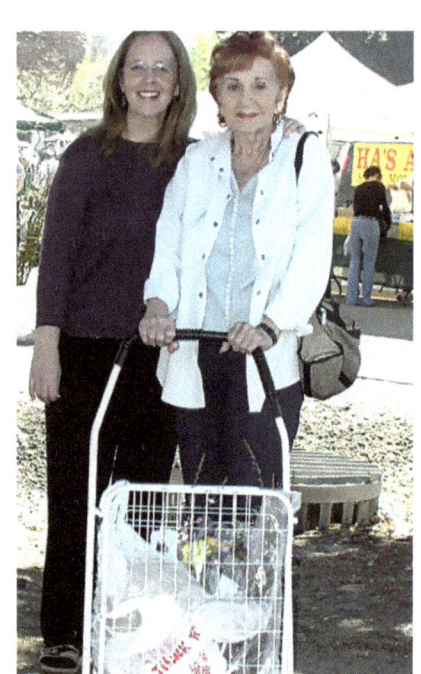

My mom at the Farmers Market, quite a few years ago.

On that particular morning, my mom had a brilliant idea: we should take along her "Brooklyn style" basket on wheels, which she dubbed her *vehgala* (some sort of Yiddishism). So, we were no longer burdened to schlep the many small bags from table to table; the *vehgala* carried it all effortlessly. Here are a few of the recipes that were created to honor the market and the organic producers.

CHOPPED SALAD WITH TEMPEH

Serves 4 to 6

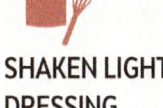

SHAKEN LIGHT DRESSING

This is an easy dressing to make in a jar. Just add the ingredients, close the lid and give it a good shake.

- ½ C Olive oil
- ¼ C Apple wine vinegar
- Fresh pepper and salt to taste
- Dash of Aleppo chili pepper, to taste
- Drizzle of honey or agave syrup.
- 1 t brown, whole seed mustard
- ½ t lemon zest
- Pinch turmeric
- Dash of dulse flakes (optional)
- 2 T cilantro or parsley, fresh, chopped very small

There is nothing as tender and fresh as organic baby greens; they come in all varieties and are just simply adorable. It's nice to mix them with a bit of crunchy romaine lettuce to balance their soft texture.

When bell peppers are in season, it's fun to choose from the pepper color palette—yellow, orange, green or red. The great thing about getting them from the market is the ability to select a bag containing a variety of colors.

Fresh cucumbers should still have the little bumps on them and actually snap when you bend them in half. Tomatoes are my favorite summertime fling, coming in a myriad of colors and shapes. There is also a large assortment of cherry tomatoes (some really small), grape tomatoes (super sweet), baby Romas (ideal for roasting) and the funny looking multi-colored heirloom varieties. Try the vegan feta recipe below for a dairy free alternative.

2 C organic mixed greens, torn
1 C organic romaine lettuce, chopped
1 C mixed colored peppers, chopped
1 C cucumber, sliced thin
1 carrot, shredded
1 C tomatoes, de-seeded, chopped
1 corn on the cob, roasted, remove kernels
½ C feta cheese (vegan option)
½ C fresh mozzarella cheese, chopped
½ C olives, pitted and chopped in half

Fried Tempeh

1 T olive oil
1 C tempeh, cubed
1 T tamari
¼ t ginger powder
¼ t turmeric

1. HEAT oil, add tempeh, tamari, ginger, and turmeric powder.
2. FRY on medium heat until golden.
3. COOL in a bowl.

Vegan Feta

14 oz. firm tofu, pressed
1 T nutritional yeast
1 T white miso paste
½ C coconut oil, melted
2 T lemon juice
1 T apple cider vinegar
1 t salt & 1 t onion powder

1. PRESS tofu to remove excess water.
2. PLACE in blender with nutritional yeast, miso, oil, lemon juice, vinegar, salt and onion powder.
3. PUREE until very smooth, scraping down the sides.
4. PLACE in bowl, cover and put in the fridge, allow it to firm up overnight, then cut into feta-like cubes.

CRANBERRY/ORANGE RELISH

Serves 6 to 8

GMENSY

HOW TO MAKE GINGER JUICE

To make ginger juice begin by peeling and grating several slices of ginger. Wrap the gratings in cheesecloth before squeezing. As long as the ginger is fresh, and not dried out there should be no problem squeezing out enough juice.

The seasonal organic oranges and lemons are incomparable. They are candy-sweet and incredibly juicy. These fruits don't have the polished orange presentation that you often find in supermarkets.

Cranberries have thick skins and a waxy appearance. This wax-like surface causes pesticides to "cling" to the berries, which is why it's so important to buy them organic, if at all possible. They are quite a bit more expensive than those commercially grown since there are only a handful of organic cranberry bogs throughout the country.

You can use this relish as a condiment with almost any stir fry dish and rice that you make. It adds a sweet and tart bite to any meal. This recipe uses the natural sweetness of apricots and raisins, rather than extra sugar, to balance the tartness of the cranberries.

3 C fresh organic cranberries (12 oz. bag)
1½ C organic turbinado sugar, 1 C honey (lavender or orange blossom honey goes very well) or agave syrup
1 C chopped dried apricots (cut with oiled kitchen shears)
1 C golden raisins
¼ t salt
½ t cinnamon
½ t cardamom
1 C orange juice, freshly squeezed
1 T grated orange rind
1 T grated lemon rind
1 t ginger juice

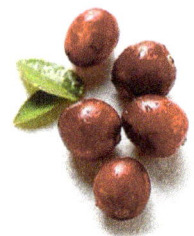

1. MIX all the ingredients together in a heavy bottom large pot.
2. STIR over medium heat until the sugar is dissolved.
3. INCREASE heat, cover and boil until cranberries burst (approximately 8 minutes), stirring occasionally.
4. POUR mixture into a bowl.
5. COVER and refrigerate until cold (mixture will thicken as it cools down).

ZESTY ZUCCHINI STIR FRY

Serves 4 to 6 GMENSY

Organic zucchini goes really well with lemon zest and red peppers. It's a simple and quick stir fry that I often cook as my weekly staple. I tend to add fresh ginger and turmeric to most of my veggie and rice dishes—both are healthy powerhouses.

2 T olive oil
1 chili pepper, fresh or dried, de-seeded and chopped
1 onion, sliced
2 red or yellow peppers, chopped
1 t ginger, freshly grated
½ t turmeric and ½ t cumin powder
4 zucchinis, chopped
1 t fresh thyme, remove from stem and crush to release oil
2 t lemon zest
1 T salt and pepper
Stir fry ½ C firm tofu in a separate pan, with a little oil, salt and freshly ground black pepper; this adds protein to this dish (optional).

1. HEAT oil; add crushed red chili flakes or fresh chopped chili pepper.
2. STIR FRY onion and red peppers until almost soft.
3. ADD ginger, turmeric, cumin, zucchini, thyme, zest, salt, and pepper and continue to fry for 4 to 5 minutes, until zucchini is crisp tender.
4. ADD stir-fried tofu, toss until well coated.
5. COVER stir fry an additional 5 to 7 minutes; until zucchini is tender.

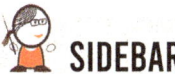 **SIDEBAR**   **THE HISTORY OF ZUCCHINI**

The various summer squashes are native to the Americas and belong to the family of curcurbita. Archaeologists have traced their origins to Mexico, dating back from 7,000 to 5,500 B.C.E., when they were an integral part of the ancient diet of maize, beans, and soft squashes. That pre-Columbian food trio is still the mainstay of the Mexican cuisine and is known today as the "three sisters." Zucchini eventually found its way to Italy and was promptly named zucchino. The colonists of New England adopted the name squash, a word derived from several Native American words for the vegetable which meant "something eaten raw." If zucchini is left on the vine or bush too long, the fruit becomes enormous, the seeds large and tough, and may even become inedible.

Vegetables and Tofu

SESAME BROWN RICE AND RED SCALLIONS

Serves 4 to 6

G M E N Y

A summer specialty at the Vista Farmers Market is a bunch of red scallions. They have a delightful color and add a unique flavor, especially to brown rice. Long grain basmati brown rice has fewer carbohydrates and yet retains all the health benefits and fiber.

1 C organic basmati brown long grain rice
2 C water or vegetable broth
½ t salt
2 T olive oil
1 t sesame oil (optional)
¼ C cilantro, fresh, chopped small
¼ C brown sesame seeds
1 T tamari or Himalayan salt
1 t ginger, freshly grated
½ t turmeric
4 red scallions, diced along with their green tops

1. COMBINE water, rice, and salt in pot with a tight-fitting lid. Bring to a rousing boil and then lower heat to very low.
2. COOK for 45 minutes to 1 hour, until all the liquid is absorbed. Do not stir or lift lid during the cooking process. When the rice is cooked, remove lid, and let the excess steam evaporate to cool rice, so it doesn't get soggy.
3. HEAT oil and add sesame seeds, brown for a few minutes.
4. ADD tamari, ginger, turmeric, and scallions and stir fry until scallions are tender, about 4 to 5 minutes.
5. ADD cooled rice and mix well.
6. SPRINKLE chopped cilantro on top.

 SIDEBAR   SCALLION: WHAT'S IN A NAME

The words scallion and shallot are related and can be traced back to the Greek askolonion, as described by the Greek writer Theophrastus. The name *scallion* seems to originate from the Philistine town of Ashkelon in Palestine/Israel even though shallots came from farther eastern Europe.

SUMMER TOMATOES

"It's difficult to think anything but pleasant thoughts while eating a homegrown tomato."
—Lewis Grizzard

OUR SUMMER GARDENS HAVE EVOLVED THROUGHOUT THE YEARS OF MY LIFE, going from acres of land to a single, humble tomato plant. Whatever is growing at the moment is a joy to behold, whether it is a tiny seed, vegetable or herb plant. I must say I enjoy observing the simple miracle of watching a plant unfolding, leaf by leaf, flower by flower, fruit by fruit.

One particular tomato plant holds a special place in my heart. It was in 1985, after returning from India and setting up our house from scratch. It was early summer, and the season was entering warm, lumbering days. We rented a townhouse in the Finger Lakes region of New York State, and I took a graphic design job at a local newspaper. There was a small area on the side of the townhouse that contained an empty and long forgotten flower bed. I visualized tomatoes growing there, but had to wait until my first paycheck to be able to buy the plants and soil. So, I spent the time getting the little spot and its tired soil ready for those plants. I tilled the area on my hands and knees, using a large serving spoon, while meticulously removing all of the tiny stones. The two weeks I waited for my paycheck seemed like an eternity.

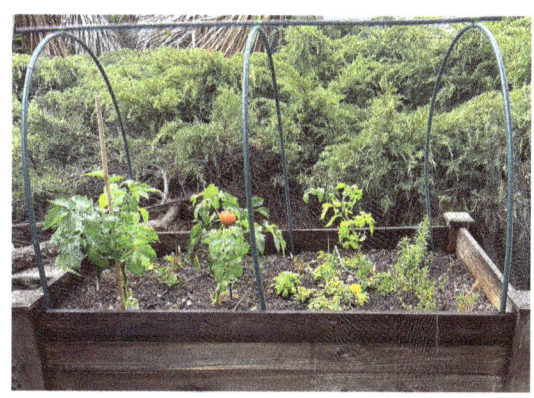

My tiny raised garden, growing a few tomatoes and herbs on a small patio, even today.

Then, I ran to the local store and bought three small tomato plants and some good garden soil. Getting those plants into the ground, stepping back, and seeing them sway in the summer breeze was something—even to this day—I will never forget. Every evening after work, I'd water them with a soup pot. I spent the summer watching the plants transform from yellow flowers to small green tomatoes to perfectly vine-ripened brilliant red spheres. How simply and lovely it can be to watch a tomato grow.

CHETNA'S TOMATO MOZZARELLA SALAD

Serves 2 to 4

GMENSY

My friend Chetna makes this simple but elegant salad quite often when I stopped by for dinner. She knows I like a light meal at night, and this is perfect for a refreshing summer treat when fresh tomatoes and basil from the local farmer's market are at their best.

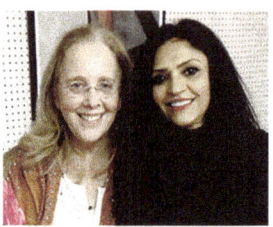

Chetna

1 C fresh mozzarella cheese, cut into small pieces, you could use a cheese substitute or casein-free mozzarella
2 C cherry tomatoes (different sizes and colors are nice), cut in half
½ C black olives, pitted and cut small
½ C cucumber, de-seeded, cut small
5 to 6 basil leaves, chiffonade

Dressing
½ lemon, juiced
1 t lemon zest
1 T olive oil
2 T balsamic vinegar
½ t salt and generous helping of freshly ground pepper

1. MIX salad ingredients, top with shaken dressing just before serving.

 SIDEBAR   **THE INTERESTING HISTORY OF TOMATOES**

Because tomatoes can be traced back to the early Aztecs in southern Mexico (700 A.D.), it is believed that the tomato is native to the Americas. Though it was not until the 16th century that European explorers were introduced to this vegetable. These travelers brought the tomato home with them, and it soon became adopted in kitchens throughout southern Europe. The British admired the tomato for its beauty but believe that it was poisonous, as its appearance was similar to that of the wolf peach. The tomato was not regarded as a kitchen vegetable until shortly before the Civil War. However, from that point forward, it became a staple throughout the world. For sometime, there was a debate over the nature of the tomato: was it a fruit or vegetable? Until the late 1800s, the tomato was classified as a fruit in order to avoid taxation. This was changed after a court ruling stated that the tomato is a vegetable and should be taxed accordingly.

RED PEPPER-LENTIL-TOMATO BLENDED SOUP

Serves 6 to 8   GMENSY

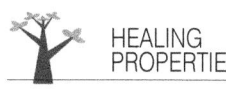 **HEALING PROPERTIES**

Tomato
- Contains lycopene, which has anti-cancer and cardiovascular benefits
- Acts as an anti-inflammatory
- Has blood thinning properties
- May protect against prostate cancer, diabetes, and migraines

I love the combination of red peppers and tomatoes; the addition of lentils adds just enough protein to make this a full meal. Try this soup with whatever colored pepper (except green) you have on hand. Watch these few simple ingredients transform into a deep, elegant rainbow of liquid color.

3 red bell peppers, or various colors (red, yellow, or orange)
2 T olive oil
1 onion, thinly sliced
2 garlic cloves, peeled and sliced thin
2 C canned fire-roasted diced tomatoes, organic, if you can get it or any diced tomatoes
½ C brown lentils
8 C vegetable stock
Salt and pepper to taste
½ t ginger powder
½ C light coconut milk
A few sprigs of fresh lemon thyme

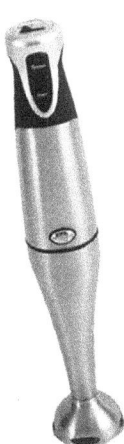

1. BROIL peppers in oven until blackened. Let them rest for ½ hour in a bowl covered with a towel. Peel, remove seeds, and chop.
2. SAUTÉ the onions in olive oil on low heat for 15 to 20 minutes until caramelized.
3. ADD the garlic. Sauté for another few minutes.
4. COMBINE the sautéed onion/garlic mixture, broiled peppers, tomatoes, lentils, salt, fresh pepper, ginger, thyme and stock in a large pot.
5. COOK gently for 45 to 60 minutes until the lentils are soft; remove thyme sprigs.
6. ADD coconut milk. Simmer for 5 minutes.
7. BLEND with hand blender, until almost smooth.

Vegetables and Tofu

ROASTED TOMATO SALSAUCE

Serves 6 to 8

GMENSY

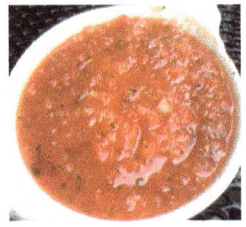

This is my favorite cooked salsa, pleasantly spicy, not too much or too little. It's great for picnics—bring along some guacamole, a big bag of corn chips, and this dip, there's not much else you need. Technically, this is both a sauce and salsa, so I've coined it as a "salsauce." This mildly spicy, sweet, yet tangy sauce can also accompany any veggie burger or tofu dish.

5 ripe large tomatoes or 8 plum tomatoes
1 red bell pepper
1 to 2 garlic cloves (do not peel)
1 pasilla pepper, deep green
½ t cumin seeds
½ t coriander seeds
1 chipotle chili in adobo sauce
1 t fresh lemon juice
¼ C cilantro
1 t salt
1 T honey or agave syrup
1 T fresh ginger, minced

1. POSITION a broiler rack about 8" from the heat.
2. BROIL the tomatoes, peppers, and garlic until well-blackened.
3. PLACE in a bowl, top with cling wrap or a moist towel and let cool about 15 minutes.
4. REMOVE blackened skin and seeds from peppers, tomatoes, and garlic peel.
5. HEAT cumin and coriander seeds in a pan, dry roasting them for about 2 minutes until brown and fragrant, then grind into a powder (you could also use about ½ t of powder if you don't want to go to the trouble of grinding it yourself).
6. PLACE all ingredients in a food processor and pulse until coarsely chopped.

THE GARLIC ROCK

Sometimes the best kitchen utensil is just outside your kitchen door. I keep a garlic rock on my counter: a smooth large stone I found outside my back door on a hillside. Find a rock that is smooth and is about the size of your palm. Look for one that is comfortable and not too heavy in the hand. When you first pick the rock, run it through the dishwasher and it's ready to use. If you don't have a dishwasher just wash it in hot soapy water with a bit of bleach.

To crush garlic: hold the rock and smash it on a clove of garlic. Pull out the skin and there you have it, crushed garlic ready to cook with.

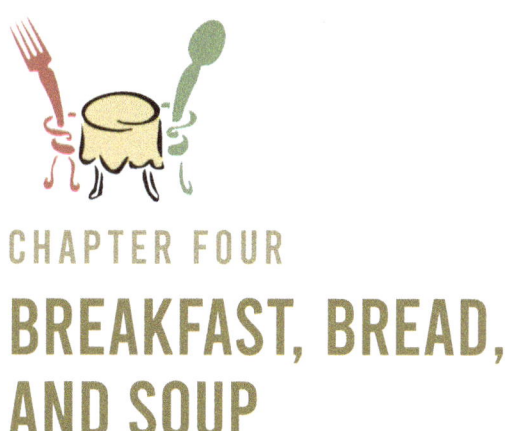

CHAPTER FOUR
BREAKFAST, BREAD, AND SOUP

THE ROOSTER'S CALL
BREAD OF LIFE
SOUP DAZE

THE ROOSTER'S CALL

DURING THE TIME WE LIVED ON A NOVA SCOTIAN FARM, a neighbor arrived at the house, presenting us with a colorful bantam rooster. We didn't have chickens, since we weren't eating eggs at the time, so he simply became a barnyard addition. We soon found out why he was given away. Besides waking us at 5:00 a.m. (which actually was rather nice), he turned out to be very grouchy and temperamental. He had the irritating habit of attacking anyone entering "his barn." As we milked the cows in the morning, we would fight off the rooster with streams of milk. It was a daily obstacle course.

When the warm milk arrived in the kitchen (often having survived the daily rooster attack) we then sat down to a breakfast of homemade maple-nut granola and fresh yogurt.

Making granola is a slowing-down adventure. You have to be around while it's baking, stir it every 15 minutes or so; then watch it transform from a semi-dense consistency into golden crispy nuggets. It created a divine aroma in the kitchen. Since those farm days, I have slimmed down the granola, which was initially made with a full cup of oil. Granola is a good rainy day afternoon project.

HOMEMADE YOGURT

Serves 4   GENSY

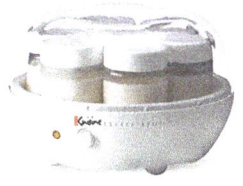

You can purchase yogurt makers, which sustain the correct temperature for you.

There is no comparison between homemade yogurt and store bought and it's so simple to make. Yogurt contains a higher concentration of solids than normal milk and will keep well in the refrigerator for about a week.

4 C skim, 1%, 2% or regular milk
¼ C non-pasteurized yogurt (to be used as a starter)

1. HEAT milk in a saucepan or double boiler to just boiling and cool immediately to 110°F. A quick nonscientific temperature test is, if you put your (clean) finger in the milk without it burning you, it is ready. [For a little sweeter yogurt, add sweetener to the milk before boiling. For a firmer texture, a little powdered milk, about 2 to 3 tablespoons, can be added also before boiling.] Heating the milk to almost boiling kills any undesirable bacteria that might be present and also changes the milk protein, giving the yogurt a firmer body and texture.
2. ADD starter culture to warmed milk.
3. MIX well, but gently, so you don't add extra air. If too much air is mixed in the starter, the culture will grow more slowly.
4. SANITIZE yogurt containers by rinsing them in boiling water.
5. POUR warm milk/culture mixture into a clean container or individual containers and cover with a lid or tin foil. Let is rest at a temperature of 110°F until firm. The finish time will vary, but it ranges between four and eight hours. Just keep checking. Immediately refrigerate.

 STARTER CULTURE AND MAINTAINING TEMPERATURE

The easiest way to obtain a starter culture is to purchase plain yogurt, with a live culture, not pasteurized. To maintain an ongoing cultures, save a small portion to use as a starter for the next batch, be sure to refrigerate the starter culture in a clean, air-tight container. Accurate temperature is probably the most important aspect, and a good stainless-steel thermometer is a handy tool to keep the yogurt at approximately 110 degrees. If it is too hot the probiotic properties will be killed. I find that if I heat the oven at 200 degrees for 2 to 3 minutes, turn off the oven and place the covered yogurt mixture inside, it will stay warm for about 4 to 6 hours. For people dedicated to making their own yogurt, a Styrofoam box fitted with a low watt light bulb may be used to maintain an even heat. You could also use a cooler, place a bottle filled with boiling water in it to heat it, and keep it warm.

Breakfast, Bread, and Soup

HOMEMADE SOY YOGURT

Serves 3 to 4   GMENY

HINT

Make sure to sterilize everything—bowl, spoons, and jars—that come into contact with your yogurt preparation so that no bacteria compete with the added probiotic (the live microorganisms that provide wonderful health benefits).

Store-bought soy or coconut yogurt cartons will not make a good starter unless they say they have live cultures in it. You can buy dairy-free probiotics from specialty stores on the Internet.

1 C cold organic soy milk (not low-fat)
2 T tapioca starch
½ t unflavored gelatin
1½ C warm organic soy milk (not low-fat), warm slowly with 1 T honey or agave, do not heat above 115 degrees
½ t dairy-free probiotic or ½ C soy live yogurt culture (you can try Nancy's Cultured Soy available in health foods stores.)

1. WHISK ½ C cold soy milk, tapioca starch and gelatin together. Then add 1 C warm soy milk and mix until very smooth.
2. COOK in a heavy pot, on low heat, stirring continuously until thickened.
3. WHISK in remaining cold and warm soy milk, let cool until it is just warm about 105 degrees. Add a live yogurt culture.
4. INCUBATE for 8 to 10 and refrigerate for 12 hours to develop flavor.

HOMEMADE COCONUT YOGURT

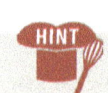

HINT

Another method to get thicker yogurt is to add 1 t of gelatin powder per quart of liquid. Sprinkle onto the cold soy or coconut milk and let sit for 5 minutes before heating.

2 (14 oz.) cans organic coconut milk
¼ C dairy-free dried milk powder
1½ T tapioca starch
½ t dairy-free probiotic

1. COMBINE coconut milk, dried milk powder and tapioca starch, whisk until very well blended.
2. HEAT slowly until the temperature comes up to 180 degrees. Use a sterilized candy thermometer to check the temperature. Turn off the heat and let it sit until it comes down to 105 to 115 degrees.
3. REMOVE ½ C of the mixture and mix with probiotic. Gently stir until well mixed. Then add the liquid back into the incubation bowl.
4. INCUBATE in a warm place for 8 to 10 hours and refrigerate for at least 4 hours.

NOVA SCOTIA MAPLE GRANOLA

Serves 6 to 8 | Preheat Oven to 325 degrees | Bake: 30 to 35 Minutes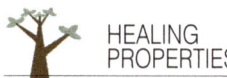

HEALING PROPERTIES

Maple Syrup
- Contains zinc and magnesium for energy and boosting the immune system
- Promotes prostate health

Using the Nova Scotia wood-burning stove, I made this every week for many years. Someone should bottle the kitchen aroma while this is baking!

½ C maple syrup

1½ t vanilla extract

¼ C avocado or coconut oil (I used ghee, since we had an abundance of butter, for a nonfat version you could use frozen apple juice concentrate)

1½ t cinnamon

4 C rolled oats

¼ C sesame, pumpkin seeds, or any nuts like walnut

2 T peanut or almond butter

1. STIR together maple syrup, vanilla and oil or juice.
2. ADD remaining ingredients and toss to coat.
3. SPREAD mixture evenly on a baking sheet.
4. BAKE until golden brown and toasty (stir a few times during baking).

LOW-FAT NUTTY AND SEEDY GRANOLA

Serves 6 to 8 | Preheat Oven to 350 Degrees | Bake: 35-45 Minutes   M E S Y

STORING GRANOLA

Store granola in a tightly sealed or vacuum sealed container at room temperature for two weeks. Granola freezes well for up to two months.

¼ C avocado oil

¼ C agave syrup

1 t vanilla extract

½ C toasted wheat germ

¼ C sesame seeds, 2 T pumpkin seeds, 1 T flax seeds, 1 T chia seeds

2 T orange zest

½ C shredded unsweetened coconut

3½ C rolled oats

½ C raw cashews and walnuts, coarsely chopped

1. COMBINE oil and syrup and heat, stirring gently. Remove from the heat and add vanilla extract.
2. MIX wheat germ, seeds, coconut, oats, cashews, and walnuts in a separate bowl.
3. ADD the warm syrup mixture and stir to coat evenly.
4. SPREAD the granola mixture onto a baking sheet.
5. BAKE until golden brown. Stir the mixture occasionally, while baking.

Breakfast, Bread, and Soup

OATMEAL AND FRUIT

Serves 4

GMENSY

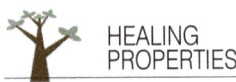 **HEALING PROPERTIES**

Oats
- Have high fiber content
- Enhance immune response to infection
- Help to stabilize blood sugar
- Contain selenium, a powerful antioxidant

I think people are naturally divided into two camps: oatmeal and non-oatmeal. I happen to be an oatmeal person. I discovered my first can of Irish steel cut oats about twenty years ago and oatmeal has never been the same since.

1 T butter or margarine
1 C steel cut oats, not quick cooking (gluten-free also available)
3 C boiling water
1 C low-fat milk, soy, almond, or rice milk
2 T maple or agave syrup
½ t cinnamon
¼ t ginger
¼ t cardamom powder
½ t salt
Fresh fruit: banana or berries

1. MELT butter or margarine in a large saucepan and add the oats.
2. STIR for 2 minutes to toast.
3. ADD the boiling water and reduce heat to a simmer. Keep at a low simmer for 20 minutes, without stirring, lid ajar.
4. ADD to pot: milk, syrup, spices, and salt and stir gently to mix, cook an additional 15 to 20 minutes until desired thickening.
5. SPOON into a serving bowl and top with fresh fruit.

 SIDEBAR   OATMEAL FACTS

Oats were one of the earliest cereals cultivated by man, known in ancient China as long ago as 7,000 B.C. It is derived from the wild red oat. And yet it was the ancient Greeks who first made porridge (cereal) from oats.

In the Scottish culinary tradition, oats became a staple as they were better suited than wheat to the short, wet growing season. It was eventually introduced into North America, especially the Northeast, by the first Scottish settlers in the early 17th century. In Vermont oatmeal has a long tradition. An old Vermont farm oatmeal recipe is: "soak whole oats overnight in cold water, salt, and maple syrup. The next morning, before beginning farm chores add ground nutmeg, cinnamon, and ginger. Place the pot over a low heat and cooked for upwards of 90 minutes. Serve after chores with cream, milk, or butter."

BREAD OF LIFE

Baking in High Altitudes

At High Elevations Increase the amount of liquid by 2 to 3 T for each cup of flour.

For 5,000 feet and above: Add 3 T extra liquid for each cup of flour. Decrease the amount of sweetener by 1 to 3 T for each cup of sweetener.

THE RHYTHM OF KNEADING DOUGH CAN OFFER A SOOTHING TIME OF INTROSPECTION—a time when all else is put aside and one's concentration is focused.

Many people feel they don't have the time to make bread. Yet, most of the work is done by the bread itself, in its own quiet moments of rising in the moist, warm air. In most cultures bread is the staple of life. It has various forms, baked in ovens or on flat surfaces on the stove or fried in vats of oil. It remains one of the simplest forms of whole food. I first began baking bread using a wood stove.

In the beginning I knew very little about how the dough should feel. I then learned that sufficient kneading made the lump of wheat feel like a smooth and pliable baby's bottom. Little by little, the dough and I got used to each other. I soon began to look forward to the nutty-sweet fragrance of bread, fresh from the oven, permeate the house.

During the last decade our carb-frenzied society almost gave up on bread entirely. Then it reappeared as a fiber-rich food. Any whole wheat bread can be made carb-friendly by adding eggs, or bean flour to boost the protein content. As with all things, there is a balance to good, wholesome bread. So, if you are going to eat bread, it might as well simply be the best, fresh from the oven, and filled with whole grains and extra ingredients like flax seeds, which add fiber; vitamins and minerals, or sprouted grains. Another great trick: slice it thin!

WHOLE GRAIN BROWN BREAD

Makes 1 Loaf | Preheat Oven to 375 Degrees | Bake: 40 to 50 Minutes   M E N S

BLOOMING ACTIVE DRY YEAST

Yeast is fragile and needs to be stored in the refrigerator. Blooming is used to test the freshness of your active dry yeast, especially if it's been around for a while. Stored yeast cells gradually die, so testing the yeast ensures that there are live yeast cells available for making a successful bread. This is also known as "proofing yeast."

Blooming is also the process where active dry yeast is prepared to be used in a recipe.

Blooming is not necessary when using instant yeast.

This is one of the first breads I ever made in my Nova Scotia wood burning oven, it soon became a staple. I love its sweetness and color and the variety of grains gives it a superior flavor. Remember, the amount of flour in any bread recipe is always approximate. The goal is to add the least amount of flour, as needed, to make it pliable, otherwise the bread will become dense. It takes a little bit of practice to know the feel of your dough. This is a high fiber and iron rich bread.

1½ C water
2¼ t active dry yeast (see Hint about yeast and salt on page 91)
1 T molasses
2 T honey
2 T melted margarine or butter
½ C sesame, chia or sunflower seeds or all three (optional)
¼ C cornmeal
½ C rolled oats
1¼ to 1½ C whole wheat pastry flour
1¼ to 1½ C unbleached white flour
1½ t salt

1. WARM water heated to 100 to 115 degrees, mix in the yeast, sweeteners, margarine or butter and let the yeast bloom (see Hint).
2. ADD seeds, cornmeal, oatmeal and 1 C of whole wheat flour. Stir vigorously with a spoon, at least 100 times, to produce a light, airy sponge.
3. STIR in salt, ¼ C whole wheat flour and 1¼ C of white flour. Add a little more whole wheat flour, until it becomes a cohesive mass, and the dough doesn't stick to the bowl. Use a little bit of white flour for dusting the kneading board.
4. TURN the dough onto the dusted board, knead until smooth. (See kneading hint on next page).
5. [FIRST RISE] Put a few drops of oil a large bowl and rotate the kneaded dough so that it's covered with a thin layer of oil. (At this point you could put it in the refrigerator overnight). Cover with cling wrap and set in a warm place for 50 to 60 minutes, until almost double in size. (See page 93, for dough proofing ideas.)

A Culinary Journey

6. [SECOND RISE] Punch the dough down with your fist. Cover and let rise again for 40 minutes.
7. SHAPE the dough. I find the simplest way is to cut the dough with a dough scraper into two equal parts. Roll each section into a ball, using as little flour as necessary to keep the dough from sticking to the board. Place two balls next to each other in an oiled bread ban. Lightly coat the top with oil and cover with a damp cloth. Let rise an additional 30 to 40 minutes, just before the rising "peaks," you want to let it finish rising in the oven.
8. PLACE a baking dish in the oven with boiling water to create steam.
9. BAKE for 15 minutes at 375 and turn down the oven to 350 to finish baking, bake until golden, you will hear a thump on the bottom when tapped.
10. REMOVE from pan(s) immediately and let cool on racks.
11. DOUBLE recipe for two loafs.

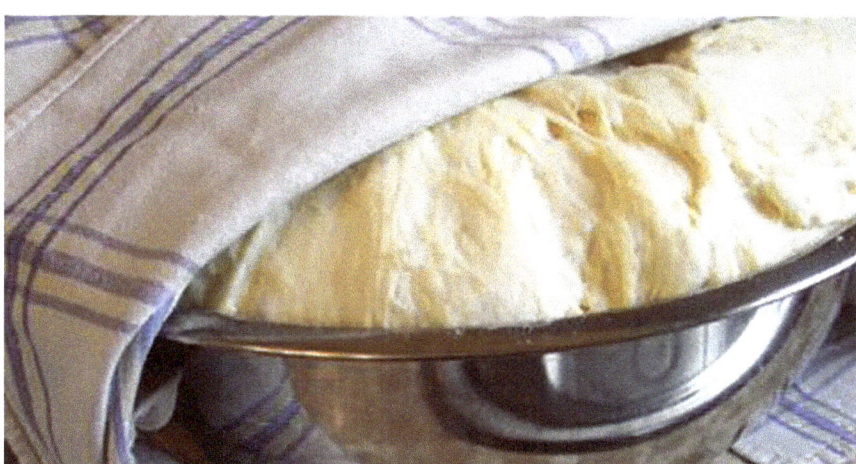

Moist Dough
On the "First Rise," make sure you keep it moist on the top, otherwise the dough will dry out.

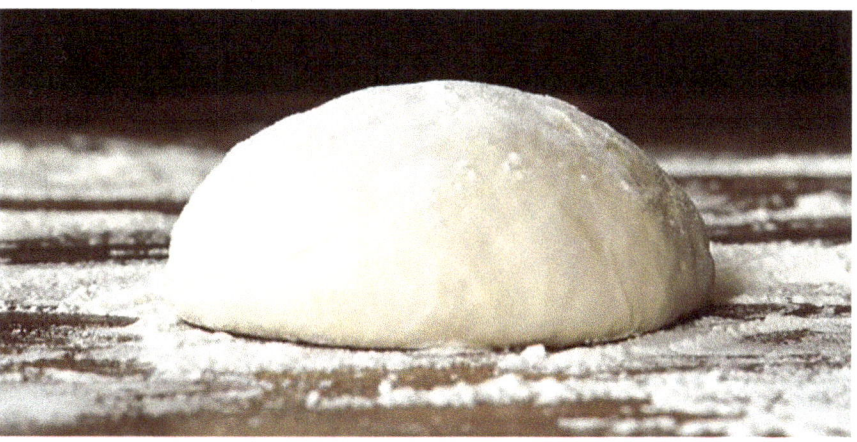

Air Vent
Shaping your dough is a fun, you have loads of options, just make sure to have a slit on the top, if you are not using the loaf balls next to each other method.

The Poetic Art of Kneading Bread

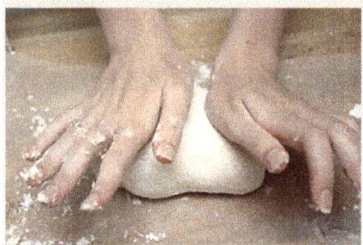

Call me crazy, but I love to knead dough.

Here's how to do it: turn the dough out onto a clean, well-floured surface, a large wooden board, marble slab, Silpat mat, or other clean working surface.

Make sure it is at a height where you are comfortable working. If the dough is very moist or sticky, sprinkle additional flour over the top. Gather the dough into a pile (a dough scraper is a good tool to have).

Begin pressing it together into a ball and with the heels of your hands working the dough, pushing forward slightly.

Fold the far edge of the dough upwards, towards you, and press it into the middle of the ball. Then rotate the dough slightly and continue this press-fold-turn kneading for at least 7 to 10 minutes.

Add just enough flour as necessary. You'll know to stop adding flour when the dough mostly stops sticking to the board. The amount will vary according to the moisture in the flour and the altitude where you are baking. You'll know you're done when you pinch the dough between your fingers, and it feels like a soft earlobe.

If it is too sticky or too dry, either add a tiny bit more flour, or a few drops of water and continue kneading.

- Time your kneading, 10 minutes can seem like a long time doing the same repetitive activity, but it's the most important aspect of bread making. Don't cut it short, it's a great exercise, too.
- A dough scraper is a handy tool to scrap up the dough as you knead and to make cleanup easier. Anything with a straight, but fairly blunt edge will do.
- Try not to tear the dough, use a gentle, but firm hand.
- Cool, dry hands are best for kneading. If your hands get warm, run them under cool water, dry them and begin kneading again.

COCONUT-APPLE BRAIDED BREAD

Makes 1 Loaf | Preheat Oven to 350 Degrees | Bake: 40 to 50 Minutes   M N S

ABOUT YEAST AND SALT

When using yeast you need to keep it away from salt, which can kill it.

Active Dry Yeast
Add yeast to warm water to bloom and foam, then add it to the rest of your wet ingredients.
In a separate bowl mix flour, salt and any other dry ingredients. Combine wet and dry ingredients together.

Instant Yeast
Add yeast to dry ingredients and then add to combined wet ingredients, or simply add yeast to one side of the bowl and salt to the other.

There is nothing quite like this light bread. The flavor, texture and beautiful appearance make this a braided centerpiece for any special occasion—a truly celebratory bread.

Dry Ingredients
3 to 3¾ unbleached white flour
2¼ t instant yeast (see "Yeast Facts" Sidebar page 200)
½ t cardamom powder

Wet Ingredients
1 can (14 oz.) coconut milk
4 T butter or margarine, melted
½ C coconut sugar or brown sugar
1 t salt
1 large egg, whisked
1 apple, peeled and shredded
1 egg, 1 T water, for basting on the top

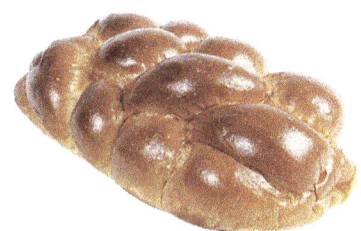

1. MIX 3 C flour, yeast and cardamom powder together in a bowl.
2. MIX first four wet ingredients together in a separate large bowl.
3. COMBINE wet to dry ingredients and stir in egg and shredded apple.
4. MIX all together, until it resembles a shaggy dough.
5. KNEAD dough (adding just enough additional flour so it is not too sticky, as needed) continue to knead for about 10 to 12 minutes.
6. PLACE in an oiled bowl and coat the top. Let it rise until doubled, about 1 to 2 hours.
7. PUNCH dough down and place onto a lightly floured surface, divide into three equal parts. Roll each piece of dough into a 20" long rope about ½" thick. Lay the three ropes side by side and pinch the ends together at the top. Braid the ropes. Pinch the ends together on the bottom and tuck underneath. Place it on a parchment paper lined baking sheet, coat top of dough with a little oil, cover and let rise 45 to 60 minutes.
8. BEAT 1 egg and water and brush on top of braid
9. BAKE until golden brown and when you tap on it you hear a thud.
10. REMOVE from pan and cool on rack.

THYME FOR SWEET POTATO ROLLS

Makes 24 Rolls | Preheat Oven to 350 Degrees | Bake: 25 to 30 Minutes   MENS

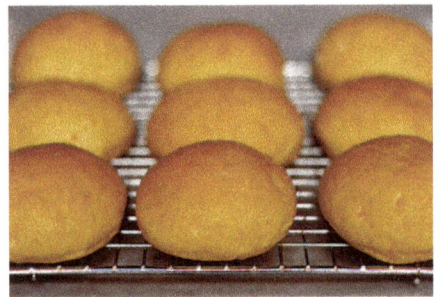

1 C sweet potatoes, baked or canned sweet potatoes
3 T margarine or butter, melted
2 eggs or ½ C soft tofu, blended with 1 T oil until smooth
3 T maple sugar or agave syrup
2¼ t active dry yeast (see Hint page 91)
1¼ C warm water, 110 to 115 degrees
1 t salt
1 T thyme, fresh, chopped small
1 C whole wheat flour and 3 to 3½ C unbleached white flour

This is my go-to recipe for Thanksgiving rolls. It's easy to start in the morning and bake an hour before you sit down to your meal. What a lovely aroma it brings to your celebration!

1. BLEND potatoes with margarine or butter, eggs, and syrup.
2. DISSOLVE yeast in ½ C warm water.
3. COMBINE potato mixture and yeast water together.
4. ADD salt and thyme to flour.
5. ADD 4 C flour to potato/yeast mixture, alternately with remaining ¾ C water, add additional flour, only if needed, until dough is not sticky.
6. TURN onto a well-floured board, knead. Place in an oil-coated bowl.
7. COVER and allow to rise one hour in a warm place.
8. DIVIDE dough into 24 pieces and form into rolls.
9. PLACE on an oil-coated baking sheet, cover with a damp cloth, and let rise again in a warm place until almost doubled in size.
10. BAKE until golden brown. Place in a wicker basket or bowl and cover with a thin cloth to keep warm.

 SIDEBAR   **FESTIVE FLAVORED BUTTER**

I first tasted the glory of flavored butter when I began making butter from our cow's cream. And it's so easy to do. Mix 1 to 2 tablespoons of herbs or spices into each stick of softened butter or margarine; roll it into a long, thin cylinder. Wrap it with cling wrap or parchment paper and chill. Then cut into ¼" rounds for individual pats of butter. Here are some flavor ideas, but make up some of your own, too:

1. **Herby**: chopped parsley, thyme and lemon zest.
2. **Zesty**: chopped cilantro and 1 canned chipotle pepper in adobo sauce.
3. **Salty**: nori and sesame seeds.
4. **Sweet**: ¼ t each of cardamom, cinnamon and ginger and 2 T agave syrup.

THE 1-2 PARADOX RICE BREAD

Makes 1 Loaf | Preheat Oven 400/350 Degrees | Bake: 45 to 50 Minutes   GMENS

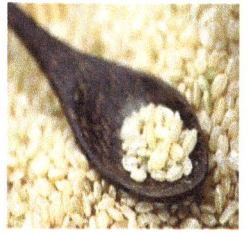

This bread goes great with zesty flavored butter (see previous page), peanut or nut butter, or any spreads.

I was first introduced to this bread in 1970 at the Paradox Bakery on St. Mark's Place in the East Village, New York City. This down to earth recipe, waited years for me to try to uncover. When I finally baked it the sweet aroma that spread throughout the house took me back decades. The bread can also be adapted very easily for people with various grain allergies or gluten sensitivities. When baked to a golden brown, the outside is crusty and the inside soft. It goes really well with zesty flavored butter (see previous page), peanut or nut butter, or any spreads. A friend describes this bread as something the 19th century Russian pilgrim in the book, The Way of a Pilgrim, *would have carried in his knapsack; a full-bodied, old world, wholesome meal in itself.*

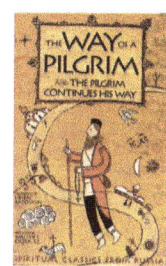

DRAFT-FREE PROOFING BREAD

Turn your oven on the absolute lowest heat possible. When it's warm, turn off the oven and place the covered dough inside to rise.

You can reheat the oven 2 to 3 times, if needed, but don't forget to turn off the oven or you'll have to start all over.

1 C warm water
½ t active dry yeast and 1 t sugar
1 C cooked brown rice
2 T agave
2 T olive oil
1½ t salt

2 C unbleached white flour (and up to an additional ½ C for kneading) or 2 C gluten-free flour blend (see Hint in next recipe)
½ C cornmeal
¼ C sesame or pumpkin seeds, or any seeds

1. ADD warm water, yeast, and sugar and let the yeast bloom.
2. ADD cooked rice, agave, and olive oil. Stir together to blend well.
3. ADD flour, cornmeal, and salt to incorporate, it will be quite sticky. Thoroughly blend all the ingredients and let it rest for 20 minutes.
4. KNEAD dough for about five minutes (if using seeds, add them now), adding small amounts of flour, as needed, so that the dough doesn't stick to the board.
5. PLACE in an oiled bowl, cover with a damp cloth or cling wrap and let it rise until double, about 2 hours (see proofing bread HINT).
6. PUNCH down and shape into two even balls and place in a greased bread pan. Oil the top of the dough and let rise for another 30 to 40 minutes, don't over rise the dough at this stage, let the final rise happen in the oven.
7. BAKE at 400 degrees for 30 minutes, then lower heat to 350 and continue baking for 15 to 20 minutes, until the top is golden.

NEW YORK GLUTEN-FREE BAGELS

Makes 8 Bagels | Preheat Oven to 375 Degrees | Bake: 25 to 30 Minutes   GMENS

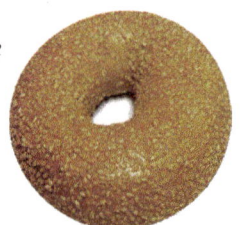

GLUTEN-FREE FLOUR BLENDS

Make a batch of this flour blend and store in a tightly covered container in the refrigerator.

General Blend

2 C brown rice flour, whirled until very fine
1 C sorghum flour
1 C tapioca starch
1 C garfava flour
2 C potato starch
2 C corn starch

Lighter Blend

2 C sorghum flour
2 C tapioca starch
2 C arrowroot flour
½ C potato starch

Life's little pleasures may include a crusty on the outside and chewy on the inside New York water bagel. Here's a chance to enjoy it on a gluten-free diet.

Dry Ingredients

3 C gluten-free flour blend (see side panel)
1 t xanthan gum
1 T flax meal
1 T dairy-free milk replacer powder (potato, rice, or soy)
1½ t salt
1 T instant yeast

Wet Ingredients

2 T agave syrup
1 t apple cider vinegar
3 T avocado oil
1¼ C warm water (105 degrees or a little less than hot)
Cornmeal for dusting
OPTIONAL: poppy seeds, sesame seeds, caramelized onions (top bagels just before baking.)

1. PREPARE a cookie sheet with parchment, coat lightly with cornmeal.
2. BLEND dry and wet ingredients in separate bowls.
3. FOLD dry ingredients into wet ingredients. Make sure to mix well, until very smooth and pliable.
4. FLOUR a large wooden board with brown rice flour. Shape the bagels placing a spoonful onto the board and create a large hole in the center with your thumb. Place each bagel on a parchment lined cooking sheet, which has been lightly sprinkled with cornmeal. Cover lightly with another piece of parchment paper that has been oiled. Put in a warm place to rise for about 30 minutes.
5. FILL a 12" skillet with water about 2" high. Add 1 T agave to the water; bring to a boil. Drop 3 bagels into the boiling water and simmer for 30 seconds on each side. Drain very well and add the next 2 batches, one batch at a time.
6. BAKE in a preheated oven, until golden. Cool on a rack.

A Culinary Journey

DELIGHTFUL GLUTEN-FREE SANDWICH BREAD

Makes 1 loaf | Preheat Oven to 350 Degrees | Bake: 38 to 42 Minutes   G M N S

GLUTEN-FREE RISING TIPS

During the second rise, don't put cling wrap on top, it may stick to the top and create ripples. Use a shower cap or invert another bread pan on the top.

During the second rise, don't over rise, let it finish rising in the oven. It calls for 45 to 60 minutes, but 45 minutes may be enough.

Once the bread is sliced, it is best to freeze separate slices in small packets and remove from the freezer, as needed.

I have tried my hand at many gluten-free bread recipes, but this one soars to another level. You have to use either an electric hand mixer or the preferred stand mixer, if you happen to have one. There is no choice, mixing by hand just won't do. It also toasts great!

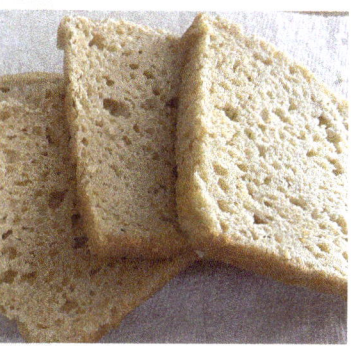

3 C any gluten-free all-purpose flour mix (if the mix contains agar agar or xanthan gum, omit the extra xanthan gum, see page 288)
3 T organic dark brown sugar
2 t active dry yeast (see Hint page 91)
1½ t salt
1¼ t xanthan gum
1 C warm milk or almond, rice, or soy milk
4 T butter or margarine, softened
3 medium eggs

1. PLACE the flour, sugar, yeast, salt, and xanthan gum in a bowl, or the bowl of your stand mixer. Mix to combined.
2. BLEND TOGETHER: slowly add the warm milk, keeping the beater on, it will at first look crumbly, but will soon come together. Then add softened butter or margarine and beat until thoroughly blended.
3. BEAT in one egg at a time, while scraping the bottom and sides of the bowl. When everything is incorporated beat at high speed for 3 minutes, to make a very smooth, thick batter.
4. FIRST RISE: Cover the bowl and let the thick batter rise for about one hour, it should pouffe up.
5. SCRAPE the bowl, which will deflate the batter slightly.
6. SECOND RISE: Scoop the dough into a generously greased loaf pan. Make the top level by using a spatula or wet fingers.
7. COVER and set in a warm place to rise, until the loaf barely comes to the top of the rim about 45 to 60 minutes
8. BAKE uncovered for 38 to 42 minutes, until golden brown. The last 15 minutes cover with tin foil, so the top won't burn. You can also bake covered with an inverted loaf pan and take it off the last 15 minutes.
9. REMOVE bread and cool completely on a rack before slicing.
10. SLICE the loaf, put about 4 to 6 slices in small freezer bags, then place those bags in one large freezer bag. It freezes well for about 3 months.

Breakfast, Bread, and Soup

SOUP DAZE

SOUP IS A UNIVERSAL FOOD; IT IS COMPRISED OF VARIOUS INGREDIENTS, spices and liquid married together. My favorite soup memory is a pot of many vegetables, various soaked beans, tomatoes, and spices simmering on top of the Nova Scotia living room wood stove in the dead of winter. The embers burned slowly within the stove to create a low, even heat. The soup cooked from morning to evening and just before it was done, a splash of apple cider vinegar was added. It was eaten with freshly baked bread and home-churned butter. A memory of eating this warm and satisfying meal, while quietly watching the snow swirl outside the bay window, is quite fresh in my mind, as if it were only days ago. Now, living in southern California, snow is a fond memory, but this soup is still a staple and favorite meal.

Roasted Sesame Tofu Soup Garnish

Add to any bowl of hot soup. Save any extra pieces in for the next day. It's great with brown rice too!

1 C firm tofu, chopped into small cubes
1 T olive oil, 1 T black sesame seed oil
1 T tamari or soy sauce
½ t ginger, fresh minced
¼ C sesame seeds (optional)

1. HEAT the oils in a frying pan and add tofu, tamari, ginger, and sesame seeds.
2. FRY on medium heat until tofu is golden brown.

PEA IN THE BONNET SOUP

Serves 6   GMENSY

HEALING PROPERTIES

Cayenne Pepper
- Has cardiovascular benefits
- Stimulates the mucus membrane lining to relieve congestion
- Boosts immunity
- Helps to kill bacteria, powerfully stimulating the cell lining of the stomach to secrete protective buffering juices that prevent ulcer formation
- Increases thermogenesis and oxygen consumption, helpful for weight loss

Make extra soup—whoever comes over to share your meal will want to take some home. It's even better the next day. Just add a little water and salt if necessary, and then reheat. If you don't like the consistency of blended soup, leave unblended, you could mash it slightly with a potato masher to blend all the ingredients. When my friend Beverly tested this recipe, she came up with this delightful name.

3 T olive oil
2 onions, chopped
2 to 4 garlic cloves, minced (less if you're not a garlic lover; more if you have a cold and want the medicinal effects of garlic)
1" fresh ginger, minced
2 celery sticks, chopped
2 small zucchinis, chopped
3 carrots, chopped
1 medium red potato, chopped
½ t cayenne pepper
½ t Hungarian paprika
2 T fresh dill, chopped or 1 t dried
1 t salt (or to taste)
1 C split peas, green
1 vegetarian bouillon cube and 6 C water or vegetable soup stock
1 T fresh dill for garnish
OPTIONAL: ½ capful liquid smoke

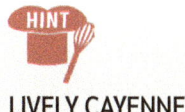

LIVELY CAYENNE

Use can add even a pinch of cayenne pepper to almost any savory dish to enliven the flavor.

1. HEAT olive oil in a large soup pan, sauté the onions until translucent.
2. ADD the garlic and ginger. Sauté for about 30 seconds, being careful not to burn the garlic.
3. ADD celery, zucchini, carrots, and red potato. Coat with oil and then add the spices and salt. Sauté vegetables until almost tender.
4. ADD 1 C rinsed split peas, bouillon cube, and water.
5. BRING TO A BOIL, then lower the heat. Cook for about 30 to 45 minutes until split peas are very tender. Add liquid smoke at the end.
6. BLEND in food processor or with hand blender until almost smooth; top with dill.

ROASTED GARLIC CARROT/GINGER SOUP

Serves 6 to 8

GMENSY

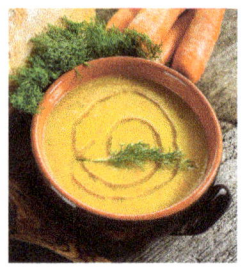

I love roasted garlic oil in soup, it gives you the benefits and flavor of garlic without the overly strong aroma. I also love to put fresh ginger in soup, it adds a zing and slight heat, along with crushed chili peppers. This is a full-bodied carrot soup with a difference!

1 T butter or coconut oil
1 T roasted garlic oil
½ t crushed chili peppers
2 T fresh ginger, grated
2 onions, peeled and chopped
6 C veggie broth
2 pounds carrots, peeled and sliced
1 t salt
½ t freshly ground pepper

1 C coconut cream
Dill for garnish

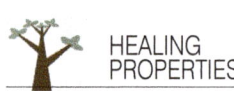

Garlic Benefits
- Boosts immunity
- Works as an anti-inflammatory
- Improves cardiovascular health
- Gives you better hair and skin
- Protects your food: Those same antibacterial properties in fresh garlic can kill the bacteria that lead to food poisoning, including salmonella and E. coli

1. MELT the butter or coconut oil and garlic oil in a saucepan.
2. ADD chili pepper and ginger fry a few moments.
3. FRY onions slowly, until translucent, do not brown.
4. ADD the rest of the ingredients except coconut cream. Bring to a boil and simmer for 20 minutes, or until carrots are very soft.
5. ADD coconut cream and simmer for another 5 minutes.
6. BLEND until smooth, you can do this in two batches.
7. DRIZZLE each bowl with garlic oil and top with a dill sprig.

SMOKY ROASTED GARLIC OIL

1 head of garlic or ½ C peeled garlic cloves, 2 C olive oil, ½ t salt, ½ t smoky paprika, ½ t dried parsley, ½ t lime zest. Mash garlic cloves in a plastic bag using a rolling pin. Stir garlic, oil, and salt together and place in a small baking pan. Make sure the garlic is submerged in the oil. Bake at 325 degrees for 40 minutes, add paprika, parsley and lime zest, bake another 20 minutes. Strain and store in the refrigerator. (Rub hands against stainless steel to remove garlic smell.)

RAMANI'S CHEESY POTATO SOUP

Serves 4   GMENSY

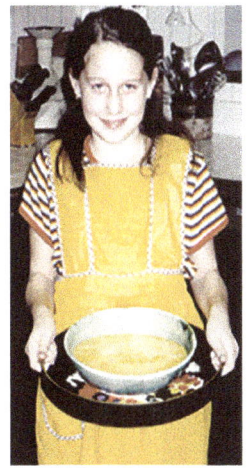

Ramani at 10, now a mother herself, still loves this soothing and comforting soup.

My then ten-year-old daughter, Ramani, and I made this soup together and she submitted the recipe for my cooking column, commenting: "I like this soup because it's easy and really good. You do need a little help from your mom, but kids can do it mostly by themselves."

2 T butter, margarine or avocado oil
2 T whole wheat pastry flour or gluten-free flour blend
½ C water or vegetable stock
2 C low-fat milk, soy, almond or rice milk and vegan cheese if you're allergic to milk (like my dad)
2 C cooked potatoes, cubed (you can also use leftover baked potatoes)
1 t salt
¾ C low or non-fat sharp cheddar cheese (or any alternative) shredded or cut into small pieces. (Be careful when shredding; this is where you can use your mom's help.)

1. MELT the butter, margarine, or oil in a saucepan.
2. ADD the flour and mix until it bubbles.
3. ADD the milk, water or stock; let it cook until it begins to thicken.
4. ADD potatoes and salt, then cook, stir for about five minutes.
5. REMOVE from the heat, sprinkle and mix the cheese into the soup.

That's it. If you want to reheat the soup, don't boil it.

 SIDEBAR   VEGAN CHEESE ALTERNATIVES

These cheeses are commonly made from soy, almond, rice milk and/or tofu. You can also try the cashew cheese recipe on page 291. Some cheeses have soy protein isolate added, as well as some type of oils like canola or soybean oil. Many include an ingredient used to boost texture, like guar gum or carrageenan. However, some use the hidden ingredient "casein," a milk protein, to make their product look, feel, and melt more like dairy cheese. Casein-free, vegan mozzarella and American singles, as well as blocks of soy cheddar, rice cheddar, and rice mozzarella are now easily available, and *Tofutti* makes casein-free soy cream cheese and sour cream. Check your labels carefully.

Breakfast, Bread, and Soup

MADAME LEPAPE'S LEEK AND POTATO SOUP

Serves 4 to 6

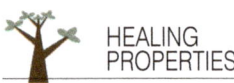

Leeks
- Contain manganese making them particularly helpful in stabilizing blood sugar
- Have been shown to protect colon cells from cancer-causing toxins

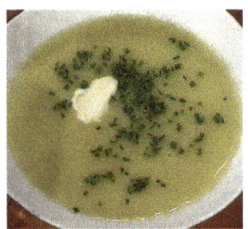

Since this is a genuine French recipe butter is preferred, though olive oil will work, too!

I asked my friend, Jeannie Salzman, for her Leek and Potato Soup recipe, an award-winning and perfectly simple recipe that she developed while living in rural France and growing a huge amount of leeks. *"When my husband and I first bought our 400-year-old farmhouse in Loire Valley, in France, I told my wonderful neighbors, Monsieur and Madame Lepape, to use our walled-in garden as a place for Marquis, their energetic wirehaired terrier, to play. Since we were back in America for months at a time, it worked out well. They in turn planted the most magnificent vegetable garden for us: rows of lettuces, tomatoes, green beans, peas, onions, carrots, celery root, garlic, chives, parsley, potatoes, and two hundred and fifty leeks. It was bountiful and beautiful! So, for the next several months, we were deliciously nourished due to the graciousness of Monsieur and Madame Lepape, and their dog, Marquis. However, being an American, I really didn't know how to use all those leeks. We tried steamed leeks, braised leeks, leek quiche and leeks in vinaigrette. But best of all was Madame Lepape's recipe for Leek and Potato Soup. It has now been many years since that first garden of Monsieur Lepape. My husband and I learned much from his wisdom and generosity, and, for many years thereafter, we also planted two hundred and fifty leeks each season. We lived through many winters sitting cozily by the fireplace, enjoying great bowls of steaming Leek and Potato Soup, and we stayed cool in summer when I served it chilled as* vichyssoise. *Leeks have become my favorite vegetable because of the depth of character they add to any dish calling for them."*
—Jeanne Salzman

4 T butter or olive oil
4 C sliced leeks, cleaned well
4 T whole wheat flour or gluten-free flour
8 C hot water or vegetable stock

4 C Yukon or Benji potatoes, peeled and cubed
1½ to 2 T salt and freshly ground pepper
Garnish each bowl: 1 t minced chives and a dollop of crème fraîche, sour cream, or coconut cream

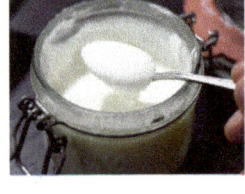

1. MELT butter or oil in a soup pot and add sliced leeks.
2. COVER and cook gently for five minutes to caramelize. Add flour and stir continually for two to three minutes.
3. ADD water or stock, potatoes, salt, and pepper.
4. SIMMER for 40 minutes.
5. PUREE with hand blender or in a food processor.
6. TOP with minced chives and cream.

JEANNE'S KABOCHA PUMPKIN SOUP

Serves 4 to 6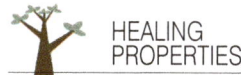

HEALING PROPERTIES

Winter Squash
- Excellent source of vitamin A and C, powerful antioxidant and anti-inflammatory
- Excellent source of fiber, helpful for irritable bowel syndrome
- Helps protect against emphysema

This recipe is also from Madame Lepape. However, since we moved to northern California, I've substituted the Kabocha (Japanese pumpkin) for the traditional acorn squash.
—Jeanne Salzman

2 C pumpkin, peeled and cubed (kabocha if possible). Simmer in boiling water for twenty minutes. (You can use canned pumpkin, but it is not as tasty as the fresh kabocha.)
1 yellow onion, sliced thin
2 T butter or margarine
4 C vegetable stock
1 T salt
Nutmeg to taste
Blue cheese, chives, or cilantro to garnish

1. COOK pumpkin until very soft.
2. SAUTÉ onion in butter or margarine for 10 minutes.
3. COMBINE pumpkin, stock, salt, nutmeg, and onions in a large pot and bring to a boil, then simmer for 10 to 15 minutes, until pumpkin is quite soft.
4. PUREE soup.
5. TOP with blue cheese, chives, or cilantro, or all three.

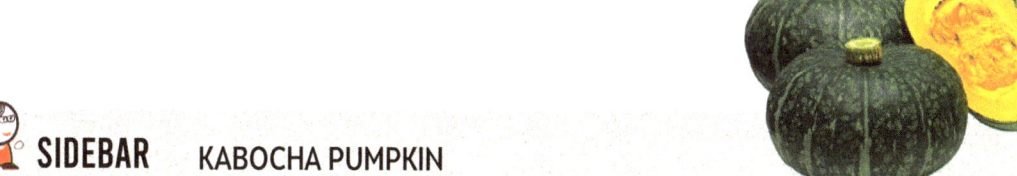

SIDEBAR   KABOCHA PUMPKIN

Also known as an Ebisu, Delica, and Hoka, the Japanese pumpkin shaped Kabocha pumpkin has a forest green skin. Kabocha pumpkins have hard, thick skins and only the flesh is eaten. Its flavor is similar to a sweet potato or pumpkin with a rich sweetness and almost fiber less flesh. It is very versatile and can be baked, steamed, puréed, braised, or left chunky in soups, or baked in puddings and pies. It is best to choose squashes that are heavy for their size. The rind should be dull and firm; avoid any with soft spots. Kabochas can be substituted in any recipe calling for acorn squash.

CHICKPEA/SWEET POTATO SOUP

Serves 4 to 6   GMENSY

This is a quick, yet complex soup, which tastes even better the next day after all of the flavor's blend together. To make it quickly and retain flavor and vitamins, I use an Instant Pot. You can, of course, also use a good soup pot and cook it until all the vegetables are soft.

2 T olive oil
1 onion, chopped
10 button mushrooms, chopped
½ red bell pepper, chopped
1 large, sweet potato, peeled and chopped
2 to 3 zucchinis, chopped
2 carrots, peeled and chopped
3 sprigs fresh parsley and 3 bay leaves

1 can chickpeas, drained and rinsed
2 veggie bouillon cubes
1 t salt
1 t ginger, freshly grated
½ t turmeric
½ t cumin powder
½ t smoky paprika
Pinch cayenne pepper
Water or soup stock
1 t balsamic vinegar

1. SAUTÉ onions, mushrooms, and pepper in oil (in the Instant Pot on the "sauté" setting) until cooked.
2. ADD the balance of the ingredients, except vinegar.
3. ADD water to just "below" the ingredients, if using an Instant Pot or pressure cooker.
4. COOK 15 minutes (on "stew" setting). [increase water to "over" ingredients for soup pot, cook 40 to 50 minutes.]
5. REMOVE parsley sprigs, bay leaves and add vinegar.
6. BLEND until almost smooth; leave it a bit chunky.

 SIDEBAR   THE WONDERFUL CHICKPEA

Are they called chickpeas, or garbanzo beans? It depends on where your culinary loyalties lie. If you're with the French and Italians, you may think of them as *chiche* and *ceci*, respectively. If you're with the Spanish, then you may know them as garbanzos and in India as chana. If you were stranded on a desert island with just one food item, the chickpea and its subtle chestnutty flavor would be an ideal companion. Chickpeas contain an almost complete nutritional balance. When a diet is weighted toward protein, fiber-rich beans and other complex carbohydrates leaves you feeling fuller sooner. Additionally, a diet high in fiber may help lower blood cholesterol and also reduce the risk of developing diabetes.

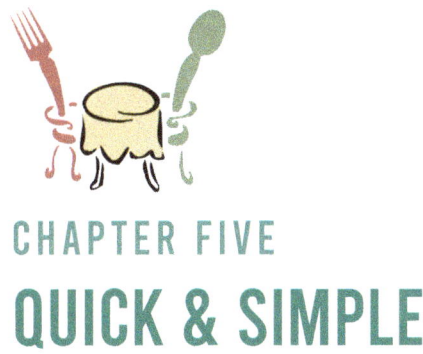

CHAPTER FIVE
QUICK & SIMPLE

THE PASTA & SAUCE PARTY
SIMPLE YET ELEGANT
A MAJ JONGG AFTERNOON

5

THE PASTA & SAUCE PARTY

*"Form does not differ from emptiness,
    emptiness does not differ from form.
That which is form is emptiness,
    that which is emptiness form."*
—The Heart Sutra

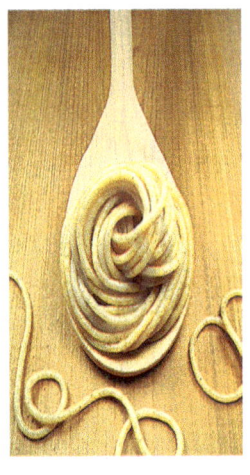

IT IS ALWAYS GOOD TO RETURN TO THE HEART, the source of all, especially when the world around us appears so much more complex. Paring a thing down to its center in all simplicity is very beneficial. In this quote from *The Heart Sutra*, an ancient Hindu text, it reminds me that emptiness and form complete and void each other in eternal nonmovement—the very circle of existence.

At the heart of one's cooking, the essence of a meal can be a simple or complex sauce. It can then be used in so many ways, especially to top the more neutral aspect of the meal: rice, pasta, bread, or grains.

One day, I had some friends over for a pasta and sauce party. We worked together to make a number of sauces, cooked the pasta, and presented them all buffet style. How simple is that!

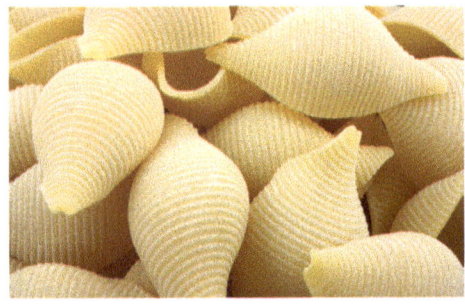

A Culinary Journey

ELEGANT EGGPLANT TOMATO SAUCE SURPRISE

Serves 4 to 6

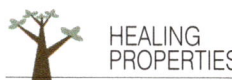

Inspired by my friend, Robin Devine (that's her real name), this sauce was born out of chopping some eggplant for another dish, with a few cups left over. Instead of tossing it in a container, we fried it up and combined it with some tomato sauce that happened to be cooking on the stove. Voila!

HEALING PROPERTIES

Tomato
- Contains significant antioxidants
- Contains lycopene with cardiovascular and anti-cancer benefits
- Aids in anti-inflammatory conditions
- Is an effective blood thinner
- Is protective against prostate cancer, diabetes and migraines

3 T olive oil
1 onion, chopped small
1 C mushrooms, chopped small
1 T ginger, fresh, grated
2 garlic cloves, chopped small
1 t salt
½ t oregano, dried
2 T fresh basil, julienned
½ t cayenne pepper
½ eggplant, chopped very small
1 t brown sugar, maple syrup or agave
1 (28 oz.) can fire-roasted, crushed tomatoes in their own juice
1 (8 oz.) can tomato paste.

1. SAUTÉ onion, mushrooms, ginger in olive oil until translucent. Add garlic and herbs and fry for a few moments.
2. ADD eggplant and stir fry until tender.
3. ADD sweetener, tomatoes, and tomato paste. Simmer for about ½ hour.
4. ADJUST salt and sweetener to taste.

ACIDIC TOMATO SAUCE SOLUTION

If your sauce starts tasting too acidic: while you're cooking, throw in a small handful of large carrots slices. You can remove them before serving. The carrots absorb some of the acid and brings a natural sweetness to the sauce.

Quick & Simple

SIMPLE LIGHT TOMATO SAUCE

Serves 4

GMENSY

20 tomatoes, Roma, halved, de-seeded
⅛ C olive oil
1 large onion, diced coarsely
2 garlic cloves, whole
1 T fresh oregano leaves, chopped
1 T fresh thyme leaves
1 C vegetable stock or water
½ t Kosher salt, fresh ground pepper

1. PLACE tomato halves on a 13" by 9" pan cut side up.
2. ADD onion, garlic, herbs, and drizzle oil on top.
3. ROAST for 40 minutes at 225 degrees, then turn the oven to 350 degrees and bake another 15 minutes.
4. REMOVE from oven and process through a food mill or in a sieve fitted over a saucepan. Discard skins and fresh herbs.
5. ADD salt and pepper, vegetable stock or water and cook covered on low heat for 30 minutes.

MISO TOMATO SAUCE

Serves 6 to 8

GMENY

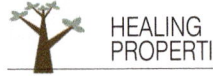 HEALING PROPERTIES

Miso
- Contains all the essential amino acids
- Contains natural digestive enzymes, Lactobacillus, and other microorganisms which aid in digestion
- Warning: contains high amounts of sodium

This is a unique version of one of my old standards. It's an easy recipe to remember because most of the ingredients are in the quantity of two. This is a generous recipe that can be stored in freezer containers to use whenever you need some extra sauce. There is no need for extra salt since the miso is sufficient. Fresh herbs work best, but you can use 1 T dried herbs in a pinch.

2 T olive oil
2 small onions, finely chopped
1 garlic clove, minced
½ C tomato paste
2 T fresh basil leaves, chopped
2 T fresh parsley, chopped
2 bay leaves (remove before serving)
2 (28 oz.) cans diced tomatoes, in their juices
2 T miso paste and 3 T water
Black pepper, freshly ground.

1. HEAT oil in large skillet and sauté onions in olive oil. Add garlic and sauté another minute.
2. ADD tomato paste, herbs, and diced tomatoes and bring to a boil. Reduce and simmer for about 15 minutes, until it begins to thicken slightly.
3. COMBINE miso and water with a whisk to blend completely. Add the miso water to the pan and simmer for an additional five minutes.

TOASTED PINE-WALNUT PESTO

Makes 2 Cups   G M E S Y

PINE NUTS

Because the buttery taste of pine nuts goes rancid quickly, buy them in stores with a quick turnover rate. Raw pine nuts should be stored in a tightly sealed container in the refrigerator where they will keep for up to 3 months. In the freezer, pine nuts will keep for up to 9 months.

Be careful when toasting pine nuts and walnuts; attention is essential. One time, I was busy in the kitchen and my toasted pine nuts burned to a crusty black. Since I only had half the amount left to make pesto, I used some walnuts I had on hand. It turned out to be a great combination, my best pesto ever! Blend together until very smooth and adjust salt to taste. Pesto can be stored in the refrigerator for two weeks.

1 garlic clove (optional)
¼ C pine nuts, dry toasted
¼ C walnuts, dry toasted
3 T olive oil
¼ warm water
¼ C Parmesan cheese or ¼ C Romano cheese or ¼ C vegan alternative
¾ t salt
¼ t freshly ground black pepper
4 C fresh basil, don't press down when measuring

1. DROP garlic through a food processor and mince.
2. ADD the rest of the ingredients and process until smooth
3. ADJUST water and cheese to create a slightly thicken consistency.

CREAMY TOFU SAUCE   G M E N Y

Makes 1½ Cups

In this basic recipe I often use tahini (sesame seed paste) but when that is not available, peanut, or sunflower butter will do just as well.

1 C fresh tofu, firm
¼ C tahini or nut butter
2 T tamari (soy sauce)
1 t ginger, freshly grated
½ C light coconut milk
2 T avocado oil

1. BLEND together until very smooth.
2. ADD tamari to taste.

Quick & Simple

TOMATO/BASIL BRUSCHETTA

Serves 4 to 6   GMENSY

SUN-DRIED TOMATOES

Slice tomatoes into ½ inch slices. Drain on paper towels and place in single layers on wire racks, on a cookie sheet. Bake at 125 degrees around 10 hours. Rotate cookie sheets a few times.

This can be made ahead, covered with aluminum foil, and refrigerated until ready to serve.

1 large loaf crusty bread (can be gluten free)
2 whole garlic cloves
2 T butter, melted or 2 T olive oil
4 to 6 sun-dried tomatoes (soak in water for 1 hour and drain)
4 to 6 fresh basil leaves, roughly chopped (for garnish)
Freshly ground pepper and flake salt (see page 311)

1. CUT bread into ¼" wedges.
2. PLACE on two cookie sheets.
3. MELT butter or oil in small pan, add garlic cloves and simmer for a few seconds, don't burn, remove cloves.
4. DRIZZLE garlic butter/oil mixture over bread.
5. TOP bread with re-hydrated sun-dried tomatoes, and basil.
6. TOP with cracked pepper and a pinch of flake salt.
7. BROIL for five to ten minutes until golden brown, just before serving.
8. REMOVE from cookie sheet and place on a large serving plate.

SIMPLE PASTA

Serves 4 to 6   GMENSY

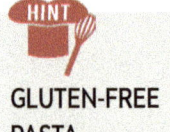

GLUTEN-FREE PASTA

- Mrs. Leepers
- Ancient Harvest
- Cappellos Grain Free, Gluten-Free Fettuccine

Just to name a few!

You can make pasta ahead of time and immerse it in boiling water for a few seconds just before serving.

½ C pasta, per portion
4 C water, per portion
½ t salt, per portion

1. BOIL water and keep it warm. When you are about to serve the meal, bring water to a boil again, add salt.
2. ADD pasta to water.
3. COOK according to recommended time shown on pasta package.
4. DRAIN thoroughly, save a few spoons of cooking water.
5. DRIZZLE cooking water and olive oil, over top of the cooked pasta.

SIMPLE YET ELEGANT

"In everything one does it is possible to foster and maintain a state of being which reflects our true destiny. When this possibility is actualized, the ordinary day is no longer ordinary. It can even become an adventure of the spirit."
—Karlfried Graf von Dürckheim

I LOVE THE PHRASE "ADVENTURE OF THE SPIRIT." It can be as simple as peeling an onion and wiping the tears from one's eyes. Since we have to eat to live and most of us have to cook to eat, we often have ample opportunity in the kitchen to be in the moment. It's a simple act and it can be as rewarding as we care to make it.

We often find ourselves with little time to prepare a meal. Through the years and necessity, I developed a number of quick and simple recipes that are truly sustaining. They are simple preparations, that free me to carry on with the endless tasks of life that crop up daily.

Couscous is a North African food made of soft, refined durum wheat that has been steamed, cracked, and dried. When combined with vegetables, this festive dish is easy to prepare and needs very little cooking. It has a fluffy, whole grain, nutty flavor.

Pressure-cooked vegetable soup can be as quick as cutting up whatever vegetables are available in the refrigerator and adding a soup base and some herbs. And with a little advance preparation, cornbread can be whisked together in ten minutes or even the night before keeping the wet and dry ingredients in separate bowls.

Simplifying life holds great rewards, even if it is one small act, one day at a time.

CONSCIOUS COUSCOUS AND VEGETABLES

Serves 4 to 6   MESY

THE COUSCOUS ALTERNATIVE

Couscous is a neutral grain with subtle nutty undertones. Couscous can be used in salads, pasta dishes, side dishes, and soups. Dry couscous can be added to soup and allowed to simmer for about 10 minutes. It is also a wonderful stuffing for the cavity of winter squashes or roasted peppers. Once the few basic techniques are mastered, the possibilities are endless.

I don't think I'll ever forget the first time I discovered couscous. Some friends dropped in unexpectedly and made a version of this recipe with some couscous that had traveled the world in their backpack. This recipe turned out to be a favorite, after being printed in the "Natural Kitchen" column, which I wrote for many years in the Inner Directions Journal.

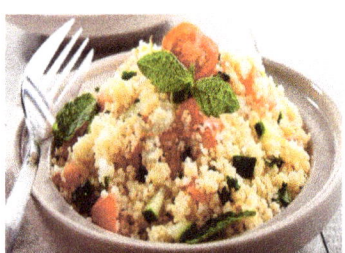

2 T olive oil and 1 T margarine or butter
1 bay leaf
1 red onion, chopped very small
1 green or red pepper, chopped very small
1 to 2 small cloves of garlic, minced
1 t ginger, freshly grated
½ C cashews or pine nuts
1 carrot, shredded
1 zucchini, shredded
½ C cherry tomatoes, quartered
2 C couscous
1¼ t salt
½ t cumin powder, (if you have time, freshly roast and grind)
¼ t turmeric
Aleppo chili pepper, generous pinch
1 T lemon zest
2 C boiling water
2 T fresh mint or basil leaves, torn

1. FRY the bay leaf, onion, pepper, garlic, ginger, and nuts in oil and margarine or butter, until soft.
2. STIR in shredded carrot, zucchini, and tomatoes. With a lid on, let the vegetables cook on a medium heat, until tender.
3. STIR in the couscous, salt, cumin, turmeric, chili, and zest and lower the heat on the stove to the absolute lowest possible setting.
4. POUR the boiling water into the pan, while stirring at the same time.
5. SIMMER for about 5 minutes, with the lid on, do not stir.
6. REMOVE from heat and let sit with the lid on for an additional 10 minutes. Fluff gently with a fork.
7. TOP with mint or basil.

NO-PRESSURE VEGGIE SOUP

Serves 4 to 6

GMENSY

OVER-SALTED SOUP

If you have a potato on hand, peel it and throw it into the over-salted soup. Let it simmer for a while, you can discard it, if you desire. The potato absorbs some of the salt. If the soup is still too salty, try adding sliced mushrooms, carrots, or tomatoes. In a curry you could also add a little coconut milk, a little lemon juice or a pinch of sugar to neutralize the saltiness.

Of course, a pressure cooker or Instant Pot works best for this quickie recipe, but it can be cooked in a heavy Dutch oven pot as well. Obviously, the main difference is the cooking time.

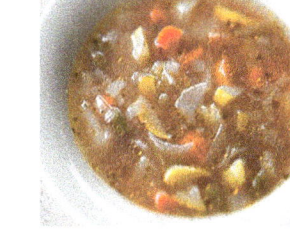

1 T olive oil
1 t salt or Braggs Liquid Aminos to taste
1 onion, chopped
Dash of cayenne pepper
2 bay leaves
Fresh herbs
4 C mixed vegetables, chopped into large chunks
½ C tomato sauce or 2 T tomato paste
½ C pasta, gluten-free pasta or cooked rice

1. ADD the oil and onions to a cooker and sauté until translucent.
2. ADD cayenne pepper and any fresh or dried herbs you have on hand (fresh dill or parsley, dried thyme, or sage work very nicely.)
3. ADD the salt and any vegetables that you have on hand to the cooker. [soup standards: garlic, carrot, celery, broccoli (stems are great for soup, peel the outer tough skin first) zucchini, parsnip, cabbage, potato, and the list goes on . . .]
4. ADD ½ C water or vegetable broth for Instant Pot, 1 C for pressure cooker, or 2 C for Dutch oven. If you are using water you can also add 1 bouillon cube. Then add the tomato sauce.
5. ADJUST pressure in your "pressure cooker," according to the particular unit, when it has stabilized, cook for 5 minutes. If you are using an "Instant Pot" set it on stew for 15 minutes or simmer in a "Dutch oven" for 30 minutes, until vegetables are tender.

OPTIONAL: After opening the pressure cooker or Instant Pot, bring the soup to a boil once again and add any pasta you have on hand. Cook until done.

 WAKING UP HERBS

To enhance the flavor of dried herbs crush them between your fingers before adding them to a dish. When using dried herbs use the ratio ½ t of dried herbs to 1 t fresh herbs.

A MAJ JONGG AFTERNOON

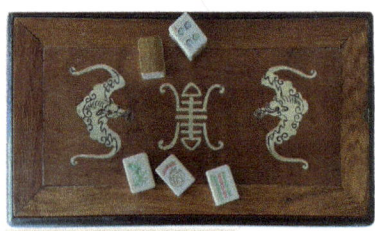

THERE ARE MANY DIFFERENT STORIES about how the game of Mah Jongg began. Many Mah Jongg theories say it started around the year 500 B.C. coinciding with the Chinese philosopher Confucius. Evidence points to the appearance of the game in several different Chinese provinces at the time when Confucius traveled extensively while teaching his new doctrines. The three "Dragon" tiles also correspond with the three cardinal virtues taught by Confucius: Benevolence, Sincerity, and Piety. Since Confucius was rumored to be fond of birds, it may explain why the name "Mah Jongg" came to be, which translates from the Chinese as, "Hemp Bird."

I first remember being fascinated with the beautiful Mah Jongg tiles around the age of seven. My aunts and grandmother would regularly play on an ancient card table that was shakily situated over the gnarled roots of a large apple tree. There, in upstate New York, the entire extended family would spend summer vacations at a rustic bungalow colony. Although I played Mah Jongg only briefly as a very young girl, I fondly remember the clicking of tiles and the hushed voices of women in housecoats. So, when a friend invited me to join their new weekly Mah Jongg group, I was thrilled. What I found is that this is not simply a game, but a teaching in meditation and concentration—one that gave my forgetful mind a real workout.

When time permits, we add a meal to the mix, and after eating it's time to return for a few more games. There are two ways to make a successful Mah Jongg meal: one is to make it ahead of time so there is not a lot of prep time the day of the party. The other is to make it simple to digest, so that the mind and body still function properly for after-meal games. Here is one of my very simple Mah Jongg meals.

I serve the Ginger Banana/Pecan Fingers a little later during the last game, with a refreshing cup of chai or coffee.

In 1939, Shanghai was one of the last possible refuges for around 10,000 Jews. Oscar Rosenzweig was one of the Shanghai exiles. He returned to Vienna from exile in 1947, bringing the Chinese game Mah Jongg with him. It is now displayed in a Museum in Vienna.

Many years ago, Matthew found a similar set online.

ROASTED VEGGIE SOUP

Serves 4 to 6

GMESY

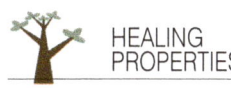

Beets
- Are bodyguards for liver cells
- Help protect against heart disease, birth defects and certain cancers, especially colon

STORING BEETS

Store beets in the refrigerator crisper, they will keep for two-four weeks. Cut the majority of the greens and their stems from the roots, so they don't extract moisture away from the root. Leave about two inches of the stem attached to prevent the roots from "bleeding." Store unwashed greens separately, where they will keep fresh for about four days.

This soup was a lovely discovery. One day I had some roasted vegetables on hand to which I simply added some soup stock and spices, and the soup came together in ten minutes. You can prepare the vegetables the day before, then make the soup quickly on the day you are going to serve it.

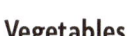

Vegetables

1 beets, peeled and chopped
2 sweet potatoes, peeled and chopped
2 zucchinis, peeled and chopped
2 carrots, chopped
1 large onion, slivered
1 red pepper, chopped
2 small garlic cloves
1 portobello mushroom, chopped
2 T olive oil
1 t kosher salt
Fresh pepper
Fresh herbs (rosemary and thyme sprigs)
½ t cumin seeds
1 t curry powder
½ t Aleppo chili
½ t ginger powder
4 C vegetable broth
1 (14.5 oz.) can fire roasted tomatoes, diced
Dash of liquid smoke (just a drop!)
3 T pine nuts, roasted

1. ADD vegetables to a large baking dish. Drizzle with 1 T olive oil, salt, and pepper, mix well to coat all the vegetables.
2. ROAST at 350 Degrees for about an hour (cover with foil for the first half hour) bake until all the vegetables are soft.
3. HEAT 1 T olive oil in a heavy-duty soup pot, sauté cumin seeds until they pop, then add curry, chili, and ginger powder, veggies (measure 5 cups), broth, and tomatoes.
4. COOK until hot and bubbly.
5. ADJUST salt and add liquid smoke.
6. MASH before serving, don't over blend. Top with roasted pine nuts for a crunch.

SAVORY POTATO PUFFS

Makes 24 Puffs | Preheat Oven to 350 Degrees | Bake: 15 to 20 Minutes

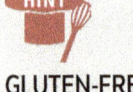

GLUTEN-FREE ALTERNATIVE

Roll ¼ C potato mixture into a tight ball, flatten slightly. Coat with a whipped whole egg, egg white, soy, or rice milk. Coat with a thin layer of cornmeal on both sides and place on a greased baking pan. Spray top with oil. Bake at 350 Degrees for 15 to 20 minutes until golden brown.

If you want to pre-cook puffs, bake for 10 minutes and finish baking just before serving. They also freeze really well when they are partially-baked.

This is a great party favorite to serve either as finger food while people are gathering, or as an extra side treat. I often make the potato/onion mixture the day before. Then, early the next day, I roll and fill the dough and half bake them. Just before the guests arrive, I finish baking and serve them piping hot.

An early memory I had while I caramelized onions was visiting Grandma Pauline in her Brooklyn walk up apartment building. The smell of cooking onions hit us as soon as we walked into the hallway. The aroma must have dwelt there for generations.

Use 4 to 5 red or Yukon gold new potatoes (medium-large). Boil until quite tender, remove skins and drain well.
1 T butter or margarine
1½ to 2 t salt (it really needs to have enough salt)
¼ t turmeric (it adds a lovely yellow color)
Freshly ground black pepper
2 baked garlic cloves (optional)
2 T vegetable or olive oil
2 medium onions, chopped extremely small
½ package frozen puff pastry dough (defrost thoroughly before using)

1. MASH potatoes with butter or margarine. Add salt, pepper, turmeric, and garlic (if you are using it) and set aside. The potato mixture should be quite thick.
2. SAUTÉ onions in oil until golden brown.
3. ADD onions to mashed potatoes, mix well. I generally use my hands at this stage.

To Make Puffs:
1. UNROLL one of the dough sections (there are usually two sections in the package) and cut into three pieces (on the length side), about 12" by 4" each.
2. ROLL each piece out on slightly floured board until it is a ⅛" thin, long rectangle.
3. FILL long center with the filling, about 1 inch high and 1 inch wide.
4. FOLD dough over the filling and pinch together until sealed.
5. CUT the whole roll into 2-inch pieces with a very sharp serrated knife.
6. BAKE until golden brown.

THE EASIEST AND BEST DARN CORNBREAD EVER!

Makes 1 Loaf | Preheat Oven to 350 Degrees | Bake: 30-35 Minutes   G M N S Y

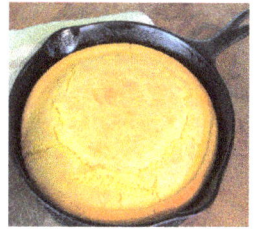

I have been making cornbread for decades. My old, batter-splashed copy of The Tassajara Bread Book *provided the initial "Three Layer Cornbread" recipe—many variations followed. This recipe has more protein to balance the carbohydrates. The very first set of pots and pans I received as a wedding present were cast iron. I dutifully learned all the required cleaning and maintenance methods for cast iron. I was ready to begin cooking until I actually filled one of the saucepans with food, which made the pan too heavy to lift off the stove. The only pan that survived through the years is an 8-inch skillet, now my cornbread baker. I have never figured out why cornbread bakes better in cast iron. It seems to work really well, as long as there is enough oil in the pan so the cornbread can be removed in one piece. The wet and dry ingredients can be prepared the night before and mixed together with the eggs just moments before you put it in the oven.*

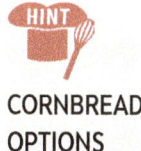

CORNBREAD OPTIONS

¼ C sunflower or pumpkin seeds; ½ C cooked corn kernels; 1 jalapeño pepper, chopped small; 1 chipotle pepper in adobo sauce, chopped small; 1 can mild green chilis, drained; cilantro, chopped very small.

BAKING IN A CAST IRON SKILLET

Add 2 T oil to pan. Place in hot oven for 5 minutes. Pour cornbread batter into sizzling pan and bake.

Dry ingredients

1 C cornmeal, ½ C whole wheat pastry flour, ½ C unbleached pastry flour [or 1 C cornmeal and 1 C light gluten-free flour blend (see page 94) mixed with 1 T gluten stabilizer (see page 310)]

2 t baking powder, ½ t baking soda, and ½ t salt

Wet ingredients

¼ C maple syrup, agave, or honey
¼ C olive oil
2 C buttermilk, low-fat milk, soy, rice, or almond milk
⅛ t nutmeg (freshly grated is best)
2 egg yolks and 2 egg whites, separated, or 4 egg whites

1. COMBINE the dry ingredients and place in a sealed container.
2. WHISK together the next five ingredients, store in refrigerator.

The day you are baking:

3. BEAT egg whites into a stiff meringue (add yolks to wet ingredients).
4. COMBINE the dry ingredients into wet ones, except for the meringue. Don't over-mix, even if there are some dry lumps.
5. FOLD in meringue using gentle strokes, then pour into a well-greased 8-inch baking pan or cast-iron skillet (see Iron Skillet Hint).
6. TOP with a little more grated nutmeg and bake. Don't overbake.

GINGER/BANANA/PECAN FINGERS

Makes 1 loaf | Preheat Oven to 350 Degrees | Bake: 30 to 35 Minutes   GMSY

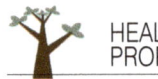

HEALING PROPERTIES

Pecans
- Have the most antioxidant capacity of any nut
- Help fight Alzheimer's, Parkinson's, cancer and heart disease
- Contain over 19 vitamins and minerals including vitamins E and A

This banana bread recipe has been with me for over three decades. The touch of ginger, lemon and aromatic spices gives this loaf a unique flavor. My favorite way to serve this bread is to cut it into long strips, pan fry with a touch of butter and serve with fresh jam on top.

Dry ingredients
1¾ C unbleached pastry flour or light gluten-free flour blend (see page 94) mixed with 1 T gluten stabilizer (see page 310)
2½ t baking powder
1 t salt

Wet ingredients
⅓ C avocado oil
⅔ C maple or ½ C agave syrup
1 t lemon zest
1½ C bananas, mashed (approximately 3)
2 egg yolks
1 t vanilla
1 t fresh ginger, minced
¼ t ground cardamom
½ t ground cinnamon

Fold-in ingredients
4 egg whites, whipped into a firm meringue
1 C pecans, chopped small

OPTIONAL: 3 T crystallized ginger, chopped small (you can cut them with oiled kitchen shears)

1. BLEND dry and wet ingredients together until very smooth in three batches.
2. FOLD in meringue or vegan version (see page 308), pecans, and ginger.
3. SPOON into a well-seasoned loaf pan.
4. BAKE until golden brown, don't overbake.

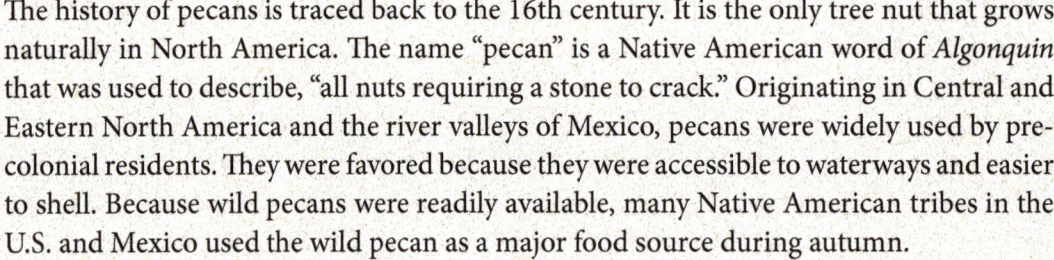

 SIDEBAR   **THE HISTORY OF PECANS**

The history of pecans is traced back to the 16th century. It is the only tree nut that grows naturally in North America. The name "pecan" is a Native American word of *Algonquin* that was used to describe, "all nuts requiring a stone to crack." Originating in Central and Eastern North America and the river valleys of Mexico, pecans were widely used by pre-colonial residents. They were favored because they were accessible to waterways and easier to shell. Because wild pecans were readily available, many Native American tribes in the U.S. and Mexico used the wild pecan as a major food source during autumn.

CHAPTER SIX
SAUCES, SALADS, DRESSINGS, AND SPICES

TOPPINGS THAT SING
DRESSINGS THE SALAD
SPICE MIXTURES
HERBS DE PROVENCE

6

TOPPINGS THAT SING

I HAVE A PASSION FOR PEANUT SAUCE. Any peanut sauce recipe I discover I save. I spent countless days reworking many of them to come up with the peanut and alternative nut sauces. They truly sing, are unique and flavorful. I often use a lower fat nut spread as its base because it has half the calories.

I love sauces in general; they can transform any dish, vegetable, or starch (such as rice, millet, buckwheat, or pasta) into a four-star meal.

Sauces provide the accent to any meal, adding depth and often an extra nutritional boost. Besides the more common peanut butter, miso, tofu or seeds are wonderful canvasses on which to build your masterpiece.

An Indian Peanut Village

I have a distinct peanut memory. It is when we were living in Chittor, South India. A friend of ours was from a family of peanut farmers. In fact, his family owned the whole village. Everyone in the village participated in some way or another in the planting and harvesting of peanuts, as well as making all its related products, especially peanut oil. The smell of roasted peanuts filled every inch of the land. Burlap bags were stacked in endless rows, and we watched with fascination as they moved from place to place with them on their heads. It put the humble legume into perspective forever.

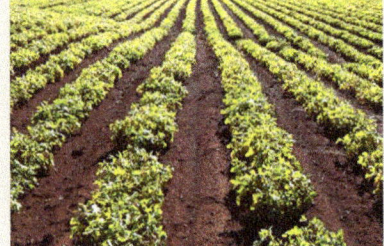

FRESH SPICY TOFU-PEANUT SAUCE

Makes 1¼ Cups GMEY

One of my all-time favorite sauces. I use freshly ground organic peanut butter for this recipe as regular peanuts are often highly saturated with chemicals.

½ C reduced-fat organic peanut butter
1 garlic clove, minced
1 T fresh ginger, minced
1 to 1¼ T Braggs Liquid Aminos
½ t crushed red pepper or ¼ t cayenne pepper
2 t lime juice
½ t lime zest
2 T honey or agave syrup
½ C tofu, silken
¼ C hot water or vegetable broth

1. BLEND together very well, adjust tamari, if needed.

This is a very versatile sauce, especially for topping brown rice. If you add a vegetable, you have a balanced meal that includes fiber and protein.

ALL PURPOSE NUTTY SAUCE

Makes 1 Cup GMESY

NUT BUTTERS

This is a surprisingly light sauce and goes well as a topping for any vegetable, salad, rice, or potato dish. It's also a great sauce for fresh vegetable rolls.

½ C reduced-fat peanut butter, almond, or sunflower butter
2 T maple syrup
3 T tamari
1 T lime juice
1 T toasted sesame oil and 2 T rice wine vinegar
½ to 1 t Sriracha chili sauce
1 garlic clove, crushed (optional)
½" ginger piece, finely grated or ½ t dried ginger
¼ C light coconut milk, add more if it's too thick

1. BLEND together very well, adjust liquid if needed.

Nut butters should be kept refrigerated to prevent rancidity and mold, for up to 3 months.

Warning: The mold aspergillus flavus produces aflatoxins, a known carcinogen.

Sauces, Salads, Dressings, and Spices

CREAMY VEGAN CASHEW SAUCE

Makes 1¼ Cups   GMESY

> Peanuts and sesame seeds are two of the most common allergens.

This is a simple, but delicious creamy sauce for many occasions: pasta, baked potatoes, veggies, or on vegan pizza.

1 C raw cashews (soak overnight, drain)
2 T nutritional yeast
1 garlic clove, minced or roasted (optional)
1 T lemon juice, freshly squeezed
½ t sea salt
½ t Aleppo chili powder
5 T water

1. BLEND together very well. Adjust water and salt. For thicker sauce, add less water.

SIMPLE MISO SAUCE

Makes 1½ Cups   GMENY

> Miso sauce is especially tasty with veggie burgers, as well as a sauce for cold soba noodle salad.

I have been making this standard recipe for decades. Tofu is a staple and because I usually keep some tahini in the refrigerator, this sauce is super easy to put together. It goes with almost any vegetable I prepare and is great with burgers too. Red miso gives this sauce a special depth.

2 T ginger, minced
2 T tahini
1 t sesame or olive oil
2 T red miso
1 C tofu, silken
½ t lemon zest
¼ to ½ t cayenne pepper
¼ to ½ C water

1. BLEND together very well.

TAHINI SHELF LIFE

Sesame butter (tahini) can be found in jars or cans. Once opened, keep refrigerated to prevent rancidity; it will keep fresh for up to 4 to 6 months.

DOUBLE SEED DIP

Makes 1½ Cups

GMENY

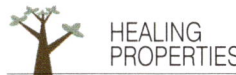

Sunflower Seeds
- Excellent source of vitamin E and selenium
- Detoxifier
- High in magnesium necessary for healthy bones and energy production

This is a unique dip or spread with a delightful nutty flavor.

Blend
3 ripe plum tomatoes, roasted, peeled and chopped
2 T sunflower seeds (soak overnight, drain)
1 C hulled pumpkin seeds (soak overnight, drain)
¼ C finely chopped cilantro and a pinch of Aleppo chili powder
1 jalapeño pepper, stemmed, roasted; remove skin and seeds and chop

Whisk
1 t mild miso and ½ t salt
1 t honey, agave or maple syrup
½ orange, freshly juiced

1. BLEND ingredients together, pour into a bowl.
2. WHISK together, and add to seed mixture, adjust seasoning.

SWEET AND SOUR MANGO/GINGER CHUTNEY

Makes 2 Cups

GMENSY

This is great as a condiment for any Indian meal.

This is an updated version of the famous Major Grey's Chutney. *In mango season, I am always looking for ways to include this amazing fruit in meals. After cutting the mango into pieces, you have the large pit to content with, so take each pit in your hands and squeeze tightly, strain, and voila! You have enough mango juice for this delightful sauce!*

1 T avocado oil
1 C red onion, chopped small
2½ C mangos, cubed
3 T fresh ginger, minced
1 garlic clove, minced
½ t salt

½ C lemon juice
1 t lemon zest
¼ C mango juice
3 T maple or agave syrup
2 T apple cider vinegar

1. HEAT oil and sauté onions until translucent.
2. ADD mango, ginger, and garlic; cook together for 7 minutes.
3. STIR in remaining ingredients and cook for 20 minutes, until thick.

Sauces, Salads, Dressings, and Spices

EASY COCONUT SAUCE

Makes 1 Cup

G M E N S Y

This is an instant sauce. It can be doubled for a larger crowd.

> You could use this sauce as a base for a Thai-style vegetable curry.

1 coconut milk
¼ C non or low-fat milk or water, rice, almond, or soy milk
1 t Cream of Wheat or rice
½ t curry powder, ½ t ground ginger, ¼ t ground cumin
¼ t ground cardamom
½ t salt and freshly ground pepper to taste.

1. SIMMER on low heat until slightly thickened, about 5 minutes.

TRIPLE-SMOKED BARBECUE SAUCE

Makes 1 Cup

G M E N Y

Making a sauce hot, sweet, smoky, and tangy is a tall order, but this has it all.

> This barbecue sauce is great for marinating vegetables and tofu for grilling.

1 T olive oil
1 onion, chopped small
½ C red cider vinegar
1 C tomato sauce
2 T unsulphered dark molasses
2 T maple or agave syrup
2 T tamari

1 T Dijon-style mustard
1 t smoky paprika
½ t liquid smoke
1 t canned chipotle pepper, de-seeded, in adobo sauce
1 garlic clove, minced
2 T Worcestershire sauce

1. SAUTÉ onion in olive oil, add all the ingredients, and simmer on low heat for about 20 minutes, until thickened.

 SIDEBAR   **THE WORCESTERSHIRE SAUCE STORY**

Worcestershire sauce was originally a recipe brought to Britain from India, by Lord Marcus Sandys, ex-Governor of Bengal. One day in 1835, he appeared at the door of a prosperous chemist's emporium, John Lea and William Perrins, in Worcester, and asked them to make up a batch of sauce from his recipe. When they did this the resulting fiery mixture was too much to handle for Lea and Perrins, and the barrel they made of it was consigned to the cellar. Much later, in the midst of a spring cleaning, they came across the barrel and decided to taste it again before throwing it out. Strangely, the mixture had mellowed into a unique, thick and rich sauce and Worcestershire was born!

GREEN TEA DIPPING SAUCE, TWO WAYS

Makes 1¼ Cups   GMENY

 HEALING PROPERTIES

Green Tea
- May help to guard against various types of cancer
- Aids in lowering cholesterol levels
- Fights inflammation and may help to prevent arthritic-type symptoms
- Protects liver cells by triggering the immune system and protects against toxins
- Promotes oral health

This is a great sauce for Asian-inspired dishes.

This is a unique Zen-like, light gingery sauce that uses green tea as its base.

1 C brewed green tea, cooled
3 T olive oil
1 T lemon juice
½ t lemon zest
½ t fresh ginger, minced
¼ to ½ t red chili flakes
1 T yellow miso

1. BLEND together very well.

Another version which is a bit more intense and concentrated, and slightly sweet. You can also marinade veggies for an added depth of flavor.

1 T green tea leaves and 3.5 oz. of hot water
1 t honey or agave syrup
2 long pieces of lemon peel, sliced thin
2 t rice wine vinegar
1 t salt
Freshly ground black pepper
2 t avocado oil

1. INFUSE the tea leaves in the hot water (see brewing recipe below), then strain.
2. ADD honey or agave and bring to a boil, then simmer until the liquid is reduced almost by half.
3. ADD lemon peel and leave to infuse until cold.
4. REMOVE lemon peel, add the oil, vinegar, salt and pepper to the liquid and whisk together briskly.

 BREWING GREEN TEA

To brew the tea correctly, cool down 1 C boiled water down to 158 to 176 degrees. Yes, use a thermometer. Add 2 t loose green tea or 1 green tea bags. Brew tea for 2 minutes. Discard leaves or tea bag immediately, or it will become bitter.

Sauces, Salads, Dressings, and Spices

DRESSING THE SALAD

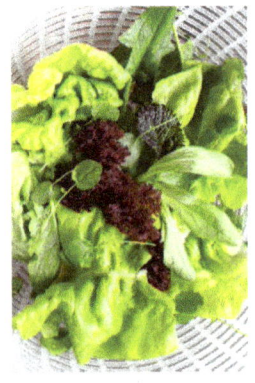

IS THERE ANYTHING MORE SIMPLE, ESSENTIAL, OR SATISFYING THEN A MIXED GREEN SALAD? Any greens can be used. Baby organic greens are wonderful. Add whatever other veggies you like to the greens and all you need is the dressing, as simple as a splash of lemon and dash of salt. I especially love to top a salad with toasted nuts. Pine nuts, sunflower seeds, or walnuts are great.

SALAD VARIETIES

GREEN SALAD
The "green salad" is most often composed of leafy vegetables such as lettuce varieties, spinach, or rocket (arugula) and is often a side dish.

BOUND SALAD
Bound salads can be composed (arranged) or tossed (put in a bowl and mixed with a thick dressing) like a potato salad. They are often assembled with a sauce, such as mayonnaise or vegenaise.

MAIN COURSE SALADS
Main course salads often include a protein like tofu, tempeh or beans. Popular main course salads include caesar, chef, and Cobb.

FRUIT SALADS
Fruit salads are made with any variety of fruit and can be topped with a yogurt or cream-style dressing.

DESSERT SALADS
Dessert salads can replace the usual sugary end of the meal. It can be a simple gelatin-type of molded salad topped with whipped or tofu cream or an ambrosia salad that uses a lot of tropical flavors.

DAD'S SALAD BAR

Serves 4 to 6

GMENSY

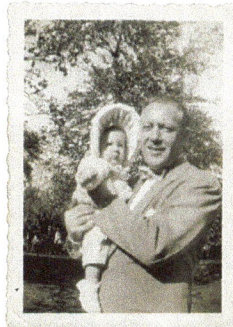

With my dad, I'm just a few years younger

When we lived in Sarasota, Florida, my parents were living on the east coast in Fort Lauderdale. They would often pop in for a weekend. Invariably my dad would ask me to make him this salad, which we called, "Dad's Salad Bar." He loved a salad where all the vegetables were cut small, while my mom preferred big cut vegetables. It was a big dilemma. Also, he didn't like scallions and radishes and she did, so they could never come to a consensus. So, I made a mini salad bar, beginning with a base of lettuce, and separate bowls of cut up vegetables, with various dressings and toppings to pick and choose from. It worked out great—a personalized salad for each of them!

Veggie Salad Bar Suggestions:
Artichoke hearts: the jarred ones with water work great
Avocado: sliced
Beets: roasted and chopped (you can use canned beets as well, drain)
Carrots: shredded or chopped
Broccoli: lightly steamed
Celery: cut small
Corn: fresh cobs roasted, and kernels cut from the cob
Cucumbers or pickles: chopped
Eggs: hard boiled, sliced
Fruit: grapes, blueberries, strawberries
Jicama: chopped into cubes
Mushrooms: chopped small
Olives: black or green, pits removed
Onions: chopped small
Radishes: diced
Red or yellow peppers: chopped small (roasted are good too)
Scallions: chopped with the green tops
String beans: cooked, chilled, and chopped
Tomatoes: de-seeded, cut small or cherry tomatoes cut in half

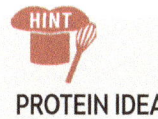

PROTEIN IDEAS FOR SALAD

- Stir-fry tofu or tempeh with soy sauce, paprika and ginger powder.
- Edamame, steamed & chilled
- Seeds and nuts.
- Cheese: feta, fresh mozzarella, cottage (or alternative cheeses)
- Seitan (wheat gluten): many varieties.

Topping Suggestions:
Croutons, any type of bread you have on hand, or crushed corn chips
Fresh herbs: cilantro, dill, basil or parsley
Parmesan cheese

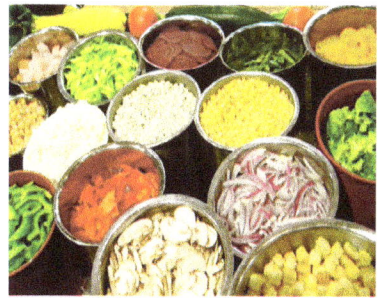

Sauces, Salads, Dressings, and Spices

ORIENTAL GINGER DRESSING

Makes 1 Cup

G M E N Y

HEALING PROPERTIES

Celery
- Contains an active compound called pthalides, which relax the muscles of the arteries that regulate blood pressure
- Works as a diuretic, regulating fluid balance, stimulating urine production, thus helping to rid the body of excess fluid

What makes this oriental dressing unique is the chopped celery, which gives this dressing a crunchy freshness, while the ginger and lemon gives it the zing.

2 T ginger, freshly grated
1 T celery, very finely chopped
3 T rice wine vinegar
2 T water or celery juice (use a lemon squeezer to extract)
2 T olive oil
2 t maple syrup
1 t lemon juice and ¼ t lemon zest
1 T yellow miso
1 t tamari
Freshly ground black pepper

1. BLEND in either a blender or mix by shaking in a jar until smooth.

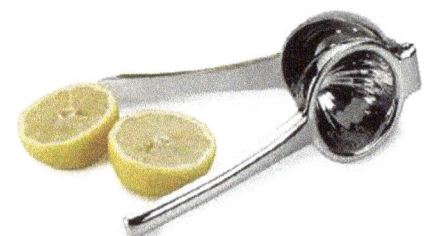

EVERYDAY HERB DRESSING

Makes 1 Cup

G M E N S Y

KITCHEN BOUQUET

Snip the ends of the herbs, store in a glass jar with enough water to touch the stems, but not the leaves. This works for parsley, thyme, rosemary, basil, and mint.

¾ C olive oil
4 T apple cider vinegar
1 t fresh parsley, dill, basil, or cilantro, chopped very small
1 garlic clove, minced
1 T lemon juice
½ t lemon zest
1 T prepared mustard
½ t kosher salt
½ t paprika
1 T maple syrup
Freshly ground pepper

1. PLACE in a glass jar with a secure lid.
2. SHAKE vigorously until well mixed.

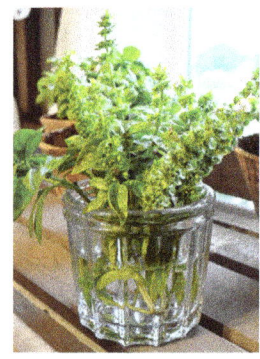

A Culinary Journey

MISO/CARROT DRESSING

Makes 1 Cup   GMENY

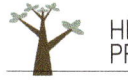 **HEALING PROPERTIES**

Vinegar
- Helps to break down calcium deposits in joints while re-mineralizing bones
- Helps prevent digestive and urinary tract infections
- Helps to replace potassium depletion
- Fights germs and infections

This low-fat, orange-hued dressing can be made a day ahead and actually tastes better when the flavors are allowed to marry.

2 carrots, small, very finely grated
1 garlic clove, minced (optional)
¾" piece of fresh ginger or ½ t dried ginger
¾ C fresh carrot juice
2 T white miso (mix in carrot juice until a smooth paste)
2 T rice wine vinegar
1 T olive oil
1 T honey
2 t basil, chopped very small
2 t cilantro, chopped very small

1. BLEND first eight ingredients until smooth.
2. ADD basil and cilantro.

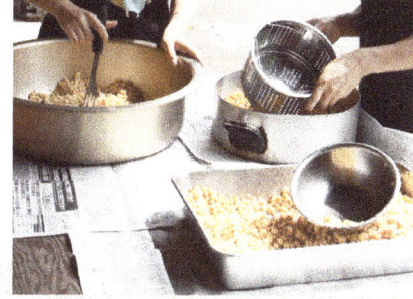
Making Miso

 SIDEBAR   MISO

Miso was introduced to Japan from China. Initially, fermented foods like miso were treated as a luxury by Buddhist monks and noblemen. It eventually became their daily staple during the Nara Period (710-784 A.D.). Later, in the Muromachi Period (1392-1573 A.D.), it became a common food. Miso was first made of soybeans, salt, and water, but over time grains such as rice and barley were included. Like fine wines, each type of miso has a distinct flavor, color, and aroma. It is also known as a non-allergenic food due to the extended maturation period in which enzymes break down the proteins in soybeans, which may otherwise cause allergies. Miso is reputed to have remarkable medicinal qualities. It contains dipicolonic acid, an alkaloid that chelates heavy metals, such as radioactive strontium, and discharges them from the body. The most remarkable evidence of the protective qualities of miso against exposure to radiation was published by Professor Akihiro Ito, at Hiroshima University's Atomic Radioactivity Medical Lab. Truckloads of miso were sent to Chernobyl, where it proved to help protect those exposed to radiation.

Sauces, Salads, Dressings, and Spices

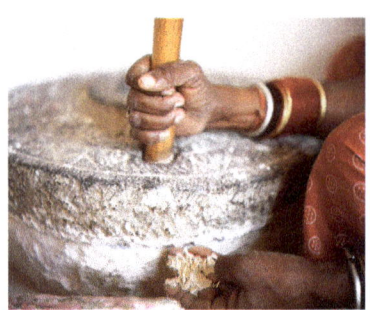

The sound of stone against stone rhythmically crushing the spices, along with their pungent smells, even now sends me into an Indian time. warp.

SPICE MIXTURES

Rules for Making Spice Mixes

1. Use only the freshest spices possible.
2. If you roast the spices, make sure that they cool down completely before grinding them into a powder and storing them.
3. Use an airtight jar and label each mixture; similar spices like cumin and coriander look alike.
4. Date the jar. Spice mixtures lose their punch after a while (make just enough for about four to six months).

SPICES FORM THE HEART OF THE KITCHEN, giving depth to the blank canvas that begins each new recipe. Spices also play an important role in maintaining health. Ginger and cumin aid digestion; turmeric acts as one of nature's most powerful cleansers. I have often made my own spices by simply dry-roasting cumin seeds and pounding them in my well-worn stone mortar-and-pestle, until it becomes fragrant smoky cumin powder.

Spices need to wake up and bloom, so in general you'll need to either dry roast or heat with a bit of oil before you add anything else.

In the Indian households I visited, I fondly remember watching *masala* (spice mixtures) being made in the early hours of the morning. The mixture of spices was an aromatic blend: fresh ginger, whole turmeric root, seeds of both cumin and coriander, freshly roasted, green chilis, and a bit of water—all deftly pounded into a potent paste.

A while back, I realized how making your own spice mixture can be very helpful. When some long-time acquaintances visited us from India, I made a unique dish that required a special spice mixture. Usually, I bought sambar powder at an Indian grocery store. However, our guests did not eat anything with chilis! So I had to make my own powder, using the same ratio of spices but without the chilis. This was my first time making this powder from scratch.

I often make my own garam masala because I prefer less cinnamon and black pepper, and more cardamom. Spice mixtures are simple to prepare and are like perfume to the senses.

HERB AND SPICE COMBINATIONS

Beans (dried): cumin, cayenne, chili, parsley, pepper, sage, savory, thyme

Breads: anise, basil, caraway, cardamom, cinnamon, coriander, cumin, dill, garlic, lemon peel, orange peel, oregano, poppy seeds, rosemary, saffron, sage, thyme

Cheese: basil, caraway, celery seed, chervil, chilis, chives, coriander, cumin, dill, garlic, horseradish, lemon peel, marjoram, mint, mustard, nutmeg, paprika, parsley, pepper, sage, tarragon, thyme

Corn: chilis, curry, dill, marjoram, parsley, savory, thyme

Eggs: basil, chervil, chilis, chives, curry, dill, fennel, ginger, lemon peel, marjoram, oregano, paprika, parsley, pepper, sage, tarragon, thyme

Fruits: allspice, anise, cardamom, cinnamon, cloves, coriander, ginger, mint

Potatoes: basil, caraway, celery seed, chervil, chives, coriander, dill, marjoram, oregano, paprika, parsley, poppy seed, rosemary, tarragon, thyme

Salad Dressings: basil, celery seed, chives, dill, fennel, garlic, horseradish, marjoram, mustard, oregano, paprika, parsley, pepper, rosemary, saffron, tarragon, thyme

Salads: basil, caraway, chives, dill, garlic, lemon peel, lovage, marjoram, mint, oregano, parsley, rosemary, tarragon, thyme

Soups: basil, bay, chervil, chilis, chives, cumin, dill, fennel, garlic, marjoram, parsley, pepper, rosemary, sage, savory, thyme

Tomatoes: basil, bay, celery seed, cinnamon, chilis, curry, dill, fennel, garlic, ginger, gumbo filé, lemongrass, marjoram, oregano, parsley, rosemary, savory, tarragon, thyme

Sweets: allspice, angelica, anise, cardamom, cinnamon, cloves, fennel, ginger, lemon peel, mace, nutmeg, mint, orange peel, rosemary

A really good organic Indian spice company is www.pureindianfoods.com

The company has been around since 1889 and has a great blog with recipes and Ayurvedic information.

COMPLEMENTARY HERBS AND SPICES

A simple way to figure out which herbs and spices complement each other is to work with herb families. Once you have established the blends you like, you can test them by mixing them with small amounts of a mild cheese, cream cheese, or a small piece of tofu. Allow the blend to marinate for at least an hour, then sample the blend, noting which combination of flavors you most enjoy. Then, make a larger portion of the herb or spice blend and store it in a tight-fitting jar. Be sure to label the blend with the ingredients so you'll know how to duplicate or modify them when you go to make a new batch.

BLEND IDEAS

Traditional Bouquet Garnish:
basil, bay, oregano, parsley

Basic Herbal:
basil, marjoram, rosemary, thyme

Spicy Blend:
chili peppers, cilantro, cumin, garlic

Pungent Blend:
celery seed, chili peppers, cumin, curry, ginger, black pepper

Spicy/Sweet Blend:
cinnamon, ginger, black pepper, star anise

Sweet Blend:
allspice, star anise, cinnamon, cloves, nutmeg

Mexican Blend:
chipotle chili powder, cumin, coriander, oregano, salt

Mediterranean Blend:
oregano, basil, thyme, paprika, cumin, sage, onion powder, black pepper, salt, brown sugar.

JOAN'S CURRY POWDER BLEND

Makes 1 Cup

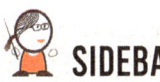 **SIDEBAR**

A CHILI HISTORY

Chili Peppers are native to Mexico and Central America. Traces of chilis have been found in bowls in Ecuador, dating back 6,100 years and wild chilis have been a part of the diet in the Americas since about 7,500 B.C.E. They were introduced to South Asia in the 1500s. Few could have imagined the impact of Columbus' discovery of a spice so pungent that it rivaled the better known black pepper native to South Asia.

The origin of the word curry is the stuff of legends, but most pundits believe it is derived from the Tamil word kari, *which means "spiced sauce." The word* kari *also refers to an aromatic herb called* karipalai, *which is used to flavor foods in the southern and western parts of India. Originally, the spice blend* kari podi, *or curry powder, contained only the curry leaf and a few spices, such as black pepper and ground gram beans known as urad dal. In time, the spice blend evolved to include various other spices and developed its deeply complex and rich character, interpreted differently throughout the many regions of the colorful Indian landscape. This is my version.*

3 T whole coriander seeds
2 T whole cumin seeds
1 T urad dhal
1 T fenugreek seeds
1 t white or black peppercorns
12 whole green cardamom pods, hull (make sure the seeds are very fresh. If they are not a robust black but a dry grey, discard them; hulled the measurement is about 1 T)
1 to 9 dried whole red chilis, broken into bits. The amount of chilis can be mild to atomic. (I generally use 3)
1 t fennel seeds
32 curry leaves, highly recommended, often only available in Indian spice stores, or if you live in a warm climate you can grow your own (optional)
2 T turmeric powder
2 T ground ginger powder
½ t paprika, for depth of color (optional)

1. COMBINE coriander, cumin, urad dhal, fenugreek, peppercorn, cardamom, chili, fennel seeds and curry leaves in a fry pan.
2. ROAST the spices over medium-high heat, stirring until they are lightly colored, about 5 minutes.
3. REMOVE and cool spice-mixture completely before grinding into a powder in a coffee grinder, or mortar and pestle.
4. ADD the rest of the ground spices.
5. TRANSFER the curry powder into a jar, cover tightly, and store in a cool dark place.

Sauces, Salads, Dressings, and Spices

GARAM MASALA

Makes 1 Cup | Preheat Oven to 200 Degrees | Bake: 30 Minutes   GMENSY

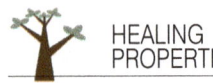 **HEALING PROPERTIES**

Cinnamon
- Contains cinnamaldehyde, which acts like as stimulant
- Good for fighting flu symptoms
- Improves the body's ability to utilize blood sugar
- Smelling cinnamon has been studied for possible positive effects on brain function

Potato/Cauliflower and Chickpea Curry are two of the many dishes that use this wonderful blend, it's also often used in North Indian cuisine. Garam Masala may be stored at room temperature in an airtight container and will retain its full flavor for up to 5 months.

5 cinnamon sticks in 3-inch pieces
1 C whole cardamom pods, preferably green
½ C whole cloves
½ C whole cumin seeds
¼ C whole coriander seeds
¼ C whole black peppercorns

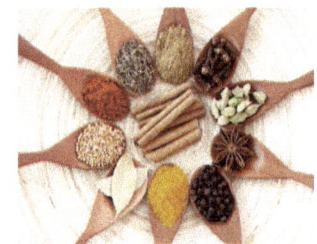

1. SPREAD the spices in one layer in a large shallow roasting pan.
2. ROAST for 20 to 30 minutes on the bottom shelf of the oven, on a low temperature. Stir 2 or 3 times with a large wooden spoon and turn the pan 2 to 3 times to ensure an even roast. Do not let the spices brown.
3. BREAK the cardamom pods by placing each one on a flat surface and pressing down on the pod with the ball of your thumb to snap open. Pull the pod away from the seeds inside and discard it. Set the seeds aside. Place the roasted cinnamon sticks in a plastic bag and pound them with a rolling pin or a kitchen mallet until they are finely crushed.
4. COMBINE the cardamom seeds, crushed cinnamon, cloves, cumin seeds, coriander seeds, and peppercorns in a small pan or bowl and stir them together until they are well-mixed. Grind the spices, a cup or so at a time, by pouring them into the jar of an electric blender or coffee grinder and blending at high speed for 2 or 3 minutes. Blend until they are completely pulverized and become a smooth powder. Transfer the powder to a jar or bottle with a tightly fitting lid.

 SIDEBAR   CINNAMON

Both cinnamon and cassia are the dried bark of Asian evergreens that belong to the laurel family. Sri Lanka is the major source of cinnamon and the Portuguese settled there just to exploit this abundant resource. The British followed in their quest for this important spice. Cinnamon bark is harvested twice a year during the rainy season. The inner bark is bruised, slit, and then carefully peeled off to dry; it then curls, forming cinnamon sticks.

HERBS DE PROVENCE

MANY YEARS AGO, OUR FRIEND ANNE FROM PARIS VISITED US and brought along several gifts, among them chocolates and a package of Herbs de Provence. What made this herbal combination special was that it was very finely ground. The aroma consisted of a delicate blend of extremely fresh dried herbs with a lovely touch of lavender. Our whole family had come down with a summer flu, so our friend (who arrived just in time) had to take care of us.

Because the visit was during the summer months, zucchini and eggplant were in abundance at our local farmer's market. So, Anne prepared plenty of traditional ratatouille, which topped steaming brown rice, graced slices of bread, or was slathered on crackers. What a delight! If you don't have a friend to bring you these herbs from France, you can buy them. Better yet why not try to grind them fresh yourself?

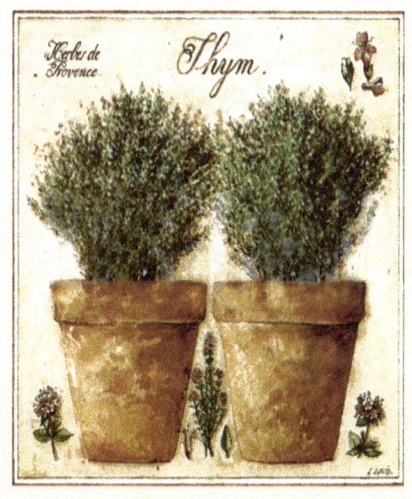

Herbs de Provence

3 T dried marjoram
3 T dried thyme
3 T dried savory
1 crushed bay leaf
1 t dried basil

1 t dried rosemary
¼ t dried lavender
½ t dried sage
½ t fennel seeds

1. COMBINE all ingredients and crush in a mortar and pestle.
2. SPOON into a small jar. Before using in a recipe, rub between your fingers to wake up the flavors. Jars of this lovely mixture makes great gifts. Makes ¾ C.

ANNE'S RATATOUILLE

Serves 4 to 6

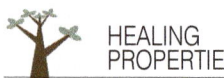

HEALING PROPERTIES

Olive Oil
- Associated with lower cholesterol levels
- Helps reduce the risk of heart attack or stroke
- May prevent brain cell damage caused by oxidative stress

3 T olive oil
2 onions (medium) or 1 large, chopped
1 red pepper, chopped
1 t fresh ginger, minced
2 to 3 garlic cloves, minced
3 zucchinis, chopped
1 eggplant, skin removed and chopped into chunks
1 T Herbs de Provence mixture (rub between your fingers)
½ t smoky paprika
½ t cayenne pepper
1 T salt
1 C tomatoes, de-seeded and chopped or ½ C tomato sauce

1. SAUTÉ onion, pepper, and ginger in olive oil for a few minutes; add garlic and fry another few minutes.
2. ADD vegetables, herbs, and salt; fry covered on medium heat until tender.
3. ADD tomatoes or sauce and cook uncovered until all the liquid has evaporated.
4. SERVE over fluffy brown rice, or with pita triangles.

HERBED BAKED PITA TRIANGLES

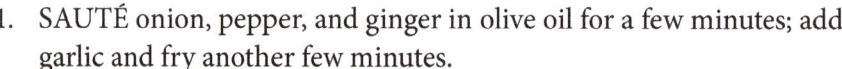

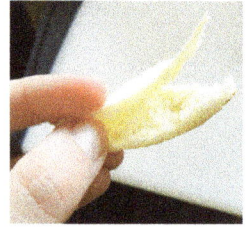

A fast and simple addition to a quick meal.

Pita bread (gluten free is available)
Olive oil spray
½ t onion powder and ½ t dried Herbs de Provence
Pinch of salt and paprika or smoked paprika

1. OPEN pita bread carefully with a sharp knife, slice into triangles, generously spray with olive oil.
2. SPRINKLE onion powder, herbs, salt and paprika over triangles. Bake in a 325-degree oven for 15 minutes, until slightly golden.

RAINY DAY HERBED SESAME-RYE CRACKERS

Makes 2 Dozen | Preheat Oven 350 Degrees | Bake: 7 to 10 Minutes   GMENSY

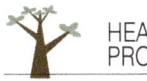 **HEALING PROPERTIES**

Rye
- Good source of fiber, high water-binding capacity, creating feeling of fullness and satiety
- Good alternative grain for diabetes, as wheat triggers a greater insulin response than rye
- Contains lignan, a phytoestrongenic ingredient that acts like a natural estrogen and helps to neutralize menopausal symptoms

Whoever thinks of making crackers? Yet they are not difficult to make (helpful for people with gluten sensitivities) and the taste is unbelievably fresh. Often crackers sit on the shelf in boxes for an inordinate amount of time, so taking the time to bake your own crackers is worth it. A rainy day is the perfect time to make them; they last quite a while in airtight containers.

Dry Ingredients
½ C whole wheat pastry flour and ½ C rye flour or 1 C gluten-free mixture
½ t baking powder
¼ C sesame seeds (substitute poppy seeds if you are allergic to sesame seeds)
1 T Herbs de Provence mixture
½ t salt

Wet Ingredients
¼ C avocado oil
1 T agave syrup or honey
¼ C fat-free or low-fat milk, soy, rice, or almond milk

1. COMBINE flour, salt, baking powder, sesame seeds and herbs.
2. ADD wet ingredients to dry ingredients, form into a smooth and pliable dough. Add a small amount of flour if dough is too sticky.
3. DIVIDE the dough into two pieces. Roll out, between wax paper, about ⅛" thick on a floured board or smooth surface.
4. TRIM the edges to make a perfect rectangle or square.
5. LOOSEN the dough on the board by slipping a long knife between the rolled dough and the board.
6. SLICE with a sharp knife, cut into cracker-size pieces, any size.
7. PLACE the crackers on an ungreased baking sheet.
8. SCORE the top with a knife or fork tine. This helps to keep them flat.
9. BAKE until golden. Don't overbake, they can burn easily.

 HINT — MAKING ALMOND MILK

To make your own almond milk, blanch or sprout 1 C almonds and remove skins. Place in a glass jar and cover with 4 cups water and close securely. Refrigerate for 1 day, no more than 2. Then pour into blender and blend until smooth. Strain the liquid from the pulp through a cheesecloth, applying pressure to squeeze out all the liquid. You can retain the almond paste pulp for other uses.

ROASTED HERBED SWEET POTATOES

Serves 4 to 6 | Preheat Oven to 450 Degrees | Bake: 25 Minutes   GMENSY

This is a great snack, made all the better with Herbs de Provence.

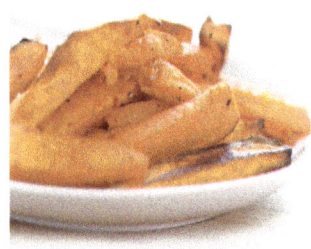

2 to 2½ pounds sweet potatoes
2 T extra-virgin olive oil, enough to coat potatoes
2 T Herbs de Provence
1 t kosher salt
Fresh pepper, to taste
½ t paprika
2 T fresh parsley, chopped
½ t rice flour (this helps crisp them)

1. LINE a cookie sheet with foil.
2. CUT sweet potatoes into wedges.
3. PLACE in a plastic bag with oil, spices, salt, pepper, paprika, parsley and rice flour, shake until fully covered over potatoes.
4. TURN out onto cookie sheet, in a single layer, turn over at least one time.
5. ROAST in a preheated oven, at least 25 minutes, until crispy.

SAVORY HERB-INFUSED RICE

GMENSY

Serves 3 to 4

This simple but very flavorful rice can be served as a side dish; it goes great with any vegetable dish.

1 C organic basmati rice
2 C vegetable stock (low sodium)
1½ t Herbs de Provence
2 T fresh cilantro, chopped
¼ t turmeric powder
¾ to 1 t sea salt or Himalayan (pink) salt and freshly ground pepper

1. COMBINE rice, stock, Herbs de Provence, cilantro, turmeric, salt and pepper, stir well.
2. SET over high heat, bring to a boil, then simmer. Stir once and then cover, cooking until all liquid is absorbed, about 20 to 25 minutes. When done, don't stir, but uncover to let the steam out, so it doesn't get mushy.

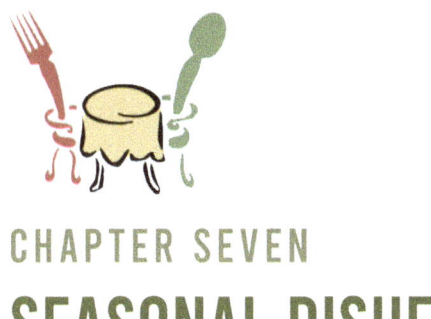

CHAPTER SEVEN
SEASONAL DISHES

SPRING LIGHTNESS
SPRING FARE
SPRING CLEANSING
NEW YEAR'S FEAST 2001
COMING TOGETHER 2003

SPRING LIGHTNESS

ONE WINTER I HAD AN INTERESTING EXPERIENCE. I fractured my ankle and spent two months healing. Each afternoon I needed to rest my ankle by elevating it and I would lie on the couch, looking out into the back garden as light streamed in through the windows.

A small blackbird with a long, tapered tail came by to visit—he came the same time every day and sat on a post. Once in a while his mate sat nearby, but mostly it was me and the blackbird, sitting and watching the fading afternoon light. Those silent, slow afternoons were when I felt the real healing taking place. Though it wasn't the dead of night, the lyrics to the Lennon/McCartney song *Blackbird* rang in my head:

"Blackbird singing in the dead of night
Take these broken wings and learn to fly
All your life
You were only waiting for this moment to arise. . ."

When spring arrived, the blackbird did not return, and there was no time or need for me to sit and watch the afternoon sun. I imagined the bird filling its nest with straw to ready itself for whatever the spring would bring. Lightness that comes from savoring each moment as it unfolds, accepting what life brings as contentedly as a little blackbird sitting on a post, without any expectation, is what that little bird continues to teach me—even in his absence.

To celebrate spring, I created a few simple and wonderfully light meals that take only moments to prepare.

TOFU NON-EGG SALAD WRAP

Serves 4 to 6

GMENY

Mustard has an excellent emulsifying ability. It can help bind a sauce wonderfully.

To maintain maximum flavor, mustard should be added late in the cooking process because heat destroys much of mustard's distinctive flavor.

This is a very quick and simple dish to prepare.

2 C firm tofu, mashed
2 T light mayonnaise or vegenaise
1 t mustard, prepared, whole-seed
1 T tamari or soy sauce
½ t turmeric powder
Dash of cayenne pepper
2 T fresh dill, chopped fine
½ C celery, chopped very small
2 tomatoes, de-seeded and cut into small chunks
4 whole wheat or corn crispy tacos or soft corn tortillas
OPTIONAL: ½ C cilantro, chopped very fine

1. MASH first seven ingredients together with a fork or in a food processor; don't overmix. Mix in celery.
2. FILL either warm tortilla or lettuce leaves with ½ C of filling; add 2 T tomatoes.
3. TOP with chopped cilantro
4. FOLD bottom up and then flap each side over each other.

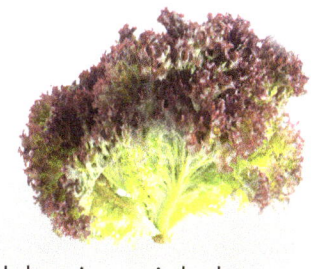

  HOW TO STORE WASHED LETTUCE LEAVES

- Remove lettuce leaves from head carefully, wash and then dry completely by using a spin basket or placing them between two paper towels.

- Unroll four paper towels, keep them all connected. Fold in half at the middle perforation, then fold each half down again on its perforation. Moisten slightly and place the paper towels into the large zipper top plastic bag. Place the lettuce in the bag, between the double-thickness layers of the paper towels. Gentle handling keeps the leaves from bruising.

- Close the zipper top, leaving about two inches open, and carefully squeeze as much air out of the bag as you can, then finish closing up the zipper top to seal it.

Seasonal Dishes

MATTHEW'S FAMOUS GUACAMOLE

Makes 1 Cup   GMENSY

Matthew is an avid avocado fan and guacamole Zen master. The eastern hills of San Diego are filled with avocado orchards due to the perfect terrain and ideal climate for growing them. This simple recipe is one that Matthew has worked on and perfected over the years.

> Ripening avocados can be quickened by placing the fruit in a brown paper bag with an apple and stored at room temperature.

1 ripe avocado
2 T lemon juice and 1 t lemon zest
½ t onion powder
½ t cumin powder
½ t salt
1 to 2 dried chilis, whole dried or 1 jalapeño (de-vein and de-seed)
1 T avocado oil
1 tomato, de-seeded and cut into very small pieces.
4 soft corn tortillas
Salsa
Shredded lettuce

1. MASH first four ingredients together with a fork or in a food processor.
2. HEAT oil and add chilis; fry until brown and add to guacamole.
3. ADD cut tomatoes.
4. SPREAD guacamole mix on tostada or warm corn tortilla.
5. TOP with salsa and lettuce.

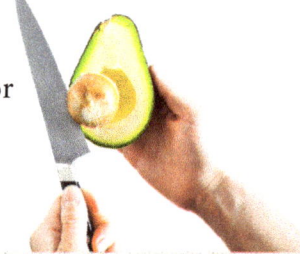

 **SIDEBAR**   **HISTORY OF THE AVOCADO**

In the 1700s English seamen discovered that the avocado could be used as a spread to soften the hardtack (hard bread) they had for meals. The avocado's reputation soon spread, and it became known as "midshipman's butter." Avocado did not achieve popularity in the United States until the early 1900s where it was first grown in Florida. Then some trees were planted in Santa Barbara, California. A California postman Rudolf Hass discovered the avocado that bears his name in 1926. His original tree is still growing in La Habra Heights, California. Little did he know that his name would be used for the most popular avocado in the world today. While other fruits gain sugar as they ripen, the avocado's sugar content decreases as it matures. Although the avocado matures on the tree, it does not begin to ripen until it is picked. The leaves of the tree supply a hormone to the fruit that inhibits the production of ethylene, the chemical responsible for ripening fruit. They often require a few days at room temperature to ripen.

ROASTED RED PEPPER, MUSHROOM, ASPARAGUS SANDWICH

Serves 4   GMENSY

STORING FETA CHEESE

Keep feta cheese in the salt brine it comes with, this way it can be stored for a long time. To decrease its saltiness, before serving soak the cheese in water or milk for a few minutes, drain.

We were very busy one day and had to put something together in moments. Some steamed asparagus spears were waiting in the refrigerator; with a few additions this sandwich revealed itself.

3 T olive oil
2 large red peppers, jarred, sliced thin
20 mushrooms, chopped
16 thin asparagus spears
1 cucumber, peeled and sliced very thin
1 C feta cheese (vegan alternative, see page 73)
½ C cilantro, chopped very small
4 whole wheat baguettes (or gluten-free option)
4 T spicy mayo, low-fat or vegan alternative

Spicy Mayo

1 C mayonnaise
1 T Sriracha chili sauce
1 t lime or lemon juice

BLEND together and store in a container in the refrigerator.

1. SAUTÉ red peppers and mushrooms in 1 T olive oil until tender.
2. STEAM asparagus until tender, 5 minutes.
3. HEAT each slice of bread by brushing it with ½ t olive oil and toasting it in the fry pan you sautéed the pepper and mushrooms in.
4. LAYER one half of the baguette with the pepper and mushroom mixture, 4 asparagus, ¼ C feta cheese, cilantro, and cucumber slices.
5. SPREAD 1 T Spicy Mayo on bottom of baguette. You can also top it with 1 T salsa fresca (recipe below.)

SALSA FRESCA

Makes 1 Cup   GMENSY

The trick to really good salsa is using very firm tomatoes. Cut the tomatoes in half and de-seed. Cooking the onions makes this salsa easier to digest.

Pulse Together (leave a little chunky)
4 tomatoes (plum are best), de-seeded and chopped
1 small onion, chopped. Option: lightly sauté in 1 T olive oil
½ jalapeño (de-seed, chop very fine)
¼ C cilantro, leaves removed from stalk
1 t lime juice and ½ t lime zest
½ t salt

SPRING FARE

SPRING IS THE TIME OF RENEWAL, a time of awakening to the rebirth of nature. The sun, which appeared hidden under winter clouds, now shines clear and bright. The seeds of nature's bounty lie dormant in the soil and wait for the warmth of the sun to release them from the earth. Both asparagus and rhubarb live through the cycle of the seasons. As perennials they hold within them the circle of life itself. They are both very selfless, too; the more you take from them, the more they give.

Eating foods according to the rhythm of nature seems quite natural. We've become used to eating any type of food, any time of the year, forgetting that nature provides us with what we need, when we need it.

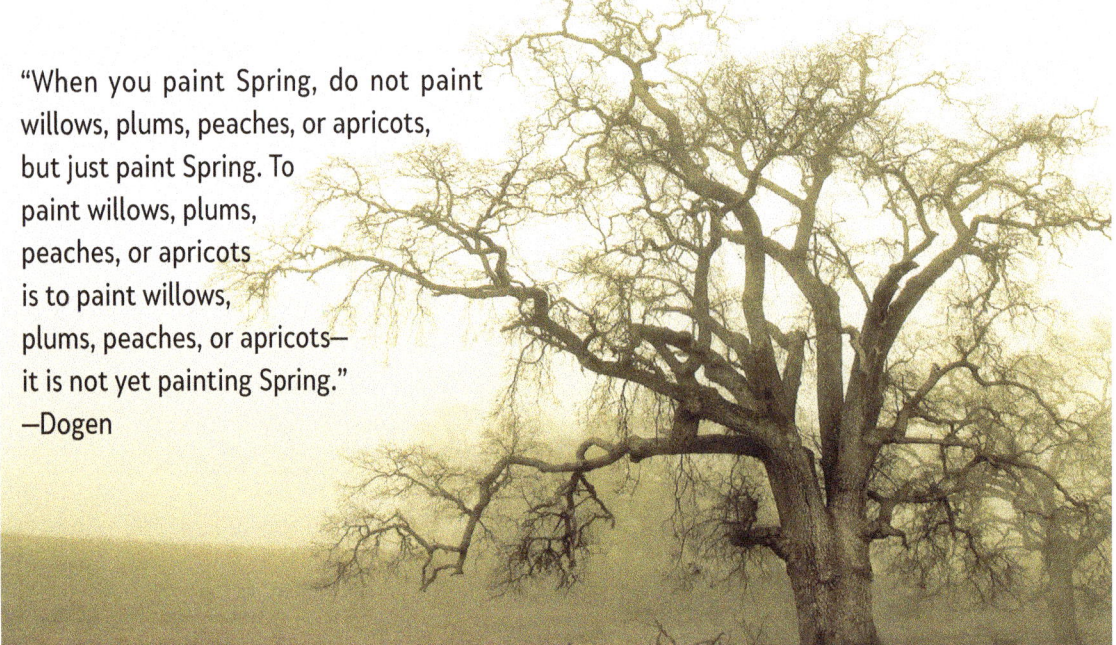

"When you paint Spring, do not paint willows, plums, peaches, or apricots, but just paint Spring. To paint willows, plums, peaches, or apricots is to paint willows, plums, peaches, or apricots— it is not yet painting Spring."
—Dogen

COUNTRY KASHA VARNISKAS: BUCKWHEAT & NOODLES

Serves 6 to 8   GMENSY

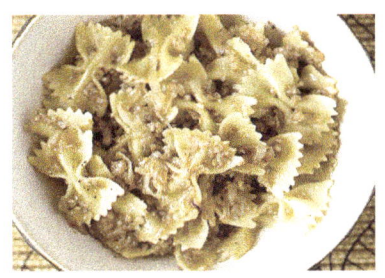

This is a special recipe for me. My mother knew that when she visited, the first thing I'd request when she entered my kitchen on one of her cooking missions was this yummy dish. Buckwheat is an ancient, non-glutinous grain—one of the healthiest known to mankind. It may take a little getting used to but trying this very basic and simple recipe is perhaps the best introduction you can get. Expect to use every burner on your stove at the same time! I often serve this dish with lightly steamed asparagus, for an earthy, spring meal. You can make extra because it freezes really well.

HEALING PROPERTIES

Buckwheat
- Contains almost 86 grams of magnesium in one cup, relaxing blood vessels, improving blood flow
- Aids in diabetes
- Is high in fiber
- Helps prevent gallstones

2 C buckwheat groats, medium grain
4 C water with 1 t salt added
2 eggs or 4 egg whites or 2 T of oil
⅛ C avocado oil and 2 T butter or margarine
2 onions, chopped very small
1½ C fresh button mushrooms, cut small
1 C bow tie noodles, cooked in ½ t salted water (Any whole grain or gluten-free noodle can be used, but bow ties are the traditional choice.)
Plenty of freshly ground black pepper

1. FRY the buckwheat groats on a low heat with beaten eggs (or substitute) until roasted, about 5 to 7 minutes. You will begin to smell a deep and husky flavor.
2. BOIL salted water while the buckwheat is roasting.
3. ADD the egg-roasted buckwheat slowly to the boiling water; stir well, then turn the heat down very low and cover the pot securely. Cook on low heat for about 15 minutes. It's finished when all of the water has evaporated. Don't stir the pot or lift the lid while it's cooking or it will get mushy; it should stay fluffy.
4. SAUTÉ the onions and mushrooms in oil/butter mixture until golden brown, while the buckwheat is cooking.
5. COOK the noodles according to directions for the particular variety you are using. These noodles are not cooked al denté but soft. When they are done cooking, drain well.
6. MIX cooled buckwheat, sautéed veggies, and cooked noodles together in a large bowl.
7. ADD plenty of black or white pepper to taste, adjust salt and mix well.

JUST-PICKED STEAMED ASPARAGUS WITH DILLY WHITE SAUCE

Serves 4 to 6

G M E N Y

STEAMED ASPARAGUS

ADD a minimal amount of water to a steam basket or a large pot.

STEAM about five minutes or until almost tender.

TOP steamed asparagus with dilly white sauce made from tofu or milk.

SCALLION PRESENTATION

Tie food together with scallions; they work well with asparagus or string beans, making a wonderful presentation.

If you have a garden and have planted the perennial asparagus, the first mark of spring is when it pops out of the ground. Most of us simply wait for it to become available in the local market. It is always best to purchase the most tender ones with tops tightly closed, firm, and deep green in color. Cut the bottom stalks off; you can save them for soup stock.

WHITE HERB SAUCE WITH TOFU

½ lb. firm tofu (about 1 C)
1 t tamari (soy sauce)
2 T oil
⅛ C fresh lemon juice
¼ to ½ C water
1 t fresh dill or ½ t dried dill or tarragon
Pinch cayenne pepper

1 T dried Herbs de Provence
1 t salt
½ t paprika
¼ t cayenne pepper

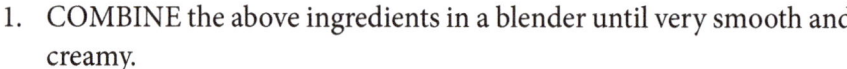

1. COMBINE the above ingredients in a blender until very smooth and creamy.
2. SERVE warm by heating sauce on a low heat; do not bring to a boil.

WHITE HERB SAUCE WITH MILK

G E N S Y

2 C low or non-fat milk
½ t salt
Dash of freshly ground pepper
3 T Cream of Rice cereal
2 T fresh dill, chopped or 1 T dried dill or tarragon

1. COMBINE milk with salt and pepper. Heat on medium heat.
2. SPRINKLE in the Cream of Rice and dill; and mix well. At the point when the milk has almost come to a full boil, lower heat.
3. COOK on medium heat for one minute.
4. REMOVE from the heat and let it stand in the pot with the lid on for 3 to 4 minutes.
5. BEAT well or mix until smooth and thickened.

A Culinary Journey

RHUBARB AND STRAWBERRY CRISP

Serves 6 to 8 | Preheat Oven to 350 Degrees | Bake: 30 to 40 Minutes   GMENSY

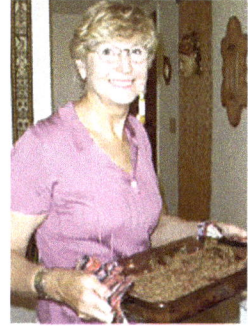

While visiting friends on a Wisconsin farm, one Spring morning we picked rhubarb in the morning dew and spent the afternoon making pies and sauce. The rare combination of sweet tartness filled every space of the house as the rhubarb bubbled from within the oven and on top of the stove. Since strawberries arrive at the same time in the year I paired them together in this very simple recipe. Here's a picture of my friend Beverly testing this recipe.

Filling
2 C red rhubarb stalks, diced
2 C strawberries, sliced, (1 pint)
2 T whole wheat flour or light gluten-free mixture
¾ to 1 C turbinado (unrefined) sugar or maple sugar, depending on how tart or sweet you like rhubarb.
½ whole vanilla bean, cut in half the long way and with a sharp knife. Scrape out the tiny seeds and pulp or use 1 t vanilla extract.
MIX together and spread in a 9" x 9" pan.

Topping
1 C whole wheat flour or gluten-free flour blend
½ C brown or maple sugar
½ C butter or margarine, cold
½ t salt

1. MIX the ingredients together into a crumbly mixture and spread on top of the filling.
2. BAKE until the top is golden brown.

WARNING

Rhubarb has laxative properties so don't overdo it. Those who tend to develop kidney stones with oxalate content should also avoid rhubarb.

 SIDEBAR   RHUBARB

While rhubarb leaves are poisonous due to their high concentration of oxalic acid the rhubarb root started out as a medicinal aid. Originally it came from northern China and was discovered by wandering Romans who named the plant after "Rha," the river along which it grew, and "barbarum," or foreign, because the territory beyond that river (today the Volga in western Russia) didn't belong to the Romans. Rhubarb is technically a vegetable, although the United States Customs Court in New York ruled it a fruit in 1947. People didn't start eating the plant's stalks until the early 1800s, probably because those who first tried the leaves became sick and died.

SPRING CLEANSING

I come into the peace of wild things who do not tax their lives with forethought or grief.

I come into the presence of still water.
And I feel above me the day-blind stars waiting with their light.

For a time I rest in the
grace of the world, and am free.
—Wendell Berry

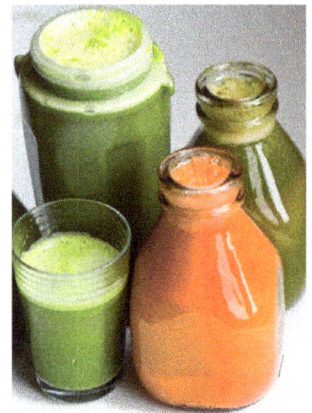

SOME OF US THINK ABOUT "FENG SHU-ING" OUR HOMES by removing the clutter and obstruction that helps release the natural flow of energy—in this way we make a fresh start. Empty space is balanced with the "things" we have accumulated. Bringing balance to our homes, we can often bring an outer and inner harmony into true focus—a harmony that is our essence, though not always apparent—like clouds covering the ever-present sun.

From time to time, this is also useful for our bodies. When cleansing one's body, anytime is a good time. But the Spring, the awakening of nature, the renewal of sunshine and warm, is as good a time as any. Throughout the year I often take a break and simply drink fresh juice all day. This invigorating juice fast is a superb cleanse.

I once spent a Spring week at a fasting center in Lemon Grove, California. I felt a sense of bodily freedom the entire week—a refreshing emptiness filled with light. Some people go to meditation retreats to bask in the silence and recharge themselves, so it is good to do the same for our bodies. Healing foods for the body—like Feng Shui for our outer life—help to greatly facilitate the natural flow of internal energy.

An invigorating juice fast is an excellent cleanse. Additionally, many wonderful cleansing foods can be added to our diet to create a healing environment that will prevent problems before they arise.

HEALING JUICE FAST

Makes 2 Cups

GMENSY

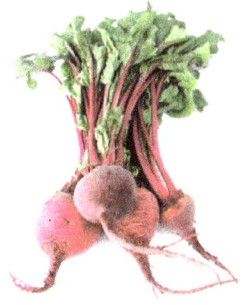

This recipe makes two large glasses of juice. Always use organic produce. When you are having a juice day, drink at least two full glasses of fresh juice and as much water as possible. If you simply can't get through the day without eating something, you can munch on carrots or celery. If you need a little sugar, eat an apple or half a banana. One or two juice days can really be a helpful break to your digestive system, which often works overtime. The second day is actually easier; I find the juice so filling and satisfying that I am usually not very hungry. It's a good idea to break the fast the following day with a simple soup recipe like the one below.

9 carrots
4 stalks of celery
1 beet, peeled
1 apple
¼" ginger, peeled

Investing in a juicer that removes the pulp from the juice may provide a lifelong boost to your overall health.

SIMPLE HEALING SOUP

Serves 4 to 6

GMENY

This is a very simple low-calorie soup, using several healing vegetables. The ginger is helpful in making the cabbage easier to digest. Make an extra pot and freeze single portions for a quick snack.

1 T olive oil
1 onion, sliced
2 garlic cloves, minced
½" ginger, minced
½ t turmeric powder

½ t oregano
½ head of cabbage, sliced thin
2 carrots, chopped small
3 celery stalks, chopped fine
2 T yellow miso

1. HEAT olive oil in a heavy-duty Dutch oven. Stir fry onions.
2. ADD garlic and ginger and fry a few moments.
3. ADD all the rest of the ingredients, with enough water to reach the top of the veggies.
4. BRING to a boil, then lower the heat to a simmer.
5. ADD miso by removing ½ C of hot broth and blending it into a smooth paste, then adding it at the end when the vegetables are tender.

Seasonal Dishes

EDAMAME SALAD WITH GOMASIO

Serves 4 to 6

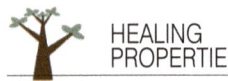

HEALING PROPERTIES

Edamame
- ½ C edamame contains 35 mg. of isoflavones, plant-based estrogen
- Contains all the essential amino acids
- Good source of fiber and essential fatty acids

Gomasio
- STIR 7 t sesame seeds and ½ t kosher or Himalayan salt in a skillet over medium heat until they are toasted and fragrant (about four minutes). Set aside to cool.
- PROCESS by pulsing in a food processor until coarsely ground; do not grind too fine. Add 2 t of dried dulse.

Soy products are a protein powerhouse. This salad blends the wonderful flavor and texture of edamame, the digestive help of ginger with the delightful sesame seed condiment and gomasio.

4 C edamame bean, fresh or frozen, shelled, and cooked
2 carrots, diced very small on an angle
¼ C tamari or soy sauce
¼ C lemon juice
1 T lemon zest
1 to 2 T ginger, minced
1 T avocado oil
4 C mixed organic greens

Edamame

1. COOK edamame until crisp-tender, shell.
2. STEAM carrots until just tender.
3. TRANSFER both edamame and carrots to a baking sheet and cool in the refrigerator.
4. WHISK tamari, lemon juice and zest, ginger, and oil in a large bowl.
5. ADD the cooled edamame/carrot mixture and toss to well coat.
6. PLACE 1 C of greens on a plate and top with edamame mixture.
7. TOP with gomasio (optional).

COOKING EDAMAME

Stove Top
1. RINSE edamame pods and into put briskly boiling water.
2. COOK 3 to 5 minutes or until tender. At this stage, you would normally notice some pods opening. Do not overcook.
3. DRAIN water, let cool; sprinkle with kosher salt and serve.

Steamer
1. RINSE fresh edamame pods and place in steamer basket.
2. PLACE basket in saucepan with water below basket.
3. COVER and bring to a full boil and steam about 5 minutes.
4. SPRINKLE on some kosher salt and serve.

CURRY TEMPEH STIR FRY

Serves 4 to 6

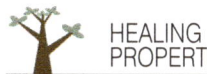

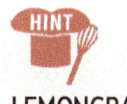

Lemongrass
- Helps lower body temperature, for flu-like symptoms
- Antibacterial and antifungal
- Anti-spasmodic properties, tonic
- Helps to combat depression

LEMONGRASS

To prepare lemongrass, peel the tough outer leaves and trim the ends. Use the bottom 4 to 6 inches where the leaves branch out. Smash before you chop or slice, to get the oil flowing. Discard the stalk, much like a bay leaf after cooking. The center portion can be eaten only if it is finely chopped.

The Indian spices—cumin, coriander and especially turmeric—all have amazing healing properties. Because tempeh is fermented, it is sometimes easier to digest than tofu and the flavor is dense, nutty, and deep. Lemongrass is a healing ingredient. You might have to make an effort to locate it in a health food store or Asian market.

1 t whole cumin seeds
1 t whole coriander seeds
¾ t turmeric
2 T avocado oil
1 (8 oz.) package tempeh
1 onion, chopped
2 garlic cloves, minced
1 jalapeño chili, seeded and chopped
1 carrot, sliced thin
1 green bell pepper, diced

2 C cauliflower florets
1 red potato, diced
4 plum tomatoes, peeled and diced
1 t fresh ginger, grated
1 T fresh lemongrass
1 t kosher salt
1 C vegetable stock
1 T fresh lime juice
½ t lime zest
4 T fresh cilantro, chopped fine

1. HEAT a dry skillet, add cumin and coriander seeds, toast until golden brown. Cool and grind in a spice mill and add turmeric.
2. BROWN tempeh on both sides in 1 T of oil, then cut into thin strips and dice into cubes.
3. ADD another 1 T oil to skillet; cook onion until tender.
4. ADD garlic and chili, and when fragrant, add the carrot, green pepper, cauliflower, and potato.
5. SPRINKLE ground spices over the vegetables and stir to coat evenly.
6. ADD tomatoes, ginger, lemongrass, stir-fried tempeh, and salt.
7. STIR FRY mixture for 3 to 4 minutes.
8. ADD stock, and when mixture starts to simmer, cover the pan, reduce the heat to low, and cook for 10 to 12 minutes or until the vegetables are tender.
9. STIR in lime juice and zest, cook until all liquid has evaporated. Sprinkle cilantro over the top before serving.

GRAPE AND DRIED FIG COBBLER

Serves 6 | Preheat Oven to 350 Degrees | Bake: 20 to 25 Minutes

GMENSY

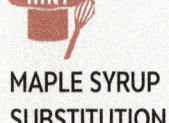

MAPLE SYRUP SUBSTITUTION

When substituting cane sugar with maple syrup, decrease baking temperature to 325 degrees.

Measuring
Syrup can hug the sides of measuring cups, be sure to scrape it all out!

Maple Syrup Grades
Use Grade A, Dark Amber, or Grade B. Late season, darker syrup, has a denser, stronger flavor for baking and cooking.

Maple Sugar
Substitute 1 Cup granulated maple sugar for ¾ Cup granulated sugar.

This is a low-sugar dessert which uses a combination of healthy fruits and nuts.

½ t fresh sage, finely minced
3 C seedless grapes—both red and green
½ C dried figs, chopped (you can use oiled kitchen shears to chop them up)
3 T maple or turbinado brown sugar
1 t lemon zest, grated
1 t lemon juice
½ C grape juice
1 t tapioca, quick cooking

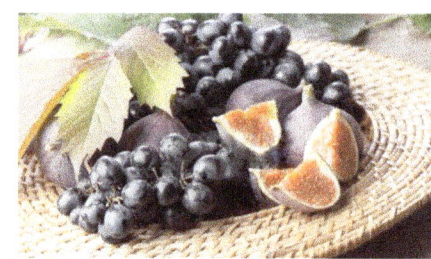

Cobbler Topping
½ t fresh sage, minced
4 T margarine, butter, or coconut oil
1¼ C whole wheat pastry flour, or gluten-free light flour
¼ C cornmeal
1½ t baking powder
½ t salt
½ C low-fat milk, almond, rice, or soy milk
¼ C maple syrup
12 macadamia nuts, toast, and crush

1. FRY sage lightly in 1 T margarine, butter or oil until fragrant.
2. COMBINE fruit, sugar, lemon juice and zest, and grape juice in an oven-safe 10" sauté or fry pan. Bring to a boil, reduce heat, and simmer 5 minutes.
3. COMBINE flour, cornmeal, baking powder, salt, and sage/butter in a processor. Add 3 T softened margarine, butter, or oil and pulse until well distributed; add milk, syrup, and pulse until just combined. Do not overmix.
4. DROP dough in large spoon-size mounds onto the fruit, allowing a little space between mounds.
5. BAKE 10 to 15 minutes, top with aluminum foil. Then uncover and bake another 10 minutes.
6. SPRINKLE with the nuts and bake for a final 5 minutes. Serve warm.

NEW YEAR'S FEAST
2001: YEAR OF THE SNAKE

> "Walk as if you are kissing the Earth with your feet."
> —THICH NHAT HANH

NEW YEAR'S EVE IS TRADITIONALLY THE TIME FOR NEW BEGINNINGS. Ideally, we should begin every moment of our life anew, experiencing each moment as a fresh start.

While moving from 2000 (The Year of the Dragon) to 2001 (The Year of the Snake), we spent the day preparing a traditional Japanese New Year's feast. Three very special Japanese friends, Sachiko, Tomiko, and June, came together to cook the dishes that their mothers and grandmothers had prepared throughout their childhood. I, along with a few close friends gathered to experience a Japanese New Year tradition.

It began the previous day with a visit to the local Japanese market. Here, we purchased several important traditional items such as burdock and lotus root, special sushi rice, *mirin*, *dashi*, seaweed, and sake. The cooking began at 10:00 a.m. and finished at 5:00 p.m. on the evening of the 31st. The first assignment given the helpers was to cut the vegetables in meticulously small pieces. The most challenging one by far was the symbolic lotus root. This hard, brown root, located in the muddy bottom of a pond, grows from one of the most beautiful flowers on earth. Gaining strength to rise above its murky surroundings, the lotus flower demonstrates that beauty can be found everywhere. The root, with its symmetrical holes running up and down its length, was to be thinly sliced. Later, Tomiko used these slices to make a delicate lotus-root salad. At the same time Sachiko was busy crafting a chestnut mountain. It began with cutting a cross-shaped slit on the top of the chestnuts then boiling them. When the chestnut meats were extracted and prepared to resemble an almost acorn squash-like preparation, Sachiko christened the mound of dessert, "Mount Fuji."

The meal ended with traditional miso soup and *mochi*. June left early to specially prepare the *mochi* in a modern, electric *mochi*-maker. *Mochi* is a sweet rice dumpling that is commonly eaten during Japanese festivals. According to June, the chewy *mochi* welcomes the New Year with happiness and blessings. Interestingly, during the day every time I would ask the meaning of any of the dishes, the three girls would say in unison: "it brings happiness and blessings."

On New Year's Day, Sachiko returned to lead a traditional Japanese Tea Ceremony. With grace and meditative movements, we all experienced a bite from a sweet teacake and then a sip of whipped green tea from a ceremonial teacup—a reminder that the art of mindful movement should be applied to all things, sweet and bitter. The combination of these simple, earthy flavors danced on our tongues—it was an ideal way to spend the first day of 2001. It was especially poignant since 2001 was to be a significant year for the world.

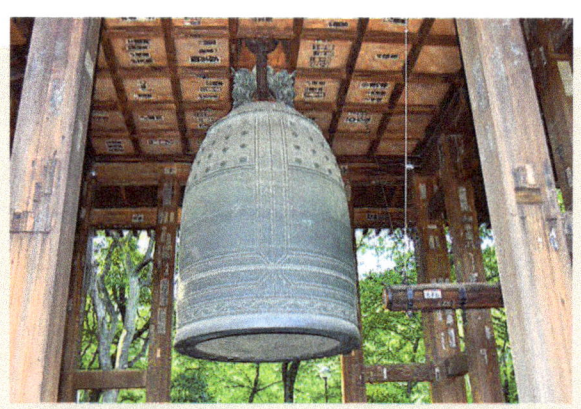

Ringing of the Bells
By Tomiko Yabumoto

In my first New Year's Eve in Japan, I went to Kyoto for the ringing of the bells (joya no kane). As I walked along the path to the temple on this cold, starry night, I thought to myself, "Now I understand why people stay in a warm home, eating noodles and watching TV." I was soon joined by others, and the stream of people swelled to a river. I forgot about the cold as we moved along like one body, travelling in the same direction, all with a common intention. There was nothing to do and nowhere to go, except to be present as "the river" carried us along. We flowed at various speeds so that on occasion my feet barely touched the ground. Our movements synchronized with the sound of the ringing bell—once, twice, and on to one hundred and eight times—an ideal way to start the New Year.

When we finally reached the temple, I was amazed by the immensity of the bell and its deep, powerful sound, which was created when one of the monks, holding a large timber, took a flying leap (of faith) and struck the bell. The sound reverberated through my body, and at that moment there was no sense of separation, like the union of form and emptiness. Afterward, we all ate toshi-koshi soba while passing the old year into the new one. Warm in body and spirit, we began the New Year with a fresh mind and happy heart.

SIMPLE AND TRADITIONAL LOTUS-ROOT SALAD

Serves 4 to 6

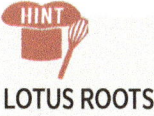

LOTUS ROOTS

Lotus roots are related to the water lily. The large seeds may be eaten raw, boiled, grilled, and also candied. The reddish-brown roots, rhizomes, are used as a vegetable, with a crisp texture and mild flavor.

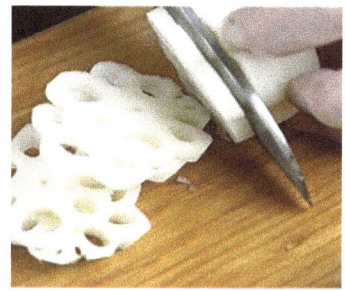

Locating the lotus root is the first challenge of this dish. You will have to go to an Asian market or find a mail order source. Cutting the lotus root as thin as humanly possible is an art form. After a few beginning disasters, you get into the momentum by calling on every ounce of concentration you can muster. Using a good quality mandolin is an alternative.

3 C lotus-root, sliced pencil-thin. Pour boiling water over them and let stand about 10 minutes (this takes the bitterness out), then drain.
1 C carrots, cut meticulously small or shredded
1" ginger, cut fine into very tiny pieces or minced

Marinade for a few hours and add to lotus root mixture:
½ C sugar and ¾ C rice vinegar (called sushi su)
1 T soy sauce
Dash salt

DELIGHTFUL TOFU-SPINACH SALAD

Serves 4 to 6

KONNYAKU ROOT

Healthy, but slimy, the "Konja Yam" (the name this tuber is known in Japan), is said to absorb toxins and called, "the broom of the stomach."

This is a bit nontraditional, but still a Tomiko family favorite. It's a fresh, delightful combination of flavors, and my personal favorite tofu dish!

2 C firm tofu, rinsed, drained, and mashed
3 T yellow miso
1 T tamari or soy sauce
1 to 2 T sugar (in a major family confession Tomiko admits that she prefers the 1 T and her grandmother the 2 T; you can decide for yourself.)
4 T sesame seeds, golden roasted and ground in a mortar and pestle
4 C spinach, cut small, steamed until just wilted, drain well

1. COMBINE all ingredients. Adjust tamari and sugar to taste.
OPTION: Top with ½ C konnyaku root (cut into thin pieces and dry roasted)

Seasonal Dishes

SWEET & SOUR SO SIMPLE BLACK BEANS

Makes 2 Cups   GMENY

RICE MIRIN

The sweetness of naturally made mirin is derived from the combination of sweet rice and koji rice (naturally fermented rice) and also includes water and sea salt.

A sweet and sour, gingery bean dish, which can end up quite thick.

1½ C black beans, soaked overnight or 2 cans cooked organic black beans, rinsed well and drained
2 to 3 T tamari
3 T honey, agave or maple sugar
2 garlic cloves, mashed
3 T rice mirin
2 to 3 T ginger, cut very small or minced

1. DRAIN soaked black beans into a large, heavy-duty pot, rinse well and cover with at least 1" of fresh water, cook until very tender, about 1½ to 2 hours.
2. ADD all the rest of the ingredients to the cooked beans.
3. COOK on very low heat, uncovered, until most of the liquids are evaporated, make sure not to burn. Taste and add more tamari if necessary.

CHESTNUT MOUNT FUJI DESSERT

Makes 1 Cake   GMEY

TOFU CREAM

1 C silken tofu
¼ C honey or
  ½ C agave
1 t vanilla extract

BLEND until very smooth.

This traditional yet simple recipe has a delicate, nutty sweetness.

4 whole sweet potatoes, peeled cut into large chunks
20 fresh chestnuts
½ C maple syrup and ½ C agave syrup
4 T margarine or butter, melted
4 T almond milk
1½ t salt

1. STEAM or roast sweet potatoes until very soft, then mash.
2. SLIT an "X" on the top of chestnuts, steam until very tender, about 15 to 25 minutes. Shell and mash.
3. MIX all ingredients together with your hands.
4. ADJUST sweetness to taste. Add enough milk to shape.
5. SHAPE into a mountain with a spatula.
6. CUT into pieces, when cooled, top with whipped tofu cream.

TRADITIONAL SOBA NOODLE NEW YEAR'S DINNER

Serves 6 to 8

DASHI JAPANESE STOCK BASE

6" piece kombu (seaweed)
3 to 4 shiitake mushrooms, dried
7 C water

Soak kombu and shiitake mushrooms in water for at least 30 minutes or overnight. Remove mushrooms. Cut off and discard stems, and slice caps.

Add mushrooms and kombu to fresh water and heat. Remove kombu just before water boils and then lower heat.

Simmer mushroom broth for at least 5 to 8 minutes, remove mushroom pieces.

To finish off New Year's Day, we made a simple soba noodle dinner. We had a lot of stock (dashi) on hand from last evenings miso soup. Ideally, the dashi should be made ahead of time. It freezes well, so you can make what you need for this recipe then freeze the rest in an ice cube tray, using a few cubes for a quick bowl of miso soup. You can buy prepared soba sauce at a Japanese grocery store, but there is nothing like the taste of fresh sauce. Soba noodles are available in a few varieties. The most common soba noodles are made from 40 to 60% buckwheat, and the balance whole wheat flour. There are two more interesting varieties of soba. The first is Jinenjo, or mountain potato. This variety helps to bind the buckwheat and is a strengthening food, rich in digestive enzymes. The other is mugwort soba, which is an aromatic bitter often used to cure general stomach upset.

COOKING SOBA — Use approximately an inch-wide handful of soba noodles per person. Since most Japanese noodles are made with salt, it is not necessary to add salt to the cooking water. In a very large pot, bring water to a full, rolling boil; use about twelve cups of water. Do not overcrowd the noodles or they will stick together. Boil about 3 to 4 minutes until noodles are al denté. Do not overcook. Rinse the noodles in two or three cold-water baths or under cold running water to prevent further cooking so noodles do not stick together. Use your hands to remove surface starch. Drain and use immediately.

SOBA SAUCE — *Serves 4 people, double for extra servings*: Combine 2½ C dashi, ½ plus 2 T dark soy sauce, 4 T mirin and 1 T sugar. Bring to a boil and remove from heat, cool to room temperature.

SERVING DINNER
Garnishes: Extra firm tofu, very small chunks; scallions, finely minced; wasabi; pickled ginger; dried seaweed, very thinly sliced; grated daikon and Japanese radishes (grate them at the last minute and squeeze out excess water; if daikon is not available, ordinary radishes will do.)
Preparation: Fill each person's bowl with cooled soba noodles, add a small amount of warm dashi. Fill a small bowl with soba sauce for each person. Add any garnishes you wish to the noodle bowl. Dip noodles into the sauce and eat.

COMING TOGETHER
2003: YEAR OF THE SHEEP

A NEW YEAR IS A PARADOX. What is truly new, what is old? Is it just a concept pointing to a flash of momentary experiences? I cooked a New Year's Eve feast for some friends that came together to share in this event. These markers, like separate frames on a film, define and sometimes transform the screening of our lives. This year was one such defining moment for me.

Most of the food preparation and cooking was done the day before. The rice dish was resting in the fridge, melding together. The spinach pockets were par-baked and finished baking on that day. The lemon tarts were made ahead and were chilling, just waiting to be topped with fresh berries. The veggies for roasting were cut and dressed that morning and simply spread out on a roasting pan to cook, an hour or so before dinner. I added a large salad that day and the evening meal came together in a flash. This way my kitchen was organized and it allowed me to spend time enjoying my guests.

After a lovely evening together sharing food and conversation, we moved to the warmth of the living room, where candles and the fireplace were aglow. Without plan we began reading excerpts from an inspiring book that was passed along from person to person. The reading filled the room with a pulsating presence. As we came to the end of the reading, we discovered a New Year had happened. It changed nothing and everything. For me, for some reason, it was to be a special moment in time. And, as it turned out, was to be our last New Year's Eve celebration in that house.

HERB-CRUSTED ROASTED VEGGIES

Makes 2 Cups | Preheat Oven to 400 Degrees   GMENSY

HERB DRESSING FOR VEGGIES

This is a simple, all-purpose dressing. Put in a mason jar and shake vigorously.

½ C olive oil
3 T balsamic vinegar
½ t kosher salt
½ t oregano, dried
½ t thyme, dried
1 T maple syrup or agave
1 T dijon mustard
Pinch Aleppo chili

Roasted vegetables have become my latest passion. They caramelize into a sweet and concentrated form of themselves and are so simple, yet elegant to make. I have learned a great lesson—not to roast them on a lower heat than what is recommended. The higher temperature seals the outside while cooking the inside. The combination of vegetables is up to you! Fresh stemmed herbs add a lot to the flavor. The selfless herbs impart their fragrance to the vegetable but since they dry out, they are discarded before serving.

3 carrots, chopped coarsely
10 small red potatoes, cut in half
2 medium red onions
1 large portobello mushroom, cut into 1" long slices
8 tiny beets or 3 large beets, peeled and chopped into 1" squares
1 jewel yam, peeled and cut into small chunks
2 to 3 garlic cloves, smashed, keep whole (remove skin)

1. CUT the vegetables and place on a lightly greased roasting pan.
2. COMBINE dressing (on right), then toss with just enough dressing to coat all the vegetables. (You can do this a few hours ahead of time.)
3. TOP vegetables with plenty of freshly ground pepper and any fresh herb sprigs.
4. ROAST until tender, cover for ½ hour and uncover, turn down heat to 350 minutes, for the last ½ hour. Stir after 30 minutes.

COOKING WITH PORTOBELLO

Refrigerate mushrooms immediately, they will keep about five days. To prevent drying or shriveling, cover gently with a damp paper towel or dampened cheesecloth. Don't store in plastic bags, this causes moisture and condensation which speeds spoilage. • The gills can be used like a truffle garnish. Scrap the gills off the underside of the cap and sprinkle them onto a dish. • Portobello stems are firmer than caps and may be sliced lengthwise, grilled, or roasted. Instead of brushing caps with oil or sauce before cooking, spray both sides with olive oil. • When sautéing, leave space around the mushrooms so they brown evenly. • Portobellos become meatier the longer they are cooked. • Cooked portobello can be frozen and will keep for several months. Place in freezer containers or bags, removing as much air as possible. (Uncooked mushrooms don't freeze well.)

Seasonal Dishes

SAFFRON/CARDAMOM THAI RICE

Serves 6 to 8

GMESY

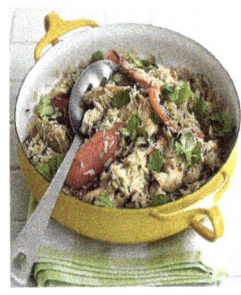

What inspired this rice was a little package of saffron and a special Thai spice combination that was given to me (Ming Tsai Blue Ginger Curry Powder). This rice cooks best in a heavy-bottomed Dutch oven-type pot. It is also best when it sits overnight, the variety of spices and layers merge together, so making it a day ahead of time is an asset.

3 T coconut oil or ghee
½ C raw cashew or pine nuts pieces
2 small or 1 large red onion, chopped very small
2 T ginger, freshly grated
1½ t salt
A few saffron threads
1 t cumin powder, roasted and ground fresh
1 t cardamom powder, ground fresh
2 T Thai spice mix, ground or paste
1 t turbinado sugar
¼ to ½ t cayenne pepper
2 C jasmine rice, rinsed and well-drained
1 roasted red pepper, jarred, chopped
1 can light coconut milk and water, totaling 4 C
1 C fresh or frozen peas
½ C shredded coconut, not sweetened
¼ C cilantro
2 T lemon juice, 1 T lemon zest

SAFFRON

Saffron is perhaps the most precious and expensive spice in the world. The filaments, are actually the dried stigmas of the saffron flower, "crocus." Each flower contains three stigmas and must be picked from each flower by hand. More than 75,000 of these flowers produce just one pound of saffron filaments. Because of saffron's strong color and intense flavor, it should be used sparingly.

1. MELT oil or ghee in a heavy-duty Dutch oven. Sauté nuts on a low heat until slightly brown. Be very careful, they burn quickly.
2. ADD onions and ginger; sauté until onions are translucent.
3. ADD salt, spices, sugar, cayenne, and zest; mix until well-coated.
4. ADD rice and stir fry for two minutes until toasted and fragrant.
5. ADD red pepper, coconut milk and water, turn heat to medium and bring to a boil. Then lower heat to the lowest possible setting and cover. Do not stir or disturb for at least 20 minutes. Check a rice grain to make sure it is cooked properly, and no water remains on the bottom.
6. ADD peas on top and let the pot sit, covered for a least 10 more minutes.
7. ADD cilantro and lemon juice on top, fluff with a fork.

SAVORY SPINACH POCKETS

Makes 24 Pockets | Preheat Oven to 350 Degrees | Bake: 20 Minutes   MENSY

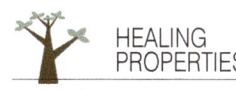

Spinach
- 13 different flavonoid compounds function as antioxidants and anti-cancer agents
- 200% of vitamin K provided daily, important for bone health
- May help prevent colon cancer
- May help protect the brain from oxidative stress and promotes brain function

This appetizer (also known as spanakopita*) was my first time working with this pesky ingredient and it was a bit like sitting in a zendo with a stick poised overhead. The filling was done in advance and waited patiently to join the filo. The actual execution of "filling the filo" is an act of pure concentration. You have to be totally unrushed and ready to abandon yourself to the act. The ultra-fine sheets can rip by merely letting your mind drift for a moment. Also, the beauty of this recipe is that is can be totally vegan.*

Spinach Filling
2 T olive oil and 1 T margarine, butter, or ghee
4 shallots, cut small and 1 clove garlic, minced
1 T ginger, freshly grated
5 to 6 C fresh spinach, chopped very small
¾ t salt
2 T Parmesan cheese (or vegan alternative)
½ C feta cheese (or vegan option, see page 73)
1 T Panko breadcrumbs
1 package frozen filo dough sheets

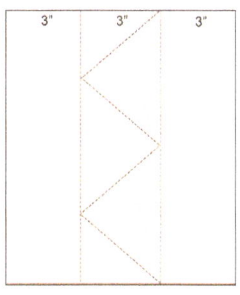

1. HEAT oil/margarine mixture and add shallots, cook until tender.
2. ADD garlic and fry for one minute. Add ginger, spinach and salt, fry 10 minutes uncovered until water is evaporated.
3. ADD cheese and breadcrumbs, mix well, cool.
4. SERVE with tzatziki (see page 169) or cashew sauce (see page 120)

Filling the Filo
1. PLACE frozen filo in the refrigerator overnight to defrost. Keep covered with a damp cloth at all times! Melt an additional 1 to 2 T margarine, butter, or ghee; keep aside.
2. CUT filo sheets into 3" strips crosswise (the long direction side of the dough).
3. COAT a single sheet with margarine or melted butter.
4. PLACE about 1 T of filling near the bottom, then fold the strip up in alternating triangle shapes, like you were folding a flag, ensuring that the dough completely encases the filling (see diagram).
5. PLACE the triangles on a baking sheet; brush the top and bottom with margarine or butter and cover with a damp cloth until all the triangles are made.
6. BAKE until golden brown. An easy way to serve them hot is to par-bake for 10 minutes, refrigerate, and then finish the last 10 minutes in the oven, just before serving.

MAPLE/LEMONY TARTS

Makes 10 to 12 Tarts | Preheat Oven to 350 Degrees | Bake: 30 to 40 Minutes   M N S Y

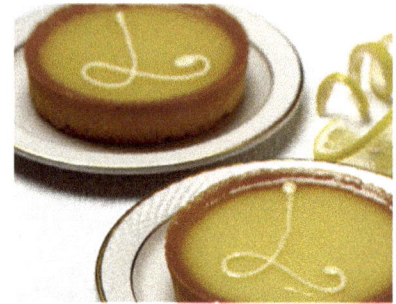

These bite-size tarts are really fun because you get to use a clean ketchup bottle to fill them into the melt-in-your mouth crust.

Tender Pie Crust
This crust can be made in advance, frozen, and defrosted just before rolling out.

2½ C unbleached white pastry flour
½ t salt
½ C margarine or butter, chilled, cut into pieces
1 egg and 4 to 6 T ice water

1. BEAT the egg with enough of the ice water to measure ½ C.
2. COMBINE flour, salt, margarine or butter. Rub or cut into the flour until it is a coarse meal.
3. POUR just enough liquid into the dry ingredients until it bunches together forming a solid dough.
4. WRAP tightly in wax paper and place in the freezer for at least 1 hour, or let it rest in the refrigerator for 2 to 3 hours.

Maple/Lemon Filling
8 oz. low or fat-free cream cheese or alternative equivalent
1 egg
½ C muscovado brown sugar, vanilla sugar or maple sugar
3 T maple or agave syrup
1 T vanilla extract or ½ of a vanilla bean, seeds scraped out lengthwise
2 T lemon zest, freshly grated

1. BLEND all ingredients together very well.
2. ROLL crust on a surface dusted with maple sugar. Cut circles using a 3" to 5" diameter cutter. Fill tart pans with the circles of crust. Crimp edges to fit into the tins. Pierce bottom of crust with a fork and bake in 350-degree oven for 5 to 6 minutes, until partially baked. Cool.
3. FILL an empty ketchup bottle with filling and squeeze into pie crust tarts until almost filled. Bake until slightly golden. Don't overbake.
4. Top with raspberries or blackberries (optional).

HINT

ALTERNATIVE SUGARS

Muscovado is produced in Mauritius and locks in the natural molasses of sugar cane.

Maple sugar is available in most stores.

You can make your own vanilla sugar (see page 295).

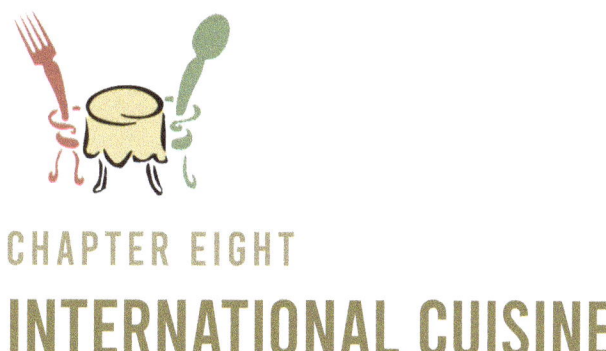

CHAPTER EIGHT
INTERNATIONAL CUISINE

GRANDMA'S SPECIALTIES

STUFFING THE PITA

A JAPANESE MEAL

MISO

GRANDMA'S SPECIALTIES

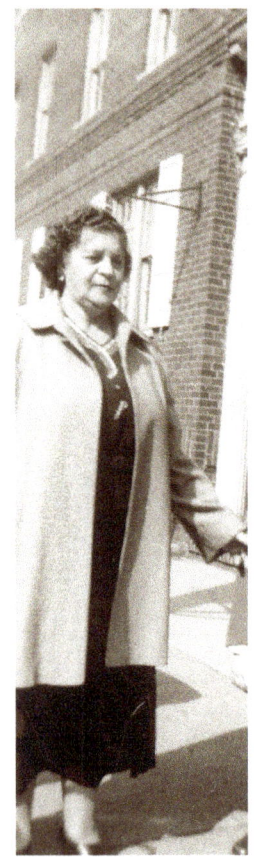

Grandma Molly

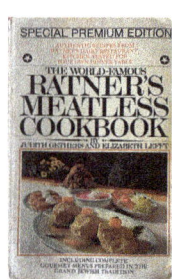

I HAD SOME EXTRA TIME ONE SATURDAY IN OCTOBER AND MY MOM and I went to the La Jolla (California) public library, a favorite haunt of mine. It is here that I've found many interesting out-of-print books. As I was looking in my usual spot, in a bin by the door—my mother exclaimed with delight. She had just found an old copy of the *Ratner's Meatless Cookbook*. If you're not from the New York area, this book and its history may not be fascinating. Having been to the famous Ratner's Restaurant in the late 1960s, when they still served hot coffee in traditional glasses, I was as delighted as my mother at this discovery. To me, Ratner's was from another era, something out of an Isaac Beshavis Singer novel, where serious philosophers spoke Yiddish and the food was earthy and filling—made from recipes passed down through generations.

There were two recipes in this book that my mother had been looking for, for over forty years, since her own mother had passed away with her secrets tucked away in her well-worn house-dress pockets. Though she had watched her mother's cooking and baking marathons (that took place during visits to our home a few times a year), she never bothered to ask her to write the recipes down. I doubt Grandma Molly would actually have been able to formulate measurements on paper. Cooking from Grandma's perspective was a combination of pure intuition and experience, a pinch here and a dab there.

Sometimes we need a little help—an experienced hand that has traveled the path before us, made some mistakes, and discovered that the recipe is simply the reed, and we are the wind that creates the culinary music. Even if we have just the right recipe, we still need our own intuition and experience to make the dish "sing."

GRANDMA'S EVERYDAY EGGPLANT SPREAD

Serves 4 to 6 | Preheat Oven to 350 Degrees | Bake: 1 hour   GMENSY

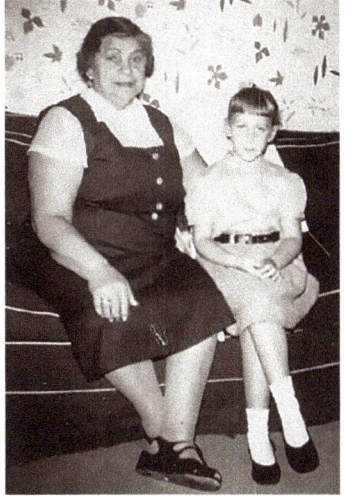

With Grandma Molly

This family recipe is simple to make and works well as a light lunch or appetizer. It combines the traditional recipe of Grandma Molly, hints from the classic Ratner's Meatless Cookbook *and my own addition of ginger and lemon zest to wake it up a bit more.*

2 medium eggplants
3 T avocado oil
2 onions, medium, chopped small
1 red pepper, finely chopped

1 t ginger, fresh minced
2 garlic cloves, chopped
Juice of ½ lemon, 1 t lemon zest
Salt and pepper to taste

1. BAKE unpeeled eggplants in oven until soft. Cool, peel, and chop finely.
2. SAUTÉ onions and red pepper in oil, until well-cooked. Add ginger and garlic near the end of cooking and fry for a few moments.
3. STIR in cooked, chopped eggplant, lemon juice and zest, salt, and pepper.
4. CHILL and serve with whole grain crackers, wedges of whole wheat bread, or warm corn tortillas.

 SIDEBAR   EGGPLANT VARIETIES

- **American eggplants** (globe eggplant) are the familiar large, dark purple, pear-shaped variety. 1 medium eggplant = 1 pound = approximately 4.5 cups of peeled and cubed eggplant.
- **Baby eggplants** are small versions of American eggplants, but sweeter with thinner skins.
- **Japanese** and **Chinese eggplants** have thinner skins and a more delicate flavor and not as many of the seeds that tend to make eggplants bitter. They're usually more slender than American eggplants, but they vary in size and shape. They range in color from lavender to pink, green, and white.
- **Italian eggplants** are smaller than American eggplants.
- **Thai eggplants** are golf-ball sized eggplants and more bitter than American eggplants. They're usually green, mixed with yellow, or white. They're often used in hot chili or curry dishes. Remove as much of the bitter seeds that you can before using.
- **White eggplants** have a tough skin, a more delicate flavor and firmer flesh.

International Cuisine

TWO UNIQUE SPREADS

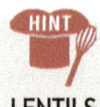

LENTILS

Brown lentils tend to get mushy if overcooked. If you want them to be firm, add a little oil to the cooking water and cook a short time, 15 minutes. You can substitute French green lentils or red lentils which are smaller and take less time to cook.

Matthew's Grandma Pauline created these spreads when her wayward vegetarian grandchildren visited her Brooklyn walk-up apartment. They were the appetizers; much more was to come, which often included a potato soup and some homemade blintzes.

LENTIL SPREAD
Serves 6 to 8

G M N S Y

½ lb. organic brown lentils
2 large onions, chopped small
8 hard-boiled eggs
3 T avocado oil
1 T sesame (tahini) or nut butter
Salt and cayenne pepper to taste

1. COOK lentils until quite soft, but not watery (fill pot with just enough water or vegetable stock to cover lentils) cook about 45 minutes, then mash well with eggs.
2. SAUTÉ onions in oil until golden brown.
3. MIX lentils, onions, sesame or nut butter, cayenne, and salt.
4. CHILL, serve with crackers, pita bread, or warm corn tortillas.

GREEN BEANS WITH CASHEWS
Serves 4 to 6

G M E S Y

3 T avocado oil
2 C onions, chopped small
1 C cashews, toasted dry
2 C string beans, steamed until quite soft
1 T lemon juice
Salt and fresh black pepper
2 T parsley or cilantro, chopped small

1. HEAT oil and sauté onions slowly until golden brown.
2. COMBINE onions with remaining ingredients in food processor.
3. BLEND until almost a smooth puree, leave just a bit chunky.
4. TOP with chopped parsley.

HEALING PROPERTIES

Green Beans
- Have a spectacular amount of vitamin K, essential for strong bones
- Good source of vitamin A and C; excellent antioxidant
- Good source of fiber
- Have almost twice as much iron as spinach

KASHA KNISH APPETIZER

Makes 24 Knishes | Preheat Oven to 350 Degrees | Bake: 20 to 30 Minutes   M N S Y

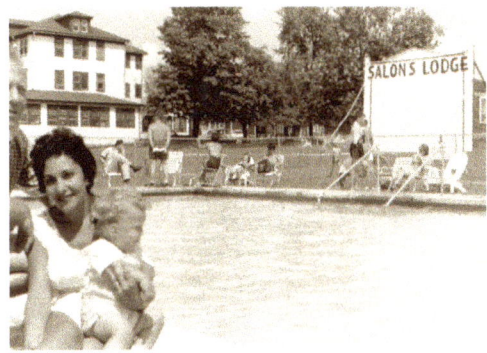

My mom and little brother at Salon's Lodge.

I have a wonderful memory of the knish man who came daily to the bungalow colony where our family vacationed for the entire summer in the early 1960s, when I was in elementary school. It was deep in the heart of the Catskill Mountains, in New York State, and was called "Salon's Lodge." The knish man traveled in a small van to all the colonies, he carried a heated box filled with fresh knishes. He visited us mid-morning as we sat under large trees that shaded the front lawn.

The knish man's visit always elicited a great deal of excitement, and Grandma Molly would send me scurrying to the communal kitchen where she left her change purse. When I ran back, she would reward us with a kasha (buckwheat) knish. My brothers and I always preferred the kasha, though most of my cousins insisted on potato only version.

Here is an easy version of Grandma's kasha knishes. The secret is in the filling. I've made it simple by using store bought puff pastry wrappers and I think even Grandma Molly would approve! If you want to pre-cook in advance, then parbake for 10 minutes and finish baking just before serving. They also freeze really well.

SAUTÉ

The term sauté means to jump. In cooking, it means to place food in a hot pan with some butter or oil and to shake the pan so the food jumps around (preventing it from burning).

Potato Filling

2 potatoes (medium) or 1 large, peeled, chopped small
2 onions (medium) chopped very small
1 t salt
2 T avocado oil and 2 T margarine or butter (grandma used schmaltz, chicken fat she rendered herself that she kept in a jar by the stove.)

Buckwheat Filling

½ C medium buckwheat groats, kasha
1 egg
1 C water
¾ t salt
1 package frozen Puff Pastry dough, defrosted

1. COOK potatoes until very tender and mash well.
2. SAUTÉ onions in oil and margarine or butter until golden brown, add onions and salt to mashed potatoes.

International Cuisine

KASHA KNISH APPETIZER (CONT'D)

3. SAUTÉ buckwheat a beated egg for about 3 minutes, until brown and it begins to emit a nutty fragrance.
4. BOIL water and add salt.
5. ADD sautéed buckwheat to boiling water stir well. Cover with a tight-fitting lid.
6. LOWER heat to lowest setting and cook 15 to 20 minutes until all liquid is absorbed. Don't lift the lid or stir while it is cooking; then uncover, fluff with a fork and let rest for 10 minutes.
7. COMBINE cooked buckwheat with potato/onion filling.

To Make Knishes
1. UNROLL 1 entire dough section and cut into three pieces (on the length side), about 12" by 4" each.
2. ROLL each piece out on floured board until it is ¼" depth rectangle.
3. FILL the long center with the filling, 1" high and 1" wide.
4. FOLD dough over the filling, pinch together until sealed at the fold.
5. CUT the whole roll into 2-inch pieces with a very sharp serrated knife.
6. BAKE 20 to 35 minutes until a lovely golden brown.

 SIDEBAR   BUCKWHEAT

Buckwheat is native to Northern Europe, as well as Asia. From the 10th through the 13th century, it was widely cultivated in China. From there, it spread to Europe and Russia in the 14th and 15th centuries and was introduced in the United States by the Dutch during the 17th century. Many people categorize buckwheat as a grain when it's a fruit seed related to rhubarb and sorrel. Its name is supposedly derived from the Dutch word *boekweit*, which means "beech wheat," since buckwheat is beechnut shaped with wheat-like characteristics. Roasted buckwheat, called "kasha," is a name from a European dish, which uses buckwheat as its base. In order to be edible, the outer hull is removed, with special milling equipment. Buckwheat is either unroasted or roasted. Unroasted buckwheat has a soft, subtle flavor and roasted buckwheat has more of an earthy, nutty taste. Its color can range from tannish pink to brown. It can also be ground into flour. The darker color is more nutritious. Because buckwheat does not contain gluten, it can be mixed with some type of gluten-containing flour (such as wheat) for baking or with gluten-free flour for a true gluten-free mixture.

GRANDMA'S RUGELACH

Makes 32 Pieces | Preheat Oven to 350 Degrees | Bake: 20 to 25 Minutes

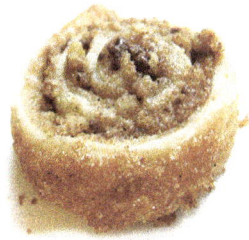

This pastry has been made in my family ever since I can remember. Grandma Molly would arrive at our house, at least twice a year, with rolling pin in hand and a collection of aprons. We would simply lead her to the kitchen, and she spent two weeks cooking and baking. The dining room table filled up with pastries and cookies as the days worn on. This recipe was coaxed out of my mom who was also an expert baker. Since she followed the intuitive recipe style, we went through the motions of measuring ingredients. This was the last thing she baked for my older brother, six months before she passed away.

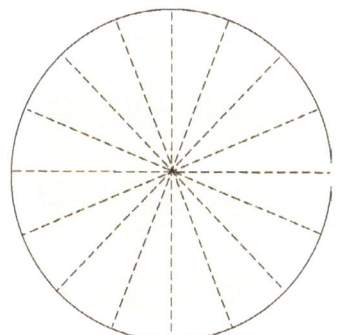

Wet Ingredients
(A shortcut is to use a frozen puff pastry dough)
1 packet active dry yeast with ½ t sugar
¾ C sweet butter or margarine
2 oz. low-fat cream cheese or alternative cheese, softened
2 eggs beaten or 1 egg and 2 egg whites

Dry Ingredients
2½ to 3 C unbleached white flour
½ C turbinado brown sugar and ½ t salt

Filling Ingredients
7½ oz. raisins soaked in brandy or fruit juice, drain well
3 oz. walnuts, chopped very small
½ C sugar and 1 T cinnamon, to taste
All fruit preserves, slightly melted (raspberry and apricot are traditional)

To Roll Out and Bake

ROLL up each triangle tightly, from the wide area to the narrow part, and place on an ungreased cookie sheet, brush each piece with beaten egg or water, sprinkle lightly with sugar and bake until golden.

1. DISSOLVE yeast in water and add sugar, let rise and bubble.
2. SOFTEN butter or margarine, add along with softened cream cheese and mix well. Add eggs, then add foamed yeast mixture. Mix flour, sugar, and salt together. Add dry to wet ingredients to form a dough. Divide into four parts, cover and refrigerate for at least 2 to 3 hours.
3. SOAK raisins in small bowl and let rest for an hour or even overnight; drain and combine sugar, cinnamon, and nuts in a separate bowl.
4. ROLL each quarter into a ¼" thick circle. Spread preserves onto each circle, leaving a ½" edge, sprinkle cinnamon sugar, raisins, and nuts on top. With a sharp knife cut 12 triangular pieces, just like you would cut a pizza (see diagram above).

International Cuisine | 167

GRANDMA PAULINE'S THUMBPRINT COOKIES

Makes 24 Cookies | Preheat Oven to 375 Degrees | Bake: 11 to 15 Minutes   MNS

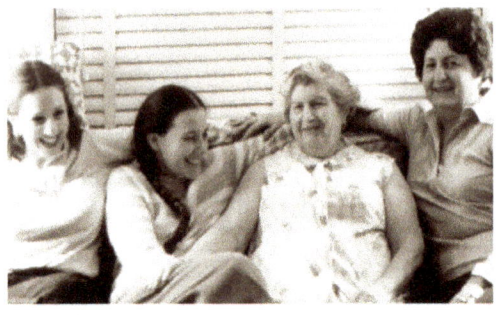

Grandma Pauline and the Greenblatt girls.

When we lived in Nova Scotia, Matthew's Grandmother Pauline, would send us a round Quaker Oatmeal box filled with these old-world thumbprint cookies. They would arrive in miraculous condition with a perfectly cut round circle of waxed paper on top. They stayed fresh through the shipping process and for the week it took us to polish them off. What makes these cookies different is that they are relatively low sugar (even more so if you omit the maple glaze). Also, the use of yeast rather than baking powder for leavening, I think, made them stay fresh for so long.

¼ C sour cream, low-fat yogurt, or soy yogurt
1 packet active dry yeast and 1 t sugar
1 egg
2 C unbleached white flour
¼ C maple sugar or brown sugar
¾ C butter or margarine
1 C all fruit preserves (strawberry, raspberry, apricot, anything will do.)

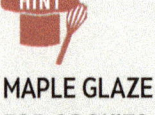

MAPLE GLAZE FOR COOKIES

1 C confectioner's sugar, sifted
¾ t vanilla extract
1 t maple syrup
1 T milk, soy or rice milk.

Combine with a whisk, adding more liquid if needed to make a semi-thin stream of glaze.

1. COMBINE yeast and sugar in a small bowl. Set aside until bubbly, about 10 minutes.
2. COMBINE bubbly yeast with sour cream or vegan alternative.
3. STIR in egg.
4. SIFT flour and sugar together in a separate large bowl and cut butter into flour until small pea-sized balls.
5. STIR sour cream mixture into flour mixture just until it comes together. Transfer to a lightly floured board and knead gently together. Make into a ball in the same way you make a pie crust.
6. WRAP in wax or parchment paper and refrigerate at least 30 minutes. You can also do this in the evening and roll them out in the morning.
7. ROLL dough out until about ¼" thick and cut into 3" rounds.
8. PLACE on an ungreased cookie sheet and use your thumb to make a large print in the middle.
9. FILL the center with 1 t of fruit preserve.
10. BAKE until golden; drizzle with glaze after they cool.

STUFFING THE PITA

Tzatziki Sauce

MIX all together and chill well.

2 C grated cucumber, remove excess water
1½ C plain yogurt, drained (you can substitute alternative yogurt)
2 T olive oil
2 T fresh mint and/or dill
1 T lemon juice
½ t cumin powder
½ t Aleppo chili
½ t salt

DURING THE SUMMER OF 1970, I FOUND MYSELF WORKING ON A KIBBUTZ in Southern Israel, about five kilometers from the Gaza Strip, at the edge of the Negeb desert. This was before the conflicts in that area. After a grueling day (that began at 5:00 a.m.) of weeding acres of green peppers and hauling bales of hay, I often spent the evenings sitting alone on a mound of sand, meditating as the desert dusk splashed its transforming sunset colors across the wide horizon, the sound of shepherds and stillness filling the air.

The hard labor and fresh air brought with it an amazingly large appetite, something I will probably never again experience in quite the same way. Since this particular Kibbutz had a rather large group of vegetarians from South America (which I found quite interesting as

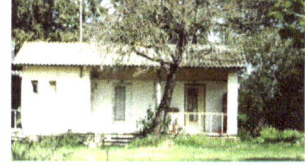
Kibbutz Bror Hayil, not far from the beach city of Ashkelon.

that area of the world is mostly known for meat eating), they offered two completely separate menus. The meals were served with freshly picked vegetables, whole grains, and tahini or tzatziki sauce.

Just experimenting with a vegetarian diet myself, each meal became both a surprise and a delight. Then during one trip outside the kibbutz into the city of Tel Aviv, I discovered the roadside falafel stand. The humble falafel, made of fresh pita bread, salad, chickpea balls, and plenty of tahini sauce was the perfect combination of flavors.

A falafel never tasted quite the same outside of Israel, although there were two places that came close: a very small restaurant called "Hershel's," located in New City, Upstate New York. The second place was a tiny (world-famous) falafel cart near 42nd Street in New York City. What made their falafel's and Tel Aviv's stand apart was the abundance of tahini sauce, amazing fluffy falafel balls, and of course warm, freshly baked pita bread.

HOMEMADE FALAFEL

Makes 6 to 8 Falafel Pitas

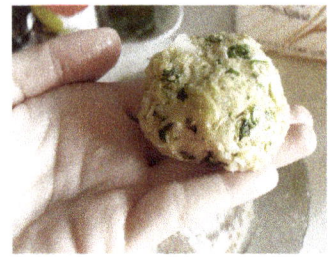

To stuff a pita, I've put together two items: a spread and my old friend, falafel. Falafels are traditional deep-fried chickpea balls, but they can also be baked with good results.

2½ C dried chickpeas, soak in water overnight, drain well
2 T parsley, freshly minced
1 clove garlic, minced
1 t salt
½ t cumin powder, ½ t coriander powder, ½ t cayenne pepper
1 t fresh ginger, minced
2½ t wheat germ or gluten-free flour blend and ½ t baking powder
1 egg, beaten (or 2 egg whites alone can be substituted, or ½ t corn starch dissolved in ¼ C water)
1 T rice flour
Oil for deep-frying.

1. COOK chickpeas in enough water to cover them, 30 minutes in an Instant Pot or at least 1 hour in a soup pot, until soft. Drain well.
2. MASH chickpeas coarsely; do not grind to a paste.
3. COMBINE the next nine ingredients.
4. CHILL chickpea batter for at least 15 to 30 minutes; longer the better.
5. SHAPE into 20 balls; flatten slightly, dip in egg or corn starch mixture, and coat lightly with rice flour.
6. FRY balls in oil until crisp. Oil should be at least 375 degrees. If the frying temperature is not hot enough the balls absorb too much oil.
7. DRAIN very well on absorbent paper or a paper bag.

To Assemble the Falafel

1. CHOP 1 C fresh greens and cucumber, very small.
2. CHOP 2 tomatoes, de-seed and cut very small.
3. HEAT pita slightly.
4. PLACE greens, cucumber, and tomato mixture on bottom of the pita and top with one large or two small falafel balls.
5. SPOON 3 T tahini sauce on top.
6. REPEAT above layer again.
7. FOLD a small square of tin foil onto the bottom of pita.
8. SERVE immediately, with plenty of napkins.

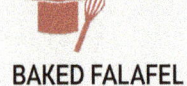

BAKED FALAFEL

Place balls on an oiled baking sheet and roll them in oil to coat all sides. Bake at 375 degrees for at least 20 minutes. Turn over at least once during baking.

TAHINI SAUCE

Blend the following ingredients together:
½ C tahini (sesame paste)
1 small garlic clove, minced
½ t salt
¼ C lemon juice
½ to ¾ C water
Pinch cayenne pepper

PUNCHY BABA GHANOUJ

Serves 4 to 6

This is a wonderful eggplant spread, often served with warm pita, corn tortillas or crackers.

1 medium eggplant, or two small
1 garlic clove, minced
½ lemon, juiced or ⅛ C lemon juice
3 T tahini
½ t hickory salt
2 T olive oil
½ t whole cumin seed
½ t ginger, ground
½ t crushed red pepper
1 T chopped parsley

1. GRILL OR BROIL Whole eggplants*
2. SCOOP the cooked eggplant into a bowl.
3. COMBINE eggplant with lemon juice, tahini, garlic, and salt.
4. HEAT olive oil in a small pan and add the cumin seed and red pepper. Heat until cumin seeds are roasted brown.
5. COMBINE spices and oil with eggplant, chill.
6. SPRINKLE parsley over eggplant spread just before serving and drizzle a little extra virgin olive oil on top.

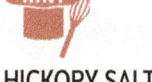

HICKORY SALT

½ C sea salt
1 T liquid smoke

Mix together and spread on a cookie sheet, allow to dry at room temperature, then rub salt between fingers to unclump. Store in a tight-fitting jar.

GRILLING EGGPLANT OPTIONS*

1. **Grill:** Pierce eggplants with a fork and grill on a rack set 5 to 6 inches over glowing coals and soaked "Char-Broil" mesquite wood chips; turn occasionally, until very soft, 30 to 40 minutes.
2. **Broil:** Place eggplants under a preheated broiler about 6 inches from heat for 30 to 40 minutes, until skin is charred.
3. **Bake:** Place eggplants in a baking pan with about ½ C water. Cut deep slits all over the eggplant to help it cook. Cover with tin foil and bake in a 350-degree oven for 40 minutes or until very tender. (Broiled and baked eggplants will not have a smoky flavor, so you could use hickory salt to impart the smoky flavor.
4. **Cool:** Transfer eggplants to a colander and when cool enough to handle, quarter lengthwise. With a small knife remove and discard as many seeds as possible. Scrape cooled eggplant into a large sieve set over a bowl, discarding skin. Drain eggplant and discard any juice.

AUTHENTIC PITA BREAD

Makes 6 Pita Breads | Preheat Oven to 425 Degrees | Bake: 10 to 12 Minutes   MENS

 **SIDEBAR**

HONEY

Honey is mankind's oldest sweetener. Bees travel as far as 40,000 miles and visit over 2 million flowers to produce a pound of honey.

Honey was found in the tombs of ancient Egyptian pharaohs, and in paintings of prehistoric men.

Though bees have been in Europe and Asia for hundreds of thousands of years, it was not until the late 1600s that bees were reintroduced into America by Europeans.

For the truly adventurous, those who wish to create an authentic Middle Eastern meal from scratch, I have included a recipe for baking your own pita. I find baking bread helps you to slow down, breathe, and let go. This basic bread, prepared since Biblical times (over open fires) is very simple to make. You have the choice of letting it rise from 3 to 11 hours. This means you could prepare the dough in the morning, let it rise all day, and bake it for dinner. Alternatively, you can prepare it in the evening, let it rise all night and bake it in the morning.

1¼ C warm water, 1 packet active dry yeast and 1 t honey
1 t olive oil
2 C whole wheat pastry flour and 1 to 1½
    C unbleached white flour or 3 to 3½
    unbleached white flour
1 t salt (see Hint of page 91)
¼ C sesame seeds, toasted (optional)
Cornmeal

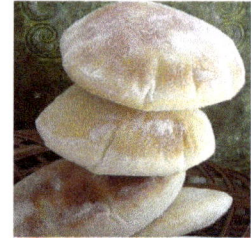

1. SPRINKLE yeast on top of warm water (115 degrees) and honey. Let it sit for 5 minutes. (If the water is too hot it will kill the yeast. If the water is too cold the yeast will not activate.)
2. ADD yeast water, oil, and salt to a large bowl.
3. MIX in whole wheat flour, ¾ C white flour and salt. (Add sesame seeds here if you are using them.) Add just enough additional white flour to make it into a solid ball.
4. KNEAD dough on a floured board for 5 to 10 minutes, until smooth.
5. PLACE in a lightly oiled bowl. Roll the dough in oil to coat all sides. Cover and let rise for 3 hours or overnight.
6. PUNCH down about 60 minutes before you want to bake it.
7. DIVIDE dough into six balls. Roll into a 6" circle, ¼" thick.
8. SPRINKLE corn meal on baking sheets. Place the pita circles on top, cover with a damp cloth and let rise about 30 to 40 minutes. With a spatula, flip the rounds of dough upside down on the baking sheet.
9. BAKE 10 to 15 minutes. To eat immediately, remove them from the baking sheet and cover with a cloth to keep soft. If you will be using them within a couple of days, cool them and store in the freezer.
10. OPEN the center of each pita gently with a sharp knife.

A JAPANESE MEAL

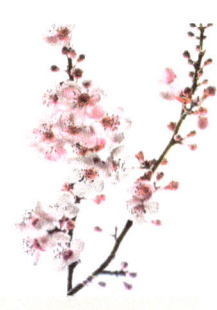

"We must cultivate beauty of character in daily life," declare the cherry-blossoms. Live to diffuse beauty, seeing the eternal, immutable Truth, in the passing and the changing—and leave the world like them, smiling, beautifying and peace-giving.
—Hari Prasad Shastri

MY FASCINATION WITH JAPAN was kindled by a small, heartfelt book, *Echoes of Japan*. It is a collection of short stories by Hari Prasad Shastri, written during his two-year visit to Japan, in 1916. During his stay, Shastri lectured at Tokyo University, witnessed cherry trees blossoming and discovered the inner significance of the Tea Ceremony. As a commentator on the *Upanishads*, he was able to distill the essence of Zen Buddhism, which is interwoven into many facets of Japanese life.

What I like about Japanese food is its simplicity. A bowl of steaming miso soup with a few vegetables floating on its surface is so very unpretentious. I was first introduced to it at a very small storefront in New York's East Village called *The Caldron*, which at the time was a kosher, macrobiotic restaurant—an interesting marriage of ideas and food. This was long before Japanese food was to become so popular. For about two dollars you could get a meal consisting of a large bowl of miso soup, salad with a myriad of sprouts, topped with sesame-tofu dressing, and a main course of stir-fried vegetables atop steaming short-grain brown rice. We'd sit at one large, long table that went from the kitchen to the door. You never knew who'd you meet, and there were always interesting people to share your meal with—a meal that was balanced, satisfying, and wholesome.

In the Kamakuna era (1185-1333 B.C.), Buddhism spread widely through Japan. To complement the Buddhist ethics of respect for all living creatures, fish and meat were avoided by monks and nuns. The simple diet evolved is known as *Kosei Shojin*. During the Edo period (1603-1861 A.D.) Zen influence flowered and the ancient capital of Kyoto became a haven for art and culinary innovations. Humble vegetables were transformed into an artistic and playful presentation of tastes, textures, and colors. Japanese food is a perfect complement to the Fall season. The warmth of miso soup combines with simple and colorful vegetable and tofu preparations.

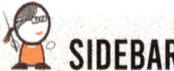 **SIDEBAR**   THE WONDER OF GINGER ROOT

Ginger is one of my all-time favorite herbs. I try to use it whenever possible. It is a perennial that originated in the jungles of Tropical Asia and is now cultivated in great quantities in Jamaica and the West Indies. The root of the ginger plant creeps and increases in tuberous joints underground. In the spring, a stalk peeks up from the root and usually grows about two feet high. The flowering stalk rises directly from the root, which gives way to a white or yellow bloom. But it is the root which is used in cooking and in the preparation of many medicinal herbs—from the Americas to India and China.

It is important to peel ginger root as thinly as possible, as the volatile oil just below the peel is the richest part of the resin. Ginger is considered a stimulant and produces a warming effect on the body. It helps treat or prevent flatulence or colic-type conditions and aids digestion in general. Adding ginger to your preparation, especially fresh ginger, always adds health benefits to your preparation.

It is important to store ginger in a dry, cool place. I usually wrap the root in tinfoil and keep it in the cheese part of the refrigerator. When I need some, I break off a piece of the root and grate it directly into the dish I am preparing. I use a tiny grater, kept just next to my stove, just for ginger. As long as the root is clean, you need not peel it. You can use the back of a spoon or a vegetable peeler to gently peel the tender skin.

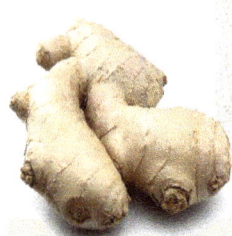

Growing Ginger in Your Home Garden

I am fascinated with the concept of growing fresh ginger. You can't grow it as easily in a cold climate; you definitely have to move it inside at the first signs of temperatures under 40 degrees. Then the dance begins of pulling it into the house on frosty days and giving it sun on warmer days. Though it can take a few years to harvest your first root, once you do, there's no stopping it. It's a beautiful fragrant plant and flower to have in the garden.

Buy some fresh ginger roots, ones that have a few developed "eyes" or growth buds. Ginger loves a sheltered spot, filtered sunlight, warm weather, humidity, and rich, moist soil; it is a tropical plant after all. You'll need really good soil, the kind that holds enough moisture, so it doesn't dry out; but it needs to be free draining, so it doesn't become waterlogged. Plant the roots 2 to 4 inches deep, with the growing buds facing up. Ginger is a slow-growing plant and can easily be overgrown by other plants that are planted near it. Fresh dug-up ginger sounds amazing. I may even give it a try myself one day!

BROCCOLI & CARROT SALAD WITH SESAME-GINGER DRESSING

Serves 4 to 6 GMENY

This is a low-fat, perfectly simple, and colorful veggie accompaniment to any meal. The ginger juice adds a special touch, spicy and fresh.

2 C broccoli florets
1 C carrots, julienne cut
3 T sesame seeds, hulled
1 T soy sauce
1 T miso
½ t toasted sesame oil
1 t mirin (sweetened rice wine)
¼ C water
1 t fresh ginger, cut small, squeezed in a garlic press to extract juice

1. STEAM the broccoli and carrots until slightly crisp, but not soft—about 5 minutes.
2. TOAST sesame seeds in a dry fry pan until golden, crush in a mortar and pestle, or on a bread board with a rolling pin.
3. WHISK 2 T crushed sesame seeds, soy sauce, miso, sesame oil, mirin, water and ginger juice together.
4. ARRANGE vegetables on a serving plate or in four individual bowls. Pour the dressing over the vegetables and sprinkle with the saved 1 T sesame seeds.

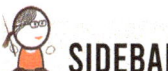 **SIDEBAR** THE MAGIC OF SESAME SEEDS

The English term sesame traces back to the Arabic *simsim*, Coptic *semsem*, and early Egyptian semsent; in fact, its earliest reference is in 3,000 BC. Sesame seeds are perhaps the world's most diverse seed. The Chinese burned sesame oil not only as a source of light but also to make soot for their ink-blocks. African slaves brought sesame seeds, which they called benné seeds, to America, where they became a popular ingredient in Southern dishes; and sesame seed oil is still one of the main sources of fat used in cooking throughout the East.

Probably the most widely known reference to this humble seed is "Open Sesame," the magic words used by Ali Baba to open the treasure cave in the classic tale, *The Thousand and One Nights*. One interpretation of this phrase suggests that it comes from the manner in which the sesame seed pods burst open with a pop, much like the sudden pop of a lock springing open.

TRADITIONAL UDON NOODLE SOUP

Serves 6 to 8

G M E N Y

SOUP BASE

- 8 " piece seaweed (kombu)
- 4 to 5 dried shiitake mushrooms
- 4 C water
- 2 onions, chopped
- 1 carrot, sliced at an angle
- 4 to 5 T soy sauce
- 1 to 2 T red miso
- 2 T mirin (sweet rice wine)

When my daughter was younger, this was and still is one of her favorite meals. The longer the noodle, the better. It's great for a meal with friends; add a fresh organic salad to balance out the meal.

Udon

14 oz. buckwheat udon noodles (not all buckwheat noodles are made of 100% buckwheat. They may be a combination of buckwheat plus other grains. Check the wrapper if you are gluten sensitive.)
1 C celery and carrots, cut into small chucks
½ C button mushrooms, cut very thin

Condiments

½ C tofu, cut very small
2 scallions, cut very small
2 T toasted sesame seeds
¼ C coriander leaves, chopped small

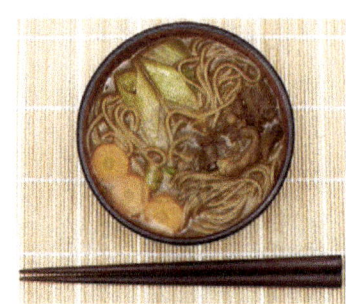

To Prepare Soup Base:
1. WIPE kombu with a paper towel, don't rinse.
2. SOAK cleaned kombu with mushrooms and seaweed in warm water for a few hours or even overnight. Drain well and remove seaweed.
3. ADD carrot, onions, and mushrooms to 4 cups of water and bring to a boil. Simmer for 20 minutes.
4. ADD soy sauce, miso, mirin, and salt to taste. Cook for an additional 5 minutes. Strain.

To Prepare Noodles (just before you are ready to serve the meal):
1. BOIL a large pot of water, add udon noodles, and return to boil.
2. SIMMER about 10 minutes until just cooked.
3. DRAIN and immediately put into cold water. (If noodles are cooked ahead of time, put them in a strainer and immerse in boiling water for a few seconds to heat. Drain well.)

To Serve:
1. DIVIDE noodles into four bowls.
2. ADD hot soup base to noodles.
3. TOP with any condiments you like.

BROILED TOFU STEAK

Serves 6 to 8

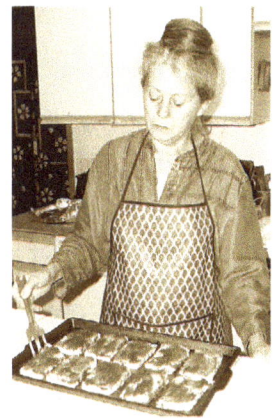

Jeanne on testing day.

This is as simple as it gets. For those who think they could never eat tofu, this is for you! When my friend Jeanne tried the recipe, she said it could be served like as a vegetable steak, along with a few side dishes.

1 lb. tofu, firm
⅓ C miso (red soybean paste)
1 T honey
2 T mirin (sweet rice wine)
¼ C water
½ t ginger, freshly grated
Sesame seeds, toasted (optional)

1. WRAP tofu tightly in a towel or cheese cloth and let sit for 30 to 40 minutes to drain out the excess water.
2. CUT tofu into 8 to 10 slices about ¼" thick.
3. WHISK next 4 ingredients together and marinade tofu slices for at least 30 minutes.
4. SPRINKLE with sesame seeds and broil under moderate heat until mixture bubbles.

 SIDEBAR   **WHAT IS MISO?**

Miso is made by combining cultured grain or soybeans, as a starter, with cooked soybeans, salt and water. This mixture is left to ferment. Various types of miso, from light to robust, can be created by varying the type of starter (rice or barley rather than soybean), by the proportions of the ingredients, by the time they are allowed to ferment, and the type of vessel it is stored in, much like making a fine wine.

Miso is reputed to have remarkable medicinal qualities. It contains dipicolonic acid, an alkaloid that chelates heavy metals, such as radioactive strontium, and discharges them from the body. The most remarkable evidence of the protective qualities of miso against exposure to radiation was published by Professor Akihiro Ito, at Hiroshima University's Atomic Radioactivity Medical Lab. Truckloads of Hatcho miso (a renowned brand created by a centuries old company, the Hatcho Miso Company) were sent to Chernobyl. The miso was deemed to protect those exposed to radiation.

MISO

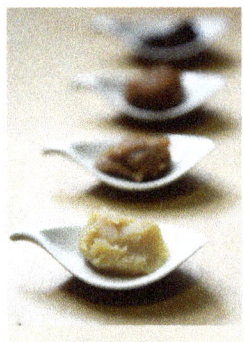

MISO ALWAYS SURPRISES ME. Strong and robust; it just has a lot of personality. I first tasted it in the 1960s at a macrobiotic restaurant on the Lower East Side of Manhattan.

Yet when I brought my first container of miso home from the store, I didn't know where to start or what to do with this strange salty mush. I felt like a new mother; at first it was truly intimidating. Many years later, returning to my macrobiotic roots, miso is no longer the "mystery container" but an old friend that is easier to use than I had ever imagined.

In fact, miso straight from the tub can be used in almost any capacity. If you are using it in a stir fry, always dilute it with a little water or broth so it doesn't get lumpy. Adding it to a vinaigrette instead of salt adds depth, and you can always make a simple miso spread which is great on grilled vegetables, tofu, or bread. You can also mellow miso by adding a little sweetness to it. Maple syrup is a good medium; so is agave syrup or a bit of rice mirin.

Types of Miso

Mugi: made from soybeans and barley; is dense and strong, aged long.

Hatcho: made from soybeans and sea salt; dark and robust, salty with a hint of sourness.

Genmai: made from soybeans and brown rice; light, mellow and sweet.

Kome: made from soybeans and white rice; red and creamy, has the highest salt content.

Natto: made from soybeans and ginger; not used in soup but as a table condiment, eaten with rice.

TOMIKO'S MISO SHOW

Serves 4 to 6   GMENY

USING MISO

- You can use miso to enhance the flavor and nutritional value of many varied dishes such as casseroles, gravies, chili, beans and stews
- You can substitute 2 T miso for 1 t salt.
- Vegetable stock seasoned with miso can easily be substituted in recipes calling for chicken or beef stock.
- 1 T of miso can be mixed into a cup of hot water for a low-calorie broth that has a surprising depth of flavor.

The possibilities of replacing miso for salt can be very creative.

There are a few culinary items that fascinate me; miso is one of them. My friend Tomiko was about to have a miso demonstration for a few friends when she stumbled and injured her foot. Bandaged and a bit wobbly, Tomiko took her place at the counter and proceeded to direct the miso show. We, her loyal followers, chopped all the ingredients. How lovely they looked all sitting in bowls waiting for the show to begin. We were soon creating the ultimate miso soup—probably the simplest and yet most amazing complete meal on the planet.

8 pieces kombu (kelp)
1 C shiitake mushrooms (dried)
6 C water or vegetable stock
Vegetables: green beans, carrots, and daikon, cut thin or small for a variety of color and taste
½ wakame, dried (seaweed)
¾ C soft tofu, cubed
¼ C red miso paste
Garnish: 4 green onions, scallions, chopped very tiny

1. WIPE the whitish powder off the seaweed (kombu) with a damp cloth, do not wash under water. Cover kombu with water and soak overnight or for at least 8 hours, drain.
2. SOAK the mushrooms (in enough water to cover) overnight or for at least 8 hours. Drain and chop small.
3. COMBINE fresh water or vegetable stock with soaked and drained kombu and shiitake and begin to cook. It is important to remove the kombu pieces just before the mixture boils. Turn down the flame and simmer until mushrooms are soft (about 20 to 30 minutes).
4. COOK vegetables by lightly steaming them.
5. RECONSTITUTE wakame by combining with warm water and let stand 15 minutes; drain.
6. CUT tofu into small cubes.
7. WHISK miso with 1 C soup stock until well incorporated.
8. ADD miso liquid back into soup along with wakame, tofu and steamed veggies. Do not bring to a boil or it will kill the beneficial enzymes.
9. TOP with green onions for garnish.

ORANGE ALMOND MISO VINAIGRETTE

Makes 1½ Cups   G M E Y

This dressing can be used for salads or as a tofu marinade. Almond butter is a great companion of miso, a good substitute for the peanut butter and together almonds and miso are protein rich.

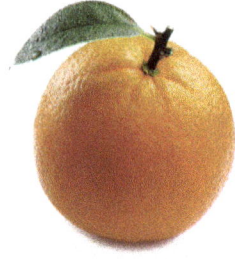

2 T light yellow miso
¼ C rice wine vinegar or mirin
1 t honey, agave, or maple syrup
2 T almond butter
Zest of 1 orange
3 T orange juice, squeezed fresh
1 T black sesame oil (optional)
⅓ C avocado oil

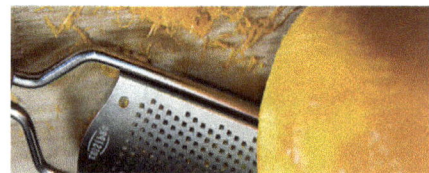

1. COMBINE miso, vinegar, sweetener, and almond butter until well-mixed.
2. PLACE over low heat and cook, stirring constantly until the mixture thickens to the consistency of original miso paste. Watch carefully, and remove from heat before it begins to boil.
3. STIR in the orange zest and orange juice.
4. WHISK in the oils.

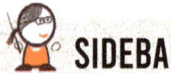 **SIDEBAR**   ALL ABOUT ALMOND BUTTER

Like other nut butters, almond butter retains the nutritional value of the almonds it comes from. It is rich in protein, fiber, and essential fatty acids and makes a good replacement for a peanut allergy. The uses for almond butter are as varied as they are for peanut butter. It can be used as a spread, mixed into sauces and dressings, eaten plain, or used as an ingredient in desserts. The flavor is actually quite similar to peanut butter, with a subtle hint of almonds.

There are a number of different styles of almond butter, starting with toasted or raw. Toasted almond butter has a richer flavor, but some people prefer the milder taste of raw almond butter. The smoothest and creamiest is made from almonds that have been blanched to remove their skins, and then finely ground. More chunky versions include almond skin and are not ground as finely. The fat in almond butter can cause it to go rancid, so it should always be kept in a cool, dry place, until it is opened and refrigerate after opening.

MISO SAUCE & SPREAD

Makes 1 Cup

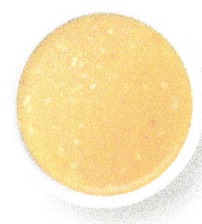

SIMPLE SESAME-MISO DIPPING SAUCE

Serve as a sauce for blanched and chilled vegetables or any raw vegetables like celery and carrot sticks.

2 T tahini (sesame paste) almond or peanut butter
2 T white miso, sweet and light
1 T lemon juice, or more to taste
1 T black sesame oil
1 to 3 T water
2 T tamari or soy sauce
2 T toasted sesame seeds

1. MIX tahini or nut butter with miso in a bowl and add lemon juice. thin sauce with a small amount of water until slightly thickened, depending how thick you want it.
2. WHISK in oil and soy sauce and top with toasted sesame seeds.

Makes 1 Cup

MISO WALNUT SPREAD

This is a thick spread, great on whole grain bread or crackers.

1 C walnuts, dry roasted
1 T robust red miso and 1 T tamari
4 T water
2 T avocado oil
¼ C scallions, finely chopped
¼ C mushrooms, chopped very small

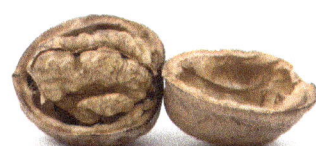

1. PLACE roasted walnuts in a food processor or blender and finely grind.
2. MIX water, miso and tamari in a small saucepan and heat, stirring the miso constantly to dissolve.
3. SAUTÉ scallions and mushrooms in oil until tender.
4. MIX cooked vegetables and ground walnuts into pot with miso mixture.
5. HEAT, stirring frequently for 2 to 3 minutes; return to blender and blend until smooth.

CLASSIC MISO STIR FRY

Serves 4 to 6

GMENY

BUYING AND STORING MISO

Miso can be found in the refrigerated section at natural food stores, and well-stocked supermarkets. Look for naturally aged brands with no additives.

It may be stored in the refrigerator for up to a year but should ideally be used within two months to take advantage of its optimal aroma and health properties.

This is a perfect, everyday dish, that you can use with whatever vegetables are on hand.

2 T avocado oil
½ t red chili flakes
½ t turmeric powder
½ t ginger powder
½ t cumin powder
½ t coriander powder
1 C firm tofu, cubed (optional)
1 red or green pepper, chopped
1 C mushrooms, chopped
3 C broccoli or cauliflower heads, chopped
1 C carrots, sliced thin
1 t tamari or soy sauce
2 T red miso mixed with ¼ C water until a thick paste

1. HEAT oil and add chili flakes; cook for a minute until they brown.
2. ADD the rest of the spices, cook 1 minute.
3. ADD tofu, peppers and mushrooms and stir fry for a few minutes. Then add broccoli or cauliflower, and carrots.
4. FRY on a medium to low heat, with the lid on, until vegetables are just about tender.
5. ADD tamari and red miso paste; fry with lid off for another two minutes.

 SIDEBAR   MISO FACTS

Miso is high in *umami*, which is the fifth basic Japanese taste described as savoriness. The longer miso is aged, the more complex its flavor. Miso is about 8 to 14 percent salt, but most of its intense and complex flavor comes from fermentation. A tablespoon of miso contains 680 mg. of sodium compared to a tablespoon of table salt at 6,589 mg. of sodium so it's a great substitute for a low-sodium diet. For recipes that require heat, it's best to add the miso at the end. Never bring to a boil.

CHAPTER NINE
GUEST RECIPES

KI'S

GARDEN TASTE

KITCHEN CONSCIOUSNESS

BAKING AT THE EDGE OF THE UNIVERSE

DASAPRAKASH

KI'S

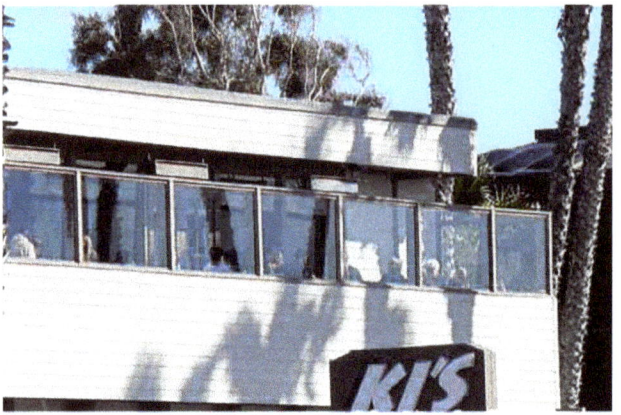

Ki's, before it was renovated.

KI'S IS A RESTAURANT PERCHED ON THE CALIFORNIA COAST between Encinitas and Del Mar, a half hour north of San Diego. Two things make this eating place unique: its beautiful location and its selection of organic specialty foods. We have held many informal meetings during sunset, lasting long after moonrise, while eating an organic salad or tofu burrito. So we were delighted when a friend set up a meeting with Ki, who was kind enough to meet with us to share a bit about herself and the history of this restaurant.

We arrived on an El Niño Saturday. The surf was wild and wonderful—it had hailed just moments before but now the sun was shining, and the clouds whirled through the sky. The outside patio had been closed because of the weather, which had happened only three times since the restaurant opened.

Ki arrived holding a plate with one of her famous millet patties, topped with her famous sunflower dressing and an avocado. Just back from Los Angeles, Ki was excited about a conference on integrated medicine she had just attended. She said she was encouraged about how doctors were beginning to truly address the mind-body relationship.

So, what made this Midwestern housewife into an innovative natural gourmet? Ki told us how as a mother she became interested in cooking. Her family moved to San Diego in 1971 so that her husband could finish his doctorate here. She also returned to school, minoring in nutrition. Always interested in health and cooking, one thing led to another, and she opened one of the earliest health food stores in San Diego County. She had a hot plate in the back of her store and began making veggie stew, which she reports is still her most popular dish today. It was a slow beginning during the early 1980s, but soon she increased her offerings. Due to its popularity, the restaurant ran out of room in the small storefront. Ki moved to the current location, continuing to develop new recipes and watch the restaurant grow year by year.

I asked Ki why she chose millet for her signature burger. She said that she remembered reading that millet was considered a "supergrain," one of only three grains that are more alkaline, making it extremely easy to digest. She had been suffering from a spastic colon and discovered that simple grains and more alkaline, non-acidic organic vegetables turned her health around. After many experiments, she and her cooks came up with Ki's Millet Burger.

We were quite astounded when we learned that the lively and vibrant redheaded woman before us was 72 years young. She attributed her vitality to her dedication to organic food that is wholesome and easily digestible. Ki bade us goodbye, suggesting we try the butternut squash burrito, brown rice, and black beans. We took her advice and sat on the upper floor enclosure, listening to the ocean pound the rocky shore, and enjoying Ki's wholesome food. She was gracious to share a few recipes from her repertoire.

GRILLED TEMPEH MARINADE

Makes 1 Cup

GMENY

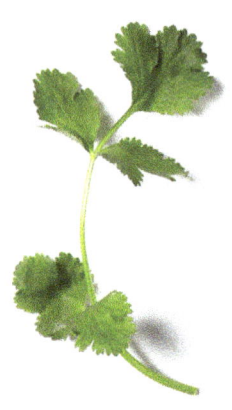

⅓ C olive oil
½ C fresh lime juice
2 T water and 2 T tamari
½ bunch cilantro
2 garlic cloves, chopped fine
1 (8 oz.) package tempeh

1. BLEND first four liquid ingredients, then add cilantro and garlic.
2. MARINATE the tempeh steaks for at least 2 hours. (If tempeh is more than ¾ inch thick, cut down the center to make thinner, and allow it to marinate in 2 hours. Tempeh should start to absorb the liquid after 1 hour and will begin to expand, and the texture should begin to soften. The more tender you like it, the longer you should marinate it.)
3. REMOVE tempeh from the liquid and grill for approximately 4 minutes on each side.
4. TOP with avocado salsa (next page).

 SIDEBAR TEMPEH

Tempeh has been a favorite food and staple source of protein in Indonesia for several hundred years. It has a firm and crunchy texture and a rich, nutty mushroom-like flavor. Although tempeh can be used in different ways, it is often sliced and fried until the surface is crisp and golden brown. It can be tossed into soups, spreads, salads, and sandwiches. Containing health-promoting ingredients, such as essential amino acids, tempeh contains all of the fiber of soybeans and grains and offers digestive benefits from the enzymes created during the fermentation process. The process is made by the controlled fermentation of cooked soybeans with a Rhizopus mold (tempeh starter). The tempeh fermentation by the Rhizopus mold binds the soybeans into a compact white cake. Tempeh fermentation also produces natural antibiotic agents, which are thought to increase the body's resistance to intestinal infections, while the fermentation leaves the desirable soy isoflavones intact.

AVOCADO SALSA

Serves 4 to 6

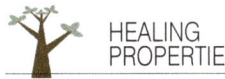

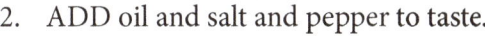

HEALING PROPERTIES

Avocado
- Contains oleic acid, which may help lower cholesterol
- Good source of potassium, helps to guard against circulatory disease
- Has high value of folate, which helps to lower risk of cardiovascular disease

2 large tomatoes, seeded and diced
1 large avocado, diced (not mashed)
½ red onion, chopped fine or oven roasted, cooled and chopped
1 lime, juiced
½ C cilantro, de-stemmed and chopped fine
1 jalapeño, medium size, de-seeded and chopped fine
1 T olive oil
Salt and pepper to taste

1. COMBINE all ingredients except oil and salt and pepper in large bowl using a wooden spoon.
2. ADD oil and salt and pepper to taste.

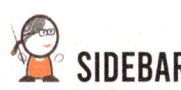

SIDEBAR   ALL ABOUT AVOCADOS

Since avocados don't start to ripen until they are picked, most avocado aficionados suggest selecting an avocado that is heavy for its size and blemish free. If you want to use it right away, it should feel firm, yet give in slightly when pressed. Although there are many varieties of avocado, those grown in California are usually smaller varieties with a dark pebbly skin that tends to get darker as it ripens. Those grown in Florida are larger with a smooth, bright green skin that usually changes little with ripening. Therefore, color is not a reliable indicator of ripeness.

To speed up ripening, place the firm avocados in a paper bag with a banana or an apple and store at room temperature. They should ripen in a day or so. For even faster ripening, a more dramatic way is to microwave each avocado for 15 seconds before putting them in the bag. Avocados can be frozen if they are puréed first. Ripen fruit until they are soft enough to yield to gentle pressure, remove the peel and pit, and puree the flesh with ½ tablespoon lemon juice for every avocado. Package the puree in firm freezer containers and use within 4 to 5 months. It is best to add the other ingredients for your guacamole to the thawed puree just before serving.

KI'S ROASTED VEGETABLES

Serves 4 to 5 | Preheat Oven to 350 Degrees | Bake: 20 to 30 Minutes   GMENSY

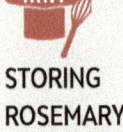

STORING ROSEMARY

Fresh rosemary should be stored in the refrigerator either in its original packaging or wrapped in a slightly damp paper towel.

3 T olive oil
1 eggplant, sliced ½" thick
2 yellow squashes, sliced lengthwise ½" thick
2 zucchinis, sliced lengthwise ½" thick
1½ pounds baby red potatoes
1 red bell pepper, julienne sliced
5 whole garlic cloves
1 red onion, julienne sliced
1 t salt and freshly ground pepper
1 t rosemary, fresh, chopped finely

1. BRUSH sheet pan lightly with 1 T olive oil and place eggplant, squash, and potatoes directly on pan.
2. SPRINKLE garlic cloves, onion, and bell pepper on top of the squash.
3. DRIZZLE or spray vegetables lightly with 2 T olive oil; sprinkle salt, pepper, and rosemary and place a separate baking pan on top as a lid.
4. BAKE until tender.

ROASTED TOFU

Serves 4 to 5 | Preheat Oven to 350 Degrees | Bake: 20 to 30 Minutes   GMENY

Wanting to find a way to introduce people to soy products, especially those who may not be able to tolerate the taste, Ki created a very simple dish—a tofu marinade that is baked. By adding tofu to burritos and salad, Ki found an easy way to get reluctant people to eat soy. This goes great on salads, soups, stir-fries, or simply as a side dish.

One cake of firm tofu cut into ½ inch cubes
3 T tamari
Dark sesame oil, a few drops (optional)
½ C vegetable broth
¼ C any prepared salad dressing and ½ C barbecue sauce
Olive oil

1. SOAK tofu 10 to 15 minutes in marinade, add to an oiled baking pan, drizzle with oil and bake until golden brown.

GARDEN TASTE

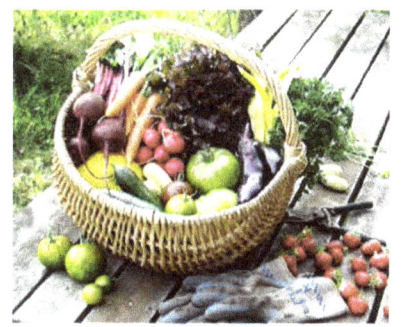

Garlic Connection

Sheila was a big proponent of using garlic in most of her recipes. Though garlic has many great health benefits, there are certain people like myself who can't easily digest fresh garlic. Roasting garlic or simply omitting it in a recipe is always an option.

ONE DAY WE DISCOVERED THIS SMALL CAFE in the seaside town of Del Mar, a half hour ride up the Pacific Coast from San Diego. The name "Garden Taste" sounded interesting. What we found was a unique and special vegan (vegetarian, dairy-free alternatives, sprouted grains) restaurant. Shredded organic carrots, beets, cucumbers, pickled ginger, and other vegetables brimmed from salad bowls, burst from burritos, and complemented garden burgers served on kamut rolls.

As the sun set on the ocean three blocks away, we visited Garden Taste to get some recipes and learn about Sheila Gabayson's philosophy on "living foods." As a customer ate a bowl of split pea soup in front of us, Sheila spoke softly about how 35 years ago she became interested in whole foods and how this interest evolved into an organic, dairy and wheat-free diet. Sheila explained why most of her dishes include sprouts—saying that sprouting transforms seeds and grains into predigested enzymes making food easier to digest. In fact, filled with life-giving oxygen, sprouts become healing food that repairs the body and gives an added boost of energy.

Organic vegetables are the core element in any Garden Taste meal; they are mostly shredded and top just about everything. Sheila was quite passionate when talking about organic vegetables and about wheat grass juice—a concentrated pure food—that goes straight into the bloodstream. She explained, "When nonorganic vegetables are made into juice the chemicals become concentrated and the juice not only loses its vitality, but is simply not healthy." The following recipes are Garden Taste classics. The restaurant has long since gone out of business. I suspect Sheila retired but the "living food" philosophy and interest in organic food has recently been embraced in mainstream stores and restaurants throughout the country.

SHEILA'S FAMOUS GARDEN TASTE ROLL

Serves 4

GMENY

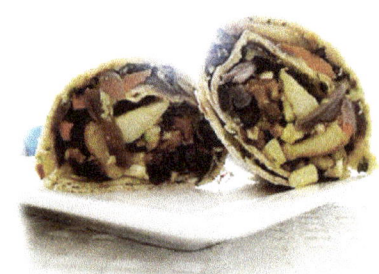

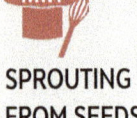

SPROUTING FROM SEEDS

Use an opaque, nonmetallic vessel, top with cheesecloth or punch holes in the top of a jar cap. Rinse 1 cup of grains or seeds and soak overnight. Drain and keep them moist by rinsing and draining a few times a day. It takes 3 to 5 days for the sprouts to begin.

Refrigerate in a sealed container. They will stay fresh for about a week.

Sunflower Seed Spread
2 C sunflower seeds, sprouted
¼ C parsley
2 garlic cloves
1 green onion, chopped
⅛ C soy sauce
⅛ C fresh lemon juice
1 t cumin powder
Pinch of cayenne pepper

1. BLEND ingredients in a food processor or blender. While blending, add a minimum amount of water to make into a spreadable consistency.

Additional ingredients for Garden Taste Roll
Shredded vegetables—carrots, beets, zucchini, cabbage, cucumber
Sprouts of any kind
Pickled ginger, available in Asian specialty or health food stores
Olives, black, chopped small
Raw sauerkraut
Sprouted whole wheat or gluten-free tortillas

1. SPREAD the sunflower seed spread generously (about ¼ C) on a heated tortilla.
2. TOP with shredded vegetables, sprouts, pickled ginger, olives, and sauerkraut.
3. ROLL up tightly and cut in half. You can use toothpicks to keep the roll in place.

 SIDEBAR   SAUERKRAUT

Fermenting cabbage produces a number of different compounds, known as isothiocyanates, which are now being studied as beneficial for cancer prevention. Previous studies have found that isothiocyanates induce precancerous cells in the digestive system to self-destruct.

CLASSIC LENTIL SOUP

Serves 4 to 6

GMENY

 **SIDEBAR**

DILL

Dill has a long history. It was used in Egypt about 5,000 years ago. The Greeks and Romans also used dill to treat ailments. It then traveled to Northern Europe in the Middle Ages to cure hiccups, while the seeds and leaves were added to sauces and pickles.

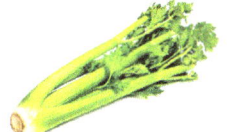

An all-time Garden Taste *favorite, we always managed to share a bowl of this soup; it is a good starter to any meal. The cumin and ginger aid digestion.*

1 C brown lentils, soaked overnight or sprouted for two days
1½ T cumin powder (for this soup it is best if you roast cumin seeds and freshly grind them).
1 T oregano, dried
1 T fresh dill, chopped
1 C celery, chopped very small
1 C carrots, shredded
1 C zucchini, shredded
2 garlic cloves, chopped
1 red onion, chopped very fine
2 t fresh ginger, grated or minced
A generous pinch of cayenne or chipotle pepper powder
2 T Braggs Liquid Aminos to taste

1. COMBINE the above ingredients except soy sauce in a large pot.
2. ADD five to six cups of water, and cook slowly until lentils are very soft, about 45 minutes.
3. ADD Braggs and simmer another five minutes. You can slightly blend for a creamier texture.

 SIDEBAR   **LENTILS**

Lentils are an ancient food, and they store really well in a cool, dry spot. In fact, they can last for up to a full year. We once invested in a 50-lb. bag of brown lentils and stored them in a small room off the farm kitchen used as a pantry. We had a bunch of lentil recipes to draw from, but even then, I'm not sure we actually used up all those lentils!

Before cooking, rinse lentils, pick out any stones and other debris. Unlike dried beans and peas, there's no need to soak them, although soaking and sprouting does aid in digestion. Lentils cook slowly if they're combined with salt or acidic ingredients, so add these at the last stage of cooking. Bigger or older lentils take longer to cook, don't cook in a pressure cooker as they can foam and may clog the valve. Yes, once I experienced the clean-up that resulted from lentils sticking to the ceiling. I will never repeat that mistake!

GARDEN TASTE SALAD WITH SESAME DRESSING

Serves 4 to 6   G M E N Y

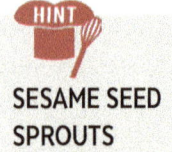

SESAME SEED SPROUTS

Only unhulled seeds will sprout. Harvest sprouts after 3 to 4 days.

On a bed of organic lettuce, add any variety of shredded organic vegetables such as carrots, zucchini, red cabbage, beets, etc. Top with this lemony wonderful blended dressing.

1 C sesame seeds, sprouted (see page 190)
2 C water
1 t soy sauce
¼ C parsley, chopped
¼ C lemon juice and ¼ t lemon zest
¼ t cumin powder
¼ t black pepper, freshly ground
¼ C green onion, chopped very small
2 garlic cloves, minced

1. MIX together and then whirl in an electric blender.

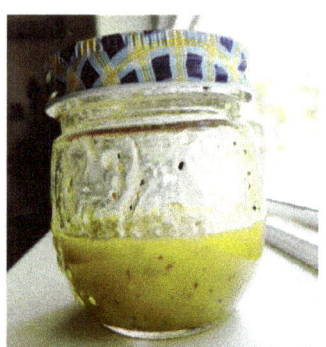

The Cold Chaser

While visiting with Sheila from Garden Taste, she mentioned a special blend she called her "cold chaser." Just before we left, Matthew ordered a cold chaser to go. It was quite spicy and unpleasant tasting, as some powerful things are . . . but what appears to be unpleasant is actually just what one needs at the moment! Combine and blend well in an electric blender.

　¾ C fresh orange juice
　1 clove garlic (2 cloves for the brave)
　⅛ C fresh lemon juice
　1 T minced ginger

KITCHEN CONSCIOUSNESS

by Ginna Bell Bragg

"When I enter the kitchen, I leave my thoughts outside the door, as a Moslem removes his shoes before entering the mosque."

THIS PARAPHRASING OF PICASSO'S FEELINGS about his studio expresses the basics of "Kitchen Consciousness," a concept conceived in my tipi at Rainbow Ranch in Calistoga and grew in my kitchen at the *Chopra Center for Well Being* (now located in La Costa, California.)

In 1991, I discovered Dr. Deepak Chopra by reading *Perfect Health*. The principles of Ayurveda, which he described clearly resonated with my heart and soul. Ayurveda is a Sanskrit word meaning the Science or Knowledge of Life. In ancient Vedic texts, the Rishis defined an approach to health based on man's link to the five elements: air, earth, fire, water, and ether. Our bodies are made of these elements, as they are the threads which hold the universe together. The idea that nutritional balance is enhanced by providing all six tastes (sweet, sour, salty, bitter, pungent, and astringent) at every meal, as well as eating the foods that best suit your unique body type, or *dosha*, made sense to me. I immediately began practicing the principles of Ayurveda in my own kitchen, taking the test to determine my body type, and embarking on the journey of discovery about the appropriate foods for my own perfect health.

At the same time, I began "loving" food, practicing the art of shedding all thought before beginning the task of cooking, and putting all my love into the process, whether cooking just for myself or for a group of 60.

I realized that, if all we are is a vibrating mass of energy and light, that energy goes into every handshake, every kiss, every act we perform. Every carrot chopped has my energy in it; every vegetable sliced can either contain my chaos or my bliss, my anger or my love.

In Oneness we can share misery or in Oneness we can share joy. Kitchen Consciousness was born out of a desire to teach assistants in the kitchen how to "become the task" of cooking: to step out of mundane thought and enter the spiritual realm. It was as if there was a specially marked box outside the door, "Leave thoughts here."

The marriage of Kitchen Consciousness and Ayurveda is a blessed one. According to Ayurveda, the ancient system of healing from India, we each inherit a proportion of three basic mind-body principles, or *doshas*, which contribute to our unique mental and physical characteristics, and are comprised of several of the five elements. Most of us have one or two most dominant, with the other one (or two) less significant. The three doshas are *Vata, Pitta* and *Kapha*.

Vata body types tend to be thin, light, and quick in thought and actions. Change is constant. When *Vata* is balanced, we are creative, enthusiastic and lively; when unbalanced, our digestion may become irregular, and we may develop anxiety or insomnia.

If *Pitta* is most dominant in our prakruti, or nature, we tend to be muscular, smart, and very determined. When balanced, a *Pitta* type is warm, intelligent, and a strong leader; if out of balance, *Pitta* can be critical, irritable and aggressive.

If *Kapha* is strongest in our nature, we are heavier of frame, think and move with leisure and are stable. In balance, *Kaphas* are calm, sweet, and loyal; in excess, *Kapha* can cause us to gain weight, be congested, and be resistant to change.

Even the briefest overview of Ayurveda would not be possible without stressing the importance of the Body Intelligence Techniques, or BITs. These little morsels of information carry great genius in their simplicity. My favorite is "Eat in a settled atmosphere." Imagine: the table is set, a lovely, luscious meal is prepared. Candles are lit and flowers fill lovely vases. You dress for dinner and enter the room, prepared to sit down with your loved ones to a family repast. Something is out of kilter . . . ah, yes; the television is on, blasting the evening news. There is some violence and aggression. Face it, news worthiness is rarely made of love, harmony, and bliss. Before you sit down to eat, be sure that the television has been put to rest for this time; otherwise, you will be ingesting the national newscast

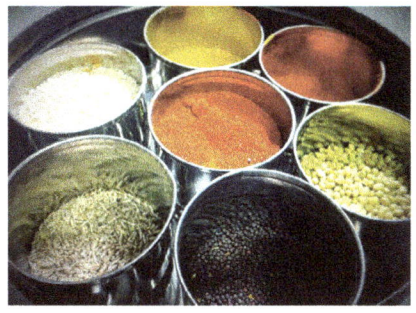

right along with your vegetarian feast.

In *A Simple Celebration*, we place emphasis on what Dr. David Simon, and I call "FLUNC" foods: Frozen, Leftover, Unnatural, Nuked, or Canned. Although the ancient rishis (sages) said that if you think about God while you are eating, you can eat anything and receive its nourishment (my paraphrase), we believe it is important to bless your body with the purest foods, as well as live your life with the purest of intentions. The most *prana*, or life force, is found in foods that are fresh, organic, and cooked with your love.

And so, enjoy these recipes from the kitchen of one who loves. Bring your mind to rest, turn off the television, light a candle, and enter the sacred space of your studio of nourishment. I promise you culinary joy, spiritual ecstasy.

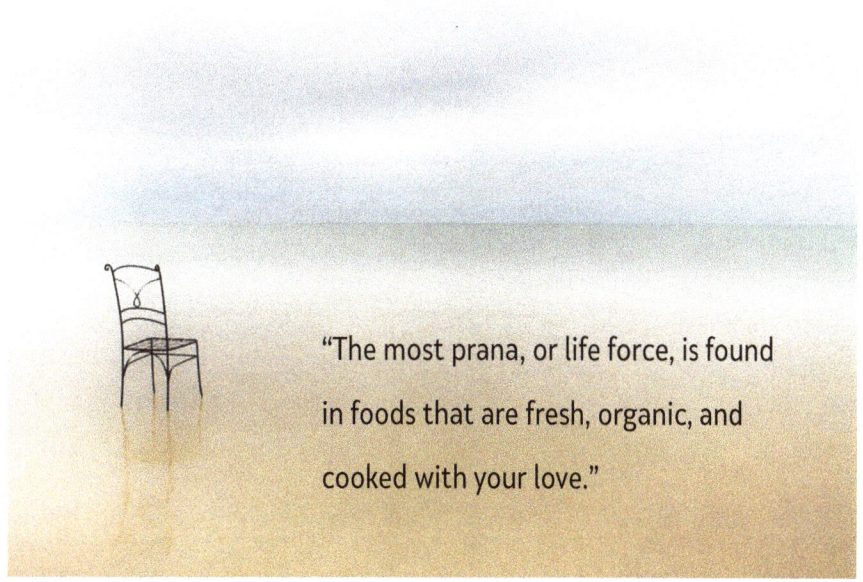

"The most prana, or life force, is found in foods that are fresh, organic, and cooked with your love."

RED LENTIL DAHL

GMENSY

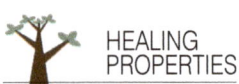

HEALING PROPERTIES

Fenugreek
- A mild laxative and for loss of appetite
- A useful aid in the treatment of diabetes

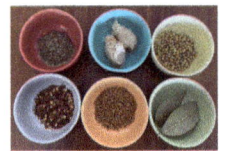

This dahl is great for a large group. Because this dish contains a lot of ingredients, being organized before you begin preparing it will make your job easier. I like to have all the spices ready before I start cooking, putting roasted and ground seeds, grated ginger, chopped raisins, and the other ingredients on hand and ready to grab in small pinch bowls.

1 quart dry red lentils (4 cups)
Enough vegetable stock to cover lentils plus 4 inches
⅛ C cumin seeds, roasted, freshly ground
⅛ C coriander seeds, roasted, freshly ground
1 t turmeric
2 T ghee or avocado oil
2 t black mustard seeds and 2 t cumin seeds
Large pinch whole fenugreek
5 cardamom pods, crushed slightly
3 cinnamon sticks and 2 bay leaves
Large pinch asafetida
1 cup leeks, chopped
2" piece fresh ginger, grated
1 C golden raisins, chopped
½ C water
2 T tomato paste
½ to 1 T salt
Chopped cilantro for garnish

Serves 8 to 10

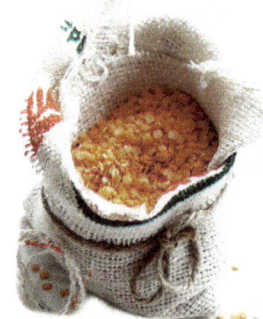

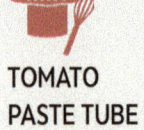

TOMATO PASTE TUBE

A simple way to have organic tomato paste on hand is to buy it as a toothpaste-style tube and use a little at a time and refrigerate the rest.

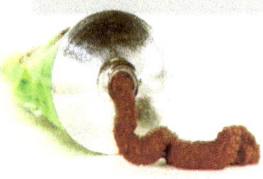

1. COOK lentils for 1 hour until they fall apart (just when the lentils begin to boil, skim foam from top until foam subsides.)
2. ADD ground cumin, coriander, and turmeric powder. Simmer 5 minutes.
3. HEAT ghee or oil in skillet and mustard seeds, cumin seeds, fenugreek, cardamom pods, bay leaves, and cinnamon sticks. Let sizzle until seeds pop. Add asafetida and leeks. Sauté until leeks are soft.
4. ADD ginger and raisins. Sauté 5 minutes.
5. ADD ½ C water, tomato paste and salt. Continue cooking 5 minutes. Introduce spice mixture to lentils, remove cinnamon sticks, bay leaves and cardamom pods before serving and top with cilantro.

WHOLE WHEAT CHAPATIS

Makes 25 to 30 Chapatis

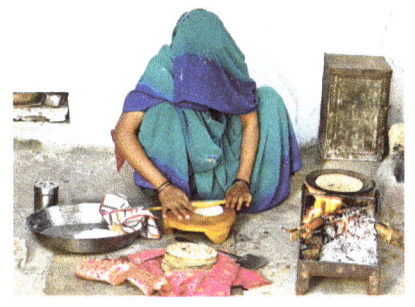

Chapatis are a good yeast-free flat bread. This lighter version is made with wheat pastry flour, but there are a variety of light, gluten-free flours you can work with, too.

2 to 2¼ C whole wheat pastry flour or gluten-free flour blend
2 t avocado oil or ghee
1¼ cups lukewarm water, approximately
1 t salt
Small bowl of extra flour

1. MIX 2 C flour and oil in a large bowl. Add water and mix into a wet dough, add more flour, only if needed. Cover and let stand for an hour. Oil hands and make small balls. Roll balls in small bowl of flour. Using a rolling pin, roll out on a floured surface to form 6-inch circles.
2. HEAT large skillet or griddle to medium.
3. COOK ½ minute on first side, and about 1 minute on second side, press down with a paper towel, to encourage it to puff.
4. SERVE immediately or keep covered with a towel, until ready to use.

 SIDEBAR CHAPATIS

Making chapatis can be quite an art form. You get used to the feel of the dough after a few tries. I start with a slightly wet dough and slowly add just enough flour to let it roll out. I remember the first time it fully popped up, it reminded me of a frog, so from that day onward I can't think of chapatis without thinking of frogs! There may be nothing as heavenly as "hot-hot" chapatis with ghee or margarine to lap up a vegetable curry. It's worth the effort and time to make them fresh. Once you get the hang of it, it's quite simple and can be made quickly. Having a second hand in the kitchen to cook them while you roll them out is an invaluable help and sends steaming hot chapatis to the table, one after the other. I often made them for dinner in South India to supplement the overabundance of rice meals. One time I noticed some monkeys watching me from the window and chatting to themselves. As luck would have it, I left the side door open for just a brief moment, but it was enough time for them to quickly prance into the cottage and steal the entire plate of warm chapatis. From the advantage of a tall limb in a tree next to the cottage, the monkey family ate the bread picking out the brown circled spots and throwing down the rest of the bread. I'm convinced I saw a smile on their faces.

TOMATO VEGETABLE SAUCE

Serves 4 to 6

GMENSY

STORING TOMATOES

For best flavor, store tomatoes at room temperature. To speed up the ripening process, place tomatoes in a brown paper bag. Refrigerate whole tomatoes only if fully ripe, and then only for a few days.

This is a great recipe for tomato harvest time when gardens everywhere are in a profusion of blossoms and often yield too many ripe tomatoes at the same time. For the best flavor, let the sauce stand at room temperature for a few hours to absorb all the flavors.

2 tablespoons ghee or olive oil
3 garlic cloves, minced
1 leek, cleaned really well, chopped
1 green pepper, minced
½ lb. mushrooms, chopped
1 bunch celery, chopped
2 zucchinis, chopped
3 carrots, shredded
6 pounds tomatoes, chopped
1 bunch parsley, chopped
1 T dried basil, 1 T dried rosemary, ground
1 t dried thyme, 1 t dried oregano
½ t nutmeg
½ to ¾ t salt

1. SAUTÉ garlic, leeks, and pepper in hot ghee or olive oil for 2 minutes.
2. ADD mushrooms, celery, zucchini, and carrots and sauté for 2 minutes.
3. ADD remaining ingredients and simmer on low heat until most of the liquid is gone, about two hours.
4. BLEND with hand mixer. Cool.
5. SERVE over fresh pasta or rice or use as a soup base.

 SIDEBAR   THE HEALTH PROPERTIES OF TOMATOES

Long considered poisonous, perhaps because the leaves and stems do indeed contain a toxic alkaloid, tomatoes are perhaps one of the healthiest and important vegetables due to their lycopene content. Lycopenes are part of the family of pigments called carotenoids, which are natural compounds that form the colors of fruits and vegetables. Research shows that lycopenes are the most powerful antioxidants in the carotenoid family. They include vitamins C and E, which are important in protecting the body from free radicals that degrade many parts of the body.

PUMPKIN PASTA SALAD

Serves 4 to 6

GMENY

PUMPKIN SEEDS

Pepitas are Mexican pumpkin seeds. They are green compared to other pumpkin seeds and sold raw or salted. For a lovely snack, buy them raw, roast them in olive oil and sprinkle with salt and a dash of cayenne pepper. If you can't find pepitas you can use raw pumpkin seeds instead.

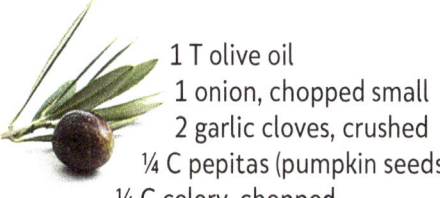

1 T olive oil
1 onion, chopped small
2 garlic cloves, crushed
¼ C pepitas (pumpkin seeds)
¼ C celery, chopped
½ C golden raisins, chopped and ¼ C Kalamata olives, pitted
1 T dry onion flakes
¼ C fresh basil, chopped and ½ C carrots, grated
3 T sun-dried tomatoes
½ C feta cheese, optional
1-pound fresh whole grain pasta, any shape, orzo works really well, as well as gluten-free varieties. Cook according to package directions.

Dressing
⅛ C oil from sun-dried tomatoes or olive oil
1 T Braggs Liquid Aminos
Dash balsamic vinegar
1 t honey
1 t lemon juice
Salt and pepper to taste

1. SAUTÉ onions, garlic, pepitas, celery, raisins, and olives in olive oil for a few minutes.
2. TOSS with remaining ingredients.
3. ADD dressing.
4. SERVE at room temperature.

 MAKE YOUR OWN SUNDRIED TOMATOES IN OIL

Cut Roma tomatoes into quarters (you can also try this with cherry tomatoes, cut in halves.) Place cut tomatoes on a baking sheet and sprinkle lightly with coarse salt. Place in oven at 175 degrees for 8 hours. Larger pieces may require more time. Cool completely and store in a glass jar filled with olive oil to cover tomatoes; they also freeze well. To freeze: place individual tomato pieces on a cookie sheet. Freeze, then remove and place in a Ziplock bag.

If you use the tomato oil in a recipe, add more oil to top the tomatoes for further preservation and storage. You can also use this flavored olive oil in many different recipes.

FRENCH BREAD

Makes 2 Loaves | Preheat Oven to 400 Degrees | Bake: 40 Minutes   M E N S

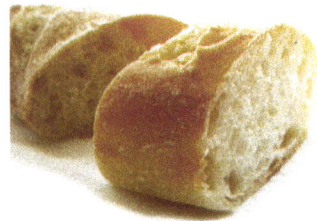

- 2 T active dry yeast (see "Yeast and Salt" Hint page 91)
- 2 T turbinado or organic raw cane juice sugar
- 4 C lukewarm water
- 8 C sifted organic, unbleached white flour, or a mixture of white and whole wheat pastry flour
- 1 T sea salt

This is a simple and basic bread. You can add herbs to the dry flour for a savory flavor. Add 1 t finely cut fresh rosemary and thyme or ½ t dried herbs, it's a perfect blend.

1. DISSOLVE yeast and sugar in 2 C of warm water. Let stand for 10 minutes.
2. STIR yeast mixture into flour and add salt.
3. ADD just enough warm water to hold dough together—it will form a soft, sticky dough. Knead in bowl for about 5 minutes.
4. COVER and let rise until double—about 2 to 4 hours. If you set it near a warm stove or oven, it will rise faster.
5. PUNCH down with your hand and divide into loaves—two medium loaf pans, or one large one. Clay loaf pans are best.
6. RISE again for 25 minutes or until risen over the top of the pans.
7. BAKE until brown and crusty.

 SIDEBAR   **YEAST FACTS**

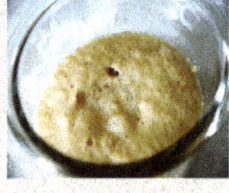

Make sure ingredients are room temperature so the yeast works quicker.

- **Instant Yeast**: is more finely ground and thus absorbs moisture faster, rapidly converting starch and sugars to carbon dioxide, the tiny bubbles that make the dough expand and stretch.
- **Active Dry Yeast**: 1 package is 2¼ t and is equal to 1 cake of compressed yeast.
- **Blooming Yeast**: You can test to see if your active dry yeast is good by adding one-half teaspoon of sugar to the yeast when stirring it into the water to dissolve. If it foams and bubbles within 10 minutes you know the yeast is alive and active.
- **Yeast Temperatures**: Yeast feeds on the sugar and starch. The temperature that is best suited to the multiplication of yeast cells and the leavening and lightening of the dough is between 70 and 90 degrees. Yeast is destroyed by heat at a temperature of 132 degrees and also by cold at approximately 40 degrees.
- **Handling Yeast**: It's important to wash your hands after using yeast. It's a live organism and you can actually pick up a yeast infection from it.

BAKING AT THE EDGE OF THE UNIVERSE

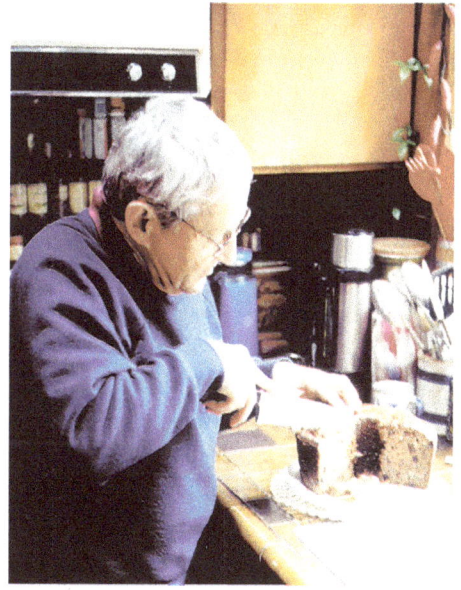

Nathan McMahon

THE SUN PEEKED THROUGH THE REDWOOD TREETOPS. It was the first warm and sunny day we experienced in our few winter days visiting Sonoma County, the Northern wine-country area in California. We inched our way along the dirt road that skirted the Armstrong State Forest on our way to Nathan's hermitage. Nathan lives among the redwoods and Northern pine, creating a self-sufficient universe for himself. It began over 50 years ago when he scraped together enough money to buy fifty acres of pristine forest amidst waterfalls and towering evergreen. He built his own house and created a garden of over 200 plants and a bamboo forest.

What struck me about Nathan was his childlike nature—filled with boundless love. Though he chose this solitary existence, throughout his life he touched people in simple, silent acts. Almost everyone in a twenty-mile radius was gifted a piece of the pear cake and jam. In his own quiet way, Nathan changed the landscape of the forest that surrounded him.

Nathan's custom-built home is filled with rough-cut timbers and brick floors. Books of every imaginable subject are tucked into every crevice of every wall. Skylights let in the slanted light that makes its way through the forest rooftop a few hours each day. The effect is that you feel you are part of the forest, not isolated from it.

As usual, Nathan offered us tea along with an array of baked goodies including his amazing pear cake! As we sampled the sweets and drank tea, Nathan played Chopin on an old piano he had dragged (almost miraculously) up the rugged slope to his home.

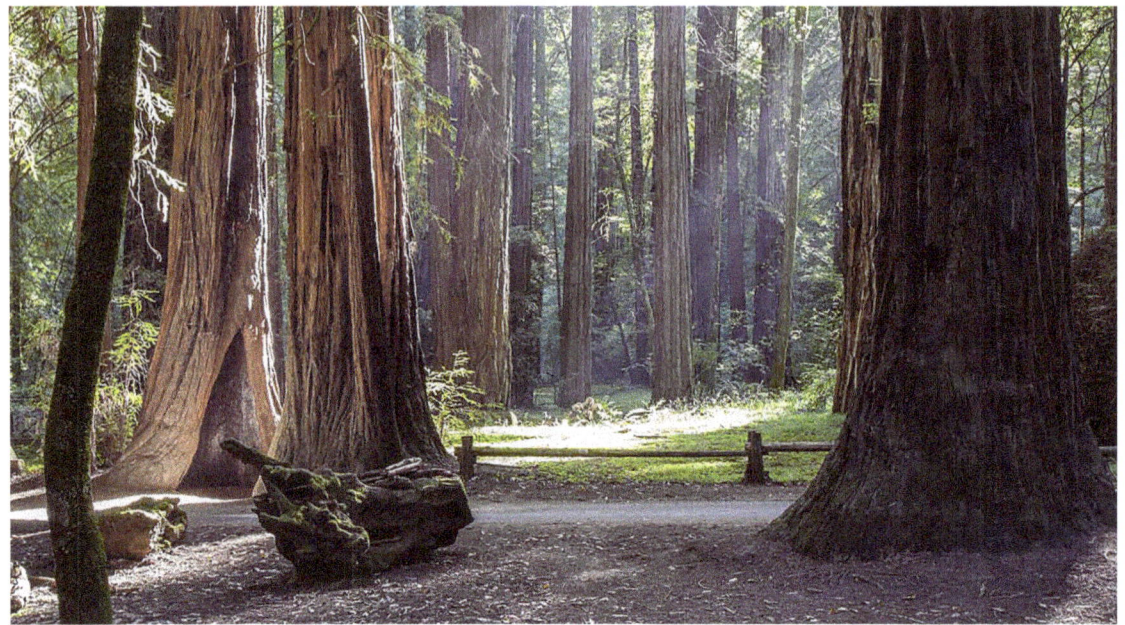

And when we left, we got a big hug and a final greeting, which Matthew dubbed, "the *bubbie* factor." It's how old-world Jewish grandmothers send off their grandchildren, with a full-fledged pinch on the cheek. It brought with it such infectious joy and love—breaking through the barriers which normally separate us. We were ushered off into the sunset, as the sleepy redwoods whispered gently in the silent presence and awe of the coming night.

COUNTRY PEAR CAKE

Makes 1 Cake | Preheat Oven to 325 Degrees | Bake: 80 Minutes   S Y

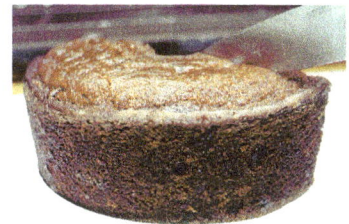

Since I raise my own pears, process them into a spiced pear sauce and can them, my original recipe is built around a quart for convenience's sake. A couple of options: buy canned pears, drain, and mash them, add a little cinnamon, nutmeg and ground cloves, and use that for fruit (or any other type of fruit sauce, for that matter) or cook up a small batch of fresh pears with the above spices ahead of time and use that for the fruit. A large can of pears will contain about 2½ cups of pears as opposed to the 4 cups in a quart, so I've reduced this recipe. It's a simple matter to increase the recipe, as this cake is wonderfully adaptable and dependable and not at all delicate or temperamental.

—Nathan McMahon

(This cake is inherently glutinous and includes butter, eggs, nuts, and wheat, which cannot be replaced, so therefore there is not an allergy-free version)

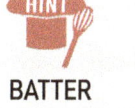

BATTER CONSISTENCY

Batter should be a thick, viscous consistency. If it is too moist, add a little flour or bake a little longer. If you're in doubt about it being done, look for the cake to show a desired bursting around the top or remove from oven when an inserted broom straw or toothpick comes out clean. Cake will seem solid when pressed on top.

1 C brown butter (heat butter gently, until it turns golden)
2 C dark brown sugar
2 large eggs
3 C unbleached white flour, sifted
1 T baking soda
½ t salt
1 t ground cloves, 1 T cinnamon, 1½ t nutmeg, freshly grated
2½ C pear sauce
2 T dark corn, dark maple syrup or dark brown rice syrup
1 C walnuts, chopped coarsely
1 C raisins

1. BLEND brown butter and sugar.
2. ADD eggs to butter/sugar mixture.
3. SIFT flour, baking soda, salt, ground cloves, cinnamon, and nutmeg.
4. MIX: 2½ C pear sauce with 2 T syrup and add alternately with butter/sugar and flour spice mixtures, stirring just enough to mix thoroughly.
5. FOLD in walnuts and raisins.
6. BAKE in a greased and floured angel food tube cake pan.
7. COOL and then remove from pan.

SPICY PERSIMMON JAM

Makes 4 Jars

GMENSY

If you live in an area where persimmons abound, chances are you know someone daunted by their abundant harvest each fall who are only too happy to share them with anyone who will take them off their hands. Persimmon jam is the ideal solution for just such a quandary. This sassy recipe adds a special twist to a traditional jam.
—NM

4 C prepared fruit
1 box pectin
2 t lemon juice
½ t lemon zest
1 t cinnamon
1 t ginger, freshly grated
½ t freshly grated nutmeg
5 C fine turbinado or maple sugar

1. COOK the soft, ripened fruit in a little water for 5 minutes, remove the skins, drain and mash, measure 4 C of fruit.
2. ADD lemon juice and zest, cinnamon, ginger, and nutmeg and sugar.
3. FOLLOW the directions for cooked peach or pear jam that come with each box of pectin.
4. REMOVE from heat once the jam is cooked; fill hot, sterilized jars.
5. COVER with sterile lid and tighten jar ring or pour melted paraffin in top of filled jar.
6. COOL lidded jars upside down and re-tighten jar rings after the lids vacuum-seal, usually after a few minutes.

CANNING FOOD

If the directions say boiling water, use rolling boiling water. • Don't begin canning in a room immediately after sweeping or dusting. Two hours should elapse before starting the canning. • Light, heat, and freezing will spoil the most carefully canned foods. • In canning at an altitude more than 1,000 feet above sea level, the time for the hot water bath should be increased 10% for each 500 feet above 1,000 feet. • Before using canned food for the table, examine every jar carefully. Do not taste to see if it is spoiled. If there is an odor somewhat resembling cheese, if there is a mushy appearance of the solid parts of the food, or if the top of the jar is blown, DISCARD the jar and its contents.

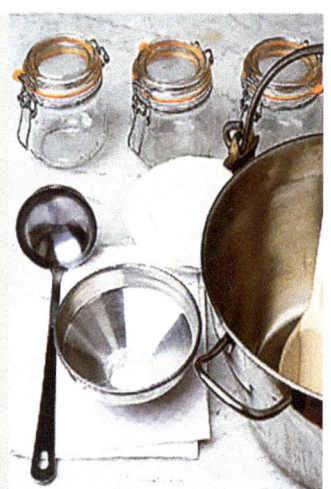

RUSSIAN RIVER SOURDOUGH RYE BREAD

Makes 4 Loaves | Preheat Oven to 350 Degrees | Bake: 50 Minutes   N S

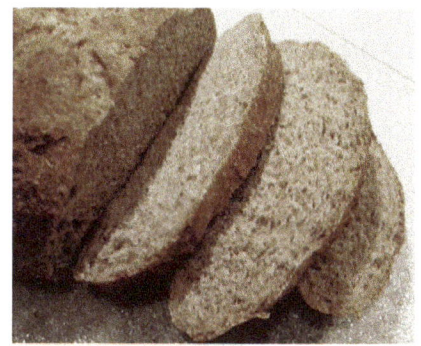

My Sourdough Recipe
Store sourdough mixture in a jar in the refrigerator for a week or two, "feeding" it about once a week by adding a little more flour and powdered milk, and occasionally with a little more yeast. As it ages and "grows," it will turn slightly sour, hence, "sourdough." Personally, I keep a couple jars of it going all the time.
—NM

This bread is inherently glutinous. Because you cannot replace the rye flour in the sourdough starter along with butter, milk powder and eggs, there is no complete allergy-free alternative for this recipe.

2 T dry yeast
2 T powdered milk
2 C unbleached white flour

1. ADD 2 T dry yeast, and 2 T of powdered milk to 2 C flour. It's easy to remember because it's all 2's.
2. ADD enough warm water to make a thick, liquid paste.

Caramel Base
The foundation for the dark, rich sweetness of a Russian Rye is a burnt caramel that is the first undertaking when making this bread. It's a simple but slightly risky process because the mixture is likely to boil violently and splatter a little, so great care must be used while attempting it.

1 C turbinado sugar, whirled in blender until fine
½ C brewed coffee
6 T butter

1. ADD 1 C sugar and slowly let it come to a boil in a deep cast-iron or heavy skillet.
2. PREPARE fresh coffee, decaffeinated, if you prefer, add to sugar. If the coffee is boiling when you add it to the golden, boiling sugar, it somewhat minimizes the splattering, but you will still need to be careful, use a big enough pan to allow for the boiling sugar to rise.
3. CONTINUE cooking at high heat until the caramel is reduced to a fairly thick caramel, by you must stir it constantly.
4. ADD butter or margarine, stir, and remove from heat to cool.

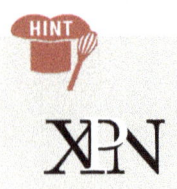

*There are several mystical "Monograms of Christ," among them, X.P.N. for the title, Our Lord Jesus Christ": intersecting letters X and P, and simply the letter N, symbol of an Avatar, the Sun elevated to the Midheaven, hence, Noon. These symbols can be found in the Catacombs in Rome and in ancient carvings in Egypt, having their mystical origin in the Hermetic Brotherhood of Luxor, Egypt. It was traditionally carved into the tops of bread loaves, as a homage to ensure their rising.

Proofing Yeast

3 C warm water
1 T sugar
3 T dry yeast
2 C sourdough starter

1. MIX 1 C *warm* water, sugar, and yeast in a very large bowl, let it froth.
2. ADD 2 C each *warm* water and sourdough starter to frothy yeast mix.
3. ADD *cooled* caramel (recipe on previous page) and stir in (if caramel is too hot, it will kill the yeast.)

Initial Dough

2 C unbleached white flour
2 C rye flour
1 C wheat bran
¾ C molasses

1. ADD initial dough ingredients to yeast sourdough starter bowl, stir well. Cover and let set until bubbly, about 40 minutes.

Finishing Dough

When mixture has reached the bubbly stage, whipping with a large spoon will develop the gluten until "ropes" or "strings" begin to appear in the dough texture. This is very important, because it will make the difference between a very dense and unappealing loaf, and one that is both substantial and airy, the hallmark of a good Russian Rye. Then, gradually add the following ingredients, stirring at first, then hand-kneading.

3 eggs
5 C rye flour
4 C white flour and ½ to 1 C whole wheat flour
2 T salt
1 egg and 1 T milk or water (for top)

1. MIX first four ingredients into initial dough bowl and knead using as little flour as possible on the bread board, until dough is smooth.
2. DIVIDE and form into 4 equal balls.
3. INCISE the top of each ball, with a sharp knife or a single razor blade*
4. BRUSH with mixture of 1 egg beaten with 1 T milk or olive oil.

If you are lucky enough to have baking tiles, place balls on a thin bed of cornmeal. I bake my loaves on top of greased pie tins until quite crusty. When baked sufficiently, loaves will resonate when lightly tapped.

DASAPRAKASH

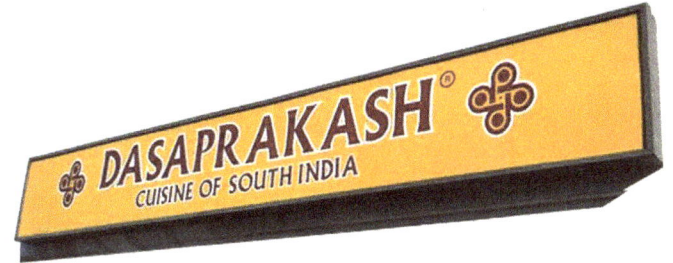

THERE ARE A FEW SPECIAL BUSINESSES IN INDIA that have become institutions. The South Indian restaurant and hotel chain *Dasaprakash* is one of them. During many excursions to the South Indian port city of Chennai, we often heard about this special hotel and restaurant chain, but never made it there.

After many years of wanting to visit Dasaprakash's new restaurant in the Southern Los Angeles area of "little India," we finally made it. After a few initial visits, over a period of a few months, we sampled authentic South Indian vegetarian cuisine. Then, one day we approached the owner—the youngest son of the founder, Madhu—who agreed to share recipes and stories with our readers. So, one afternoon, Matthew and I walked into *Dasaprakash* with camera, recorder, and a hearty appetite.

The story of *Dasaprakash* is the story of Madhu's family. Madhu's grandfather, Govinda Rao, was a very devoted Hindu who believed in its precepts of *Seva*, selfless service. As a living example of these lofty teachings, he instilled this wisdom into his sons. In fact, when Govinda Rao's two brothers renounced family life to dedicate their lives to their faith, Madhu realized he would have to make a living for the whole family. With little education, he decided that feeding people would offer a good livelihood and an opportunity to put service into practice.

Govinda began his business, naming it *Dasaprakash*. The word "dasa" means servant and "prakash" is light or illumination. He vowed to donate a portion of whatever little profits he made to those less fortunate than himself. From the start it was wildly successful, surpassing all expectations, and he was able to open the first 200-room hotel in Chennai. This was to be the forerunner of several more hotels and restaurants throughout India. Both Govinda and *Dasaprakash* grew to be legendary: the restaurant for exceptional pure vegetarian cuisine, and Govinda for the good works he performed. He fed the poor and provided funds to them for the observance of Hindu religious customs. Govinda's home in Chennai became a stopping point for religious and political leaders who grew to respect and admire him.

As *Dasaprakash* expanded, each member of the family was given their own business provided that, in whatever they did, service was never to be forsaken.

The recipes supplied by Madhu are definitely not for the casual cook. It takes dedication to find the ingredients, follow the recipe, and patiently prepare the meal. For those who do not live near a metropolitan area where most Asian grocery stores are located, you can order them online.

For the brave of heart, the time and effort are well worth it. The food you are about to experience belongs to one of the oldest continuous vegetarian traditions in the world. Since South India was spared much cultural dilution from foreign invasion, the customs, traditions, and food have been handed down from grandmother-to-mother-to-daughter for generations.

I remember staying a few days in a traditional home in Madurai where a cow resided in the courtyard of the house. Milk was taken daily from her and made into yogurt, butter, and ghee, while her dried dung was used for cooking fuel. Next to the cow unhusked rice was pounded daily for use with each meal—much the same way households prepared it 100 years ago. There is great beauty in a culture and tradition that has thrived for centuries.

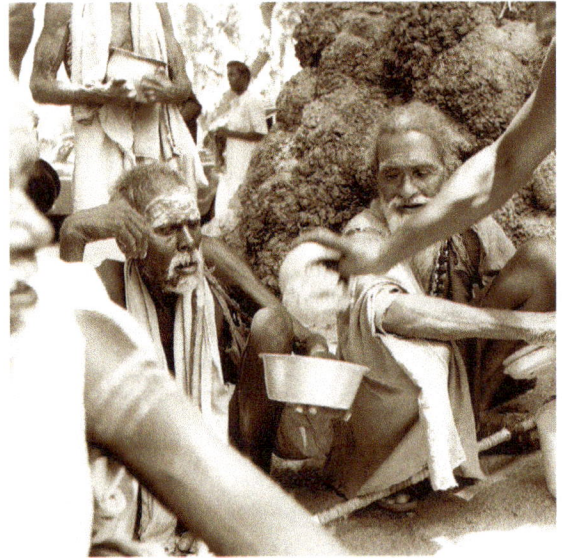

Poor feeding at Sri Ramanasramam.

I also remember the daily feeding of the poor at the hermitage in South India, Sri Ramanasramam, where we lived for a number of years. Matthew captured a moment of expectant faces lined up waiting for possibly the only food they would get for the day. They are given their food before anyone else is fed in the Ashram. The joy reflected in the faces of these simple people has had a profound and lasting effect on me. We generally take food for granted in the West. In India, food is both a blessing to prepare and to share.

Through the success of *Dasaprakash*, Govinda's family continues the tradition of public service consistent with the founder's noble vision. Though a few of years ago it closed in the Los Angeles area and is now only in India.

SAMBAR (LENTIL SOUP)

Serves 6 to 8

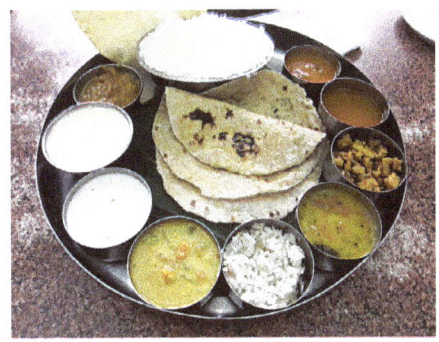

¾ C toor dhal, available at specialty markets
½ t turmeric powder
2 T ghee (see page 298 for making ghee) or avocado oil
3 medium onions, finely diced
1 to 2 t salt
2 T chopped curry leaves
2 tomatoes, diced
2 to 3 T tamarind paste or ⅛ C of fresh lemon juice
1 C chopped vegetables, either lightly steamed first (like carrot) or cooked with dhal (zucchini, string beans, potato, okra, eggplant, etc.)

Spice Paste (grind together in a blender)
1 t cumin seeds, roasted
2 to 3 green chilis, fresh
2 T coconut, finely grated, not sweetened
2 T coriander seeds, soaked for 10 minutes in water
¾ C chopped tomatoes
¼ C cilantro

Garnish
1 t ghee or avocado oil, ½ t black mustard seeds, ½ t urad dhal
10 curry leaves (optional)
Asafetida, pinch

1. COOK dhal with turmeric and salt and just enough water to cover dhal about 1". Skim the top of the water as the dhal cooks. Cook on medium heat about 40 minutes, remove before the dhal is completely dissolved. Slightly mash.
2. HEAT ghee or oil in a heavy bottom pan, add curry leaves, and sauté the onions until translucent.
3. MIX in all the other ingredients: cooked dhal, vegetables, ground spice paste along with an additional 3 to 4 cups of water.
4. BRING to a boil over medium heat, reduce heat and cook another 30 minutes until vegetables are tender and mixture is slightly thick.
5. HEAT oil in a small pan and fry mustard seeds until they pop, add dhal, curry leaves and a pinch of asafetida. Add to cooked sambar.

 SIDEBAR

THE SAMBAR STORY

One day a ruler's son in South India, Sambaji, arrived home and found his wife and daughter had left to visit her mother's village. He was famished and attempted to make rice and dhal for himself but added tamarind by mistake. It gave the dish a completely unique flavor—and sambar was born.

MIXED VEGETABLE KURMA

Serve 5 to 6

GMESY

 **HEALING PROPERTIES**

Coconut Oil
- May prevent heart disease because of its antiviral characteristics
- Its antimicrobial lipids help those with compromised immune systems
- Activates metabolism, considered anti-obesity
- Used to destroy lipid-coated viruses such as HIV, herpes, cytomegalovirus, and influenza
- Supports thyroid function and brain development

Coconut-Cashew Spice Paste
1 T coconut oil
1 onion, finely chopped
1 garlic clove, smashed
2 green chilis, de-seeded
3 cardamom pods (remove shell, crush seeds into powder)
10 to 12 cashew nuts
1" piece ginger, grated
1 t coriander powder
½ C coconut, finely shredded
2 t poppy seeds

Kurma Ingredients
1½ T coconut oil
2 onions, chopped
1 garlic clove, diced
2 tomatoes, chopped
1 T salt
1 t turmeric
5 C mixed diced vegetables potatoes, carrots, green beans, cauliflower, or peas), steam until tender.
1 C evaporated milk or coconut milk

Coconut Paste
1. HEAT oil in pan, sauté the first five ingredients.
2. ADD cashew nuts, ginger, coriander powder, coconut, poppy seeds; cook another minute, then remove from heat. Add just enough water and blend in an electric blender to form a loose paste.

Kurma
3. HEAT oil in another pan and fry onions and garlic. When translucent add tomatoes; fry them until they are broken down.
4. ADD mixed, steamed vegetables, salt, turmeric, coconut paste and evaporated or coconut milk. Cook covered on low-medium heat for 10 to 15 minutes, until thickened (don't bring to a boil).
5. SERVE AS A MEAL: Steaming rice is in the center of the plate, in separate small bowls add sambar, kurma, other stir-fried vegetables, poppadum or puri (fried chapatis), plain yogurt, and condiments.

 SIDEBAR   THE INSIDE SCOOP ON COCONUT OIL

It turns out coconut may be a good fat after all. It has a unique role in one's diet and is being researched as a beneficial oil for prevention and treatment of some heart disease. Seeing coconut oils harden into a solid state may remind us of the cholesterol-rich plaque in blood vessels. In fact, coconut-eating cultures in the tropics consistently have lower cholesterol than people in the U.S. It has also recently been discovered that it may help correct obesity, too.

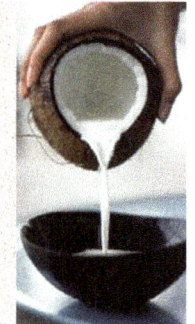

A Culinary Journey

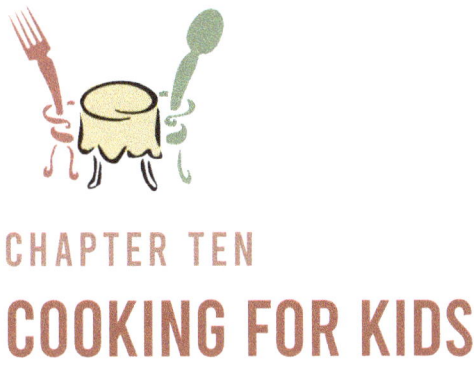

CHAPTER TEN
COOKING FOR KIDS

FUN PROJECTS IN THE KITCHEN
KIDS MEALTIME
SNACKS AND HEALTHY DESSERTS

FUN PROJECTS IN THE KITCHEN

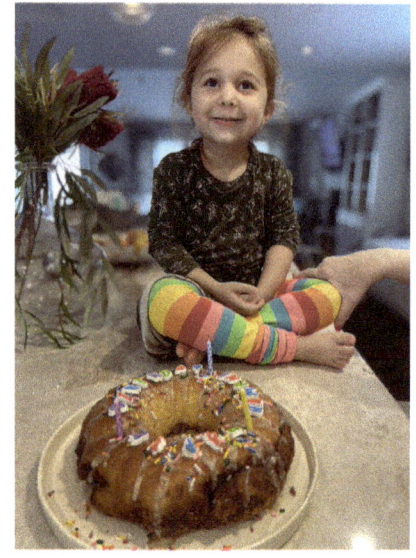

Ellie's birthday cake surprise.

THERE IS NOTHING LIKE GIVING YOUR CHILD OR GRANDCHILD the gift of discovering the love of cooking by bringing him or her into the kitchen with you. It's a delightful sharing in the fun and includes important lessons about learning patience, discipline, ingredients, and food prep. My own time with my granddaughter, Ellie, helped her to explore new foods and we enjoy the process together, at the same time.

Hiding veggies and fruit in your children's food helps to add the necessary vitamins and minerals they need, without all the fuss. My first project with Ellie was to make what we called, "Gaga Muffins." She needed a snack for preschool that was yummy and healthy, so I developed an organic, whole grain mini muffin that added broccoli, zucchini, carrot, apple and was sweetened with banana and a touch of agave.

On another occasion Ellie and I tackled a surprise birthday cake (of course made with colored sprinkles) for her mama, which you can see, pictured here. Ellie is very happy and proud of her accomplishment.

 SIDEBAR   WORKING WITH KIDS IN THE KITCHEN

When you are working with kids in the kitchen, here are two important rules:
1. KEEP sharp objects like knives out of reach, it seems quite obvious, but it doesn't hurt to repeat it. Also explain to them about sharp objects, so they understand the implications.

2. MAKE sure they understand why they shouldn't touch anything that has raw eggs in them, they love to touch and experience everything, but raw eggs can be dangerous.

THREE KID FRIENDLY ACTIVITIES

Here are a few cooking projects to inspire your child or grandchild. A personalized apron is a nice gift to create an interest in cooking and keep your child's clothes clean, at the same time.

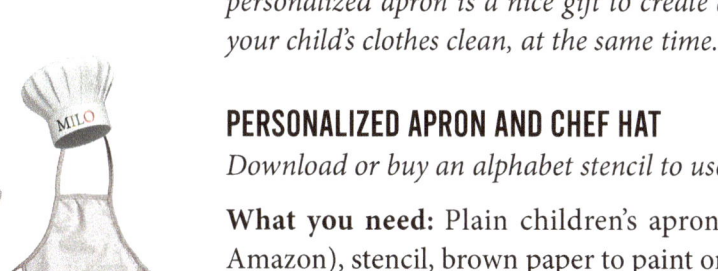

PERSONALIZED APRON AND CHEF HAT
Download or buy an alphabet stencil to use in this project.

What you need: Plain children's apron and chef's hat (available on Amazon), stencil, brown paper to paint on, Crayolo washable paint.

1. TAPE each letter stencil to form name of the child onto the apron.
2. PAINT each letter separately, with a different color.
3. DRY completely.

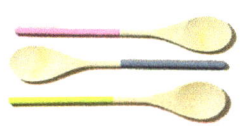

PAINTED SPOONS
Different colored spoons for specific cooking projects.

What you need: Wooden spoons (you can get them at a dollar store), brown paper to paint on, Crayolo washable paint.

1. TAPE around the center of the spoon handle.
2. PAINT the bottom of each spoon a different color.

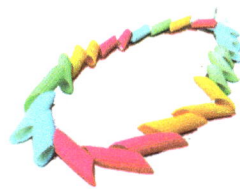

COLORED PASTA DECORATIONS OR NECKLACE
This is a colorful pasta craft

What you need: Tube pasta, brown paper to paint on, freezer bags, rubbing alcohol, food coloring, parchment paper, string for threading.

1. DIVIDE pasta into freezer bags and working with one bag at a time, add a teaspoon of rubbing alcohol to each bag (it will evaporate soon and helps the color adhere to the pasta.)
2. ADD different food colorings to each bag.
3. SPREAD colored pasta on a parchment or lined cookie sheet.
4. DRY overnight.
5. STRING colored pasta just like beads, glue them on paper for pictures or decorate Play Dough creations.

KIDS MEALTIME

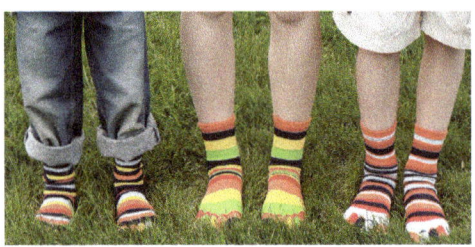

MEALTIME FOR THE TODDLER, when you want to include more vegetables in their diet, can sometimes be challenging. Different children have various degrees of tolerance for trying new foods. Involving them in the cooking process is often the key to getting them to experience a new taste. It is very important to introduce new foods early on, otherwise it will only get harder. It is even more important for vegetarian children. I raised my daughter vegetarian, and bean and cheese burritos were always a good standby and I found she gravitated to string beans and brussel sprouts, so I found creative ways to include them in her diet.

The main thing is to make sure the food is fresh, organic (if possible) varied, nutritious and tasty. One way we got Ellie to eat lunch at preschool, where sandwiches were initially on her "no" list, was to get a super large mickey mouse cookie cutter. We cut out the bread and made an almond butter and a low sugar jam (see recipe on next page) sandwich, using raisins for eyes and mouth. It did the trick!

> **HINT**
>
> **START A HERB GARDEN**
>
> You don't need a large plot of land to plant a few seeds, even a sunny windowsill will do. It helps to include your kids in the process and let them invest their time and energy in watching food grow.

Here's a few ideas to get a handle on mealtime:
1. Veggie Chili: top it with cheese and sour cream.
2. Tortellini Soup with fresh veggies.
3. Baked Parmesan Zucchini Bites.
4. Bean Burrito Bowls: brown rice, stir fried veggies, cooked black beans and cheese or vegan cheese.
5. Cauliflower Fried Rice: with scrambled eggs or tofu.
6. Alfredo Whole Wheat Pasta with Broccoli (can be made with Vegan Cashew Sauce, see page 120).

SCHOOL IDEAS

Serve 5 to 6 | Preheat Oven to 400/350 Degrees | Bake: 35 Minutes   G M N S Y

LUNCHTIME IDEAS

- A box of raisins
- Carrot and celery sticks
- Apple slices (squeeze on lemon juice, so they don't brown)
- String Cheese
- Dried fruit
- Veggie sausage (brown them slightly and cut into slices)
- Rainbow Pasta Salad
- Edamame, shelled
- Wedges of cornbread
- Lentil Balls
- Hummus and pita wedges
- Zucchini patties

You have to be creative when it comes to school lunches. My mini muffin and banana bread is perfect; it combines fruits, vegetables, and fiber. A single cornbread wedge combines many great ingredients, giving children vitamins and minerals they need for the rest of the afternoon. Most lunchrooms these days do not allow any peanut butter, due to possible allergies, luckily, we now have so many good nut butter alternatives to pair with jam.

CORNY CORNBREAD

1 T avocado oil (for cast iron pan)

Dry Ingredients
1½ C cornmeal and ½ C unbleached white flour or 2 C gluten-free flour
1 t fine sea salt
¼ C milk powder (optional)
1½ t baking powder

Wet Ingredients
2 C low-fat milk or almond milk
2 eggs, lightly beaten
¼ C olive oil

Veggie and Seed Options
½ C peas, frozen, 1 C corn kernels
2 T chia seeds, 2 T sunflower seeds

1. PUT 1 T oil in a cast iron or glass baking dish and heat in a 400-degree oven, until the oil is piping hot, at least 5 minutes.
2. COMBINE dry and wet ingredients in separate bowls. Add wet to dry ingredients, stir in veggie and seed options, just enough to combine.
3. POUR batter into the sizzling iron pan.
4. TURN the oven down to 350 Degrees and bake until golden.
5. COOL completely before cutting into wedges.

Easy Low-Sugar Strawberry Jam

4 C organic strawberries, cut small
¼ apple, grated on smallest setting, with the peel (a natural pectin)
¼ C agave syrup and 1 t lemon zest

1. COMBINE all ingredients in a heavy-duty pot.
2. COOK on low-medium heat for at least 10 minutes.
3. BLEND lightly with a potato masher.
4. COOK an additional 10 to 20 minutes on low heat, stirring (test 1 T cooked jam on an ice-cold plate, to see if it is the right consistency.)
5. REFRIGERATE immediately (stays fresh for up to 3 weeks).

LENTIL BALLS

Serve 6 to 8 | Preheat Oven to 375 Degrees | Bake: 13 to 15 Minutes   G M N S Y

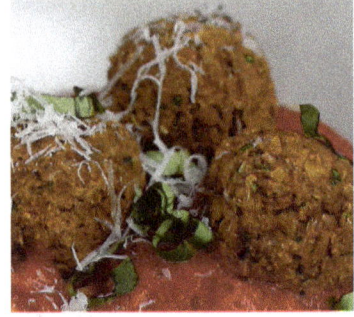

3 T olive oil, extra for coating the balls when baking
2 shallots, finely chopped
1 T kosher salt
Freshly ground pepper (optional)
½ t each dried thyme and rosemary
1 t ginger, freshly minced
¼ t smoky paprika
2 cups brown lentils, cook until soft or canned cooked lentils (drain very well)
2 T tomato paste
¼ C packed basil leaves
2 large eggs or 1 egg and 2 egg whites
½ to ¾ C whole wheat or gluten-free Panko breadcrumbs
¼ C Parmesan cheese or vegan cheese, grated

Protein Powerhouse

2 cups of cooked lentils provides 36 grams of protein, more than the same amount of chicken.

It is an excellent source of folate, iron, potassium, phosphorus, fiber, and a good source of magnesium, too!

1. DRIZZLE a pan with 2 T olive oil, place over medium high heat and add shallots.
2. SAUTÉ for about a minute until translucent.
3. ADD the dried herbs, salt and pepper, sauté for another minute or two, set aside to cool.
4. BLEND lentils in a food processor with tomato paste and basil, drizzle the remaining 1 T olive oil, pulse until smooth.
5. BEAT the eggs in a large mixing bowl. Add lentil mixture and shallot/herb mixture, combine until smooth. Then stir in Parmesan cheese and Panko breadcrumbs.
6. MIX everything together, you can use your hands, so that it is well combined. If the mixture feels too wet, add a little more breadcrumbs until the mixture is dry enough to stick together and roll into balls.
7. ROLL the lentil mixture in your hands or use a small ice cream scoop to make into small round balls, place on a greased baking sheet. Drizzle or spray the top of the balls with olive oil.
8. BAKE for about 8 to 10 minutes.
9. TURN balls, and bake for another 5 minutes, until browned.
10. SERVE on pasta and top with shredded Parmesan cheese and tomato sauce.

SIMPLE ZUCCHINI PATTIES

Serve 6 to 8

G M E N S Y

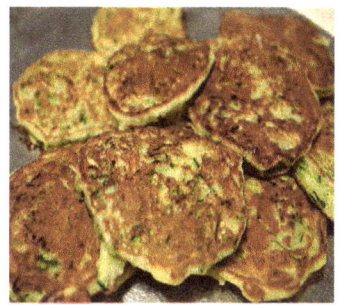

Dinner may be challenging, especially if you want to include more veggies, and if your child is a bit fussy. Here are mealtime ideas you can draw upon: Sweet Potato Fries, Steamed Edamame, Stir Fried Broccoli, Black Bean Tacos, and Lentil/Potato/Celery Soup. Though don't discount these zucchini patties, which are a great way to sneak in veggies and there are endlessly adaptable, you can use either green or yellow summer squash, sweet potatoes, carrots, or riced cauliflower. They also contain protein and fiber. They all go great with applesauce!

2 T avocado oil
2 zucchinis, shredded
1 scallion, sliced thin
1 large egg or ¼ C regular coconut milk and 1 t baking powder (see pages 307-308 for egg-free substitutes)
1 t salt
½ t pepper
¼ to ½ C whole wheat or gluten-free Panko breadcrumbs

1. COMBINE all the ingredients, if it is too wet to shape into a round paddy, add a little more Panko, until you can handle them.
2. SHAPE into 6 large or 8 small patties.
3. HEAT oil in fry pan and when it is hot add 3 patties and fry for about 3 to 4 minutes on each side, until golden brown. Keep warm by spreading out on a cookie sheet, in a low-heat oven.

 SIDEBAR   **EASY BAKED APPLESAUCE**

3 pounds peeled, organic red cooking apples (6 to 8), cut into chunks
2 t lemon juice and 1 t lemon zest
¼ to ½ C light agave syrup
½ t ground cinnamon

1. ADD the apples, lemon juice and zest into a nonreactive Dutch oven or enameled iron pot.
2. ADD agave and cinnamon, cover the pot.
3. BAKE at 350 degrees for 1½ hours, or until the apples are soft.
4. MIX with a whisk until smooth, it will be slightly chunky.

SUPER CREAMY RAINBOW SPAGHETTI AND SPIRALS

Serve 4   GENSY

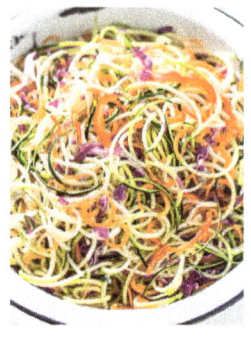

This pasta and veggie spirals, tossed with ricotta and lemon is super-easy to make in just 20 minutes. (To make it dairy free you can substitute "ricotta" for the vegan alternative on page 58.)

1 C fresh ricotta cheese, 1 lemon, juiced and zested, ½ t salt
1 C whole wheat or gluten-free spaghetti, 1" handful
½ t salt
½ C peas, frozen
1 C pine nuts (optional)
1 T extra virgin olive oil
1 shallot, sliced thin
1 C spiral zucchini, green and yellow and 1 C spiral carrot or butternut squash
½ C vegetable broth
½ C half and half or coconut cream

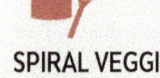

SPIRAL VEGGIE SPAGHETTI

To make any vegetable spiralized, you can buy a spiralizer or even use a mandolin, a potato peeler, or even a box grater to get the job done.

1. PLACE the ricotta, lemon juice, zest and salt in a bowl. Stir until well combined. Set aside.
2. COOK the spaghetti in a large saucepan of salted boiling water, add the peas in the last 2 minutes of cooking. Drain and set aside.
3. TOAST the pine nuts in a large frying pan over medium heat for 4 minutes or until evenly browned. Set aside.
4. ADD the oil and sauté shallot until translucent. Stir in vegetable spirals, cook an additional 3 to 4 minutes, until soft.
5. ADD the stock and cream, simmer on low heat for 5 minutes.
6. ADD drained spaghetti and peas to the vegetable spiral mixture, cover and let sit for 5 minutes before serving.
7. TOP with pine nuts and dollops of ricotta mixture.

 SIDEBAR   RICOTTA CHEESE

Ricotta is actually not a cheese, it's a creamy curd. The curd is literally cooked twice, which is the meaning of the name "ricotta," re-cooked. It is most often made from sheep, cow, goat or buffalo milk whey left over from the production of cheese. Since the casein is filtered away from the whey during the cheese making process, ricotta cheese can be suitable for persons with casein intolerance, but not a milk allergy. It is low in fat and high in protein.

SNACKS AND HEALTHY DESSERTS

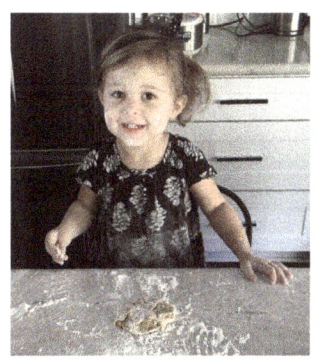

BAKING WITH ELLIE IS ALWAYS A TREAT. We have been in the kitchen together since she was two. It took a few years for her to not simply enjoy scattering flour all over both of us and the floor. Now, she can follow directions, not try to sneak a lick of the bowl with raw eggs and simply enjoy the moment when we stand in front of the oven watching our baking project transform.

Healthy snacks are easy to adapt and great to have on hand, for filling lunch boxes or simply as an in between treat that sustains the boundless energy kids have. There are a few tricks you can employ to make them less sugary and more protein and fiber rich.

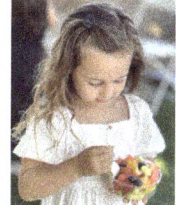

Here's just a few ideas you can add to your snack arsenal:

- Edamame
- Shredded vegetables like zucchini and carrot
- Steamed broccoli or riced cauliflower
- Chia Seeds
- Flax Seeds
- Yogurt
- Fresh fruit salad
- Agave or brown rice syrup
- Coconut or maple sugar
- Nuts
- Whole grain flours
- All fruit smoothies

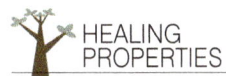

Edamame Facts
In 2005, a study published in *"The American Journal of Clinical Nutrition,"* said that edamame adds protein to your diet and is a great snack to help lessen hunger between meals, which is a benefit for children, since they can get a boost of energy and not spoil their appetite for their main meal of the day.

CREATIVE SNACK IDEAS

Healthy small portions like:
- Snap peas
- Berries
- Yogurt squeezer

- Jam filled apple stars
- Celery sticks and nut butter

Cooking for Kids

CRUNCHY TRAIL MIX

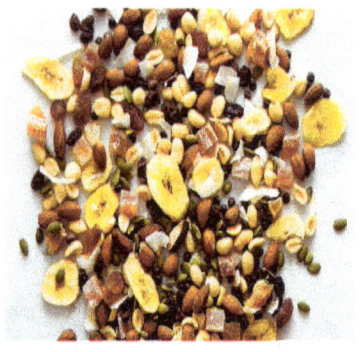

Ellie is a true snacker, when she comes home from school, she needs a quick pick-me-up. Her little brother Milo loves munching snacks too, so keeping homemade snacks available is a must. Trail mix is a super snack and a great way to involve kids, they can help putting it together. It is portable, clean, endlessly customizable and above all else good for you. You can choose from a variety of nuts, seeds, and dried fruit. They can contain healthy fats, vitamin E, copper, magnesium, and zinc, and at the same time be rich in fiber and protein!

MAKE YOUR OWN BLENDS

Simple Toddler Mix Ideas
cereal
nuts & seeds
dried fruit

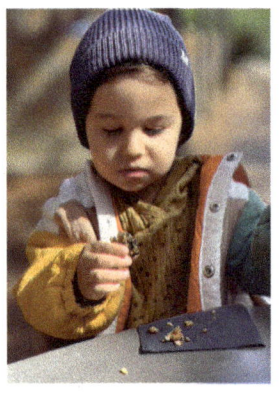

Nuts
Roasted peanuts
Almonds
Cashews
Macadamia
Pine nuts

Dried Fruit
Cranberries
Cherries
Strawberries
Blueberries
Pineapple
Apricot
Prunes
Papaya

Seeds
Pumpkin
Sunflower
Sesame, roasted
Chia

Extra
Granola
Dark chocolate or carob chips
Coconut slivers
Yogurt covered raisins
Whole wheat or gluten-free pretzels
Whole grain cereal, toasted in oven
O's cereal
Cheese crackers
Banana chips

 SIDEBAR   DRYING YOUR OWN FRUIT

Heat oven to 225 degrees. Line a baking pan with parchment paper and place fruit, cut side up, about ½ inch apart. Bake until the fruit shrivels, and edges have dried. The time varies according to the type of fruit you are drying, it is anywhere from 1½-4 hours. Transfer to a cooling rack. You can store dried fruit in an airtight container or freeze them for up to 6 weeks. You can also buy a food dehydrator.

GAGA MUFFINS

Makes 2 Dozen Muffins | Preheat Oven to 350 Degrees | Bake: 15 to 20 Minutes   G M E N S Y

SIMPLE WAYS TO REPLACE EACH EGG IN BAKING, IF YOUR CHILD IS EGG SENSITIVE

Substitute with ¼ C liquid and an extra ½ t of baking powder:
- Applesauce
- Apple juice
- Coconut Milk
- Prune Puree
- Yogurt

I created this when Ellie needed to fill her preschool lunch box with a snack. It was an instant hit, especially since we baked them together. This recipe can be made allergy-free, if necessary.

1 C organic whole wheat pastry flour and 1 C organic unbleached white flour or 2 C gluten-free flour blend mixed with 1 t xanthan gum
1 t baking powder
½ t salt
½ t cinnamon
3 T butter, margarine, or avocado oil
¼ C agave or maple syrup
2 large eggs or replacement (see Hint)
1 t vanilla extract
½ C broccoli, florets, chopped and steamed
1 small zucchini, shredded
1 carrot, shredded, ½ apple, shredded, ½ banana
¼ C applesauce, unsweetened
¼ C yogurt, plain or alternative yogurt
1 T chia seeds and/or 1 T flax seeds

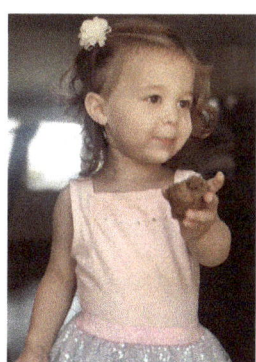

1. MIX flours, baking powder, salt, and cinnamon. Set aside.
2. SOFTEN butter or margarine.
3. MIX agave, butter, margarine, or oil, eggs, and vanilla. Beat well.
4. BLEND steamed broccoli, banana, shredded zucchini, shredded carrot, shredded apple, applesauce, and yogurt. Pulse until thoroughly mixed.
5. COMBINE the puree into the agave/butter/eggs mixture and beat until mixed. Stir in seeds.
6. ADD the dry into wet ingredients and mix until just combined.
7. SPRAY or oil mini muffin pans
8. SCOOP the mixture into the prepared muffin pan. Fill each muffin ¾ full. (I use a small ice cream scoop)
9. BAKE until the tops are slightly brown, and a toothpick comes out clean or they bounce back when you touch them with your finger.

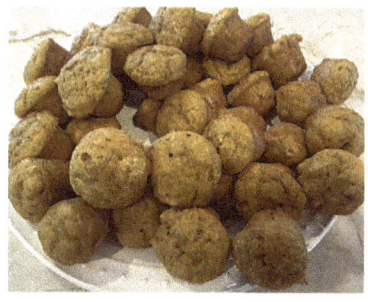

KID FRIENDLY COOKIES

Makes 38 Mini Cookies | Preheat Oven to 350 Degrees | Bake: 11 to 14 Minutes   G M E N S Y

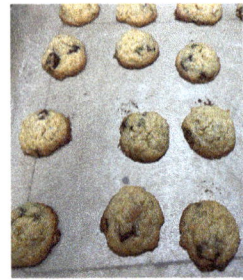

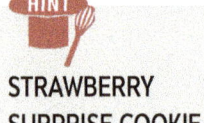

STRAWBERRY SURPRISE COOKIE

Wet Ingredients
1 egg
2 T lemon juice
½ C avocado oil
1½ t vanilla
½ C + 2 T sugar

Dry Ingredients
1 C white pastry flour and ¾ C ww flour (sift together)
1½ t baking powder
1 C chopped strawberries or ½ C strawberry jam

Mix wet and dry Ingredients separately, then combine. Stir in strawberries, chill before scooping out cookies, bake same as above.

Here's two classic small quantity cookie recipes that utilize what you have on hand in your pantry. I also tried to make them just a little bit healthier. The secret is to let the dough chill for about an hour to harden. To form the cookie, use a small ice cream scoop and don't flatten.

½ C butter or margarine
¾ C + 1 T turbinado sugar, coconut or maple sugar
¾ C white pastry flour and ½ C whole wheat pastry flour (or 1 C gluten-free flour blend) and ½ C rolled oats, sift all together
¾ t salt
1 t baking powder
1 egg, beaten or egg substitute (see page 308)
1 t vanilla extract
¼ C bittersweet chocolate or carob chunks
¼ C any nuts or seeds, chopped small (I often use pumpkin seeds)
¼ C coconut shredded (optional)

1. WHISK the flour, salt, and baking soda together.
2. MELT butter or margarine and add sugar, mix really well. Blend in egg until it's fully incorporated.
3. ADD dry ingredients to wet and stir to combine. Stir in chips, nuts and coconut. Refrigerate for at least ½ hour or even overnight.
4. SCOOP cookies and spread them out to allow for expansion.
5. BAKE until the edges are golden. Don't overbake.
6. STORE at room temperature for about 3 to 4 days.

 SIDEBAR   NATURAL SUGAR OPTIONS

Always use organic. The main thing to be aware of is when using any of the alternative sugars, like coconut or maple is that they can be replaced on a 1 to 1 cup ratio, but may need a minute or two less baking time. You can also mix and match as well, since coconut and maple sugars are a bit less sweet.

FRESH BERRY CAKE OR CUPCAKES

Makes 12 Cupcakes or 1 Cake | Preheat Oven to 350 Degrees | Bake: See Below   M N S Y

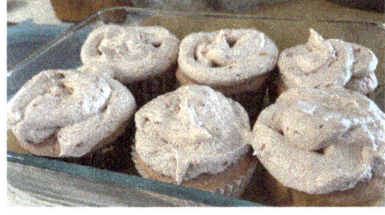

This is a special occasion cupcake. Strawberries are Ellie's absolute favs, so of course, a strawberry cupcake was our go-to flavor, but any berry will do. Ellie thought it needed some chocolate chips, so in they went. Of course, she needed to test a few herself, as she sprinkled them in. It is light, "delish," as Ellie would say, and easy-peasy to put together, she especially loved the frosting part! I developed this as a dairy-free, but not a gluten-free cupcake. Add a few candles and a birthday party can commence any time of the year.

2 eggs, separated or egg substitute (see page 308)

Dry Ingredients
1 C unbleached white flour
¾ C whole wheat pastry flour
¼ C corn starch
2 t baking powder
½ t salt

Wet Ingredients
¾ C butter or margarine
1½ C turbinado brown sugar
2 t pure vanilla extract
1 C almond milk

6 ripe berries, chop very small (reserve 1 T mashed berries, for the frosting)
¼ C dark chocolate or carob chips (optional)

1. BEAT the egg whites into a light meringue. Set aside.
2. COMBINE the dry ingredients together. In another bowl beat the butter or margarine and sugar until light and fluffy. Add the egg yolks and vanilla until well combined.
3. BLEND the dry and wet ingredients, incorporating them in intervals, until just combined.
4. FOLD in the beaten egg whites, chopped berries, and chips. The batter should be a bit thick and very smooth.
5. POUR into cupcake tins or three prepared cake pans and bake until a toothpick comes out clean.
6. BAKE 12 to 15 minutes for cupcakes and 30 to 35 minutes for cakes. Don't overbake. Cool completely on a rack, before frosting.

SIDEBAR

BERRY FROSTING

½ C margarine or butter
2 C confectioners' sugar
1 T mashed berries
Pinch salt
½ t vanilla extract

- Beat margarine until smooth, add sugar, berries, salt, and vanilla.
- Blend well until smooth. Add more sugar if it seems too thin.
- Refrigerate while cupcakes are cooling.

MINI BANANA BREAD

Makes 2 Mini Loafs | Preheat Oven to 350 Degrees | Bake: 25 to 30 minutes

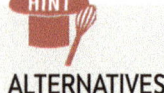

ALTERNATIVES

- You can bake these as muffins.
- You can substitute brown sugar with coconut sugar and monk fruit blend
- If you don't have yogurt or sour cream or want to go dairy free, simply add an additional ¼ C mashed banana, applesauce or canned pumpkin puree.
- Frozen bananas work as well, you simply have to defrost them, drain off any liquid and then mash.
- You can add chocolate chips or nuts, as well.

Milo loves "nanas." A great way to add ripe bananas, protein, and fiber into your kids' diet are these lightly sweetened mini loafs, one for now and one for later. You can always double the recipe to make one large loaf, but the baking time increases about 15 to 20 minutes. For this recipes eggs make this moist and light.

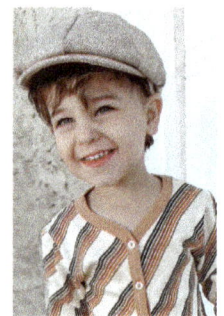

½ C whole wheat pastry flour
½ C unbleached white flour
¾ t baking powder
Pinch salt
¾ t ground cinnamon and ¼ t cardamom powder
½ t protein powder
¼ C butter or margarine, softened to room temperature
⅓ C dark brown sugar
2 medium eggs, beaten
2 T yogurt, sour cream or alternative plain yogurt
1 ripe banana, mashed
1 t vanilla extract
1 t chia seeds
1 t flax seeds

1. WHISK together flours, baking powder, salt, and cinnamon.
2. BLEND butter or margarine and sugar in a separate bowl, until creamy. Mix in eggs and vanilla, until well combined. Then add yogurt and mashed banana and beat into a smooth batter. Fold in seeds.
3. SPOON dry ingredients into wet ingredients and mix, but don't overmix.
4. ADD the batter to two prepared mini baking pans. You can cover with aluminum foil after 15 minutes, if the top begins to brown, check with a toothpick that comes out clean to be sure that it's done.
5. COOL completely in the pan, on a rack and then remove.

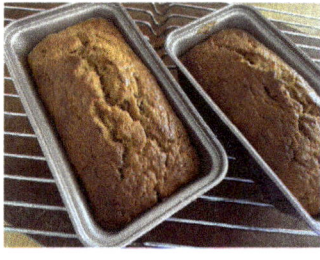

CHAPTER ELEVEN
EAST INDIAN COOKING

A DAY IN THE INDIAN KITCHEN: INDIAN VEGETABLES

AN INDIAN MEAL

SOUTH INDIAN SPECIALTIES

TIFFIN

CHUTNEY

RICE

DHAL DAY

MUMBAI KITCHEN

A DAY IN THE INDIAN KITCHEN: INDIAN VEGETABLES

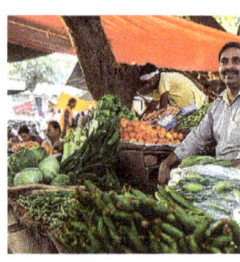

Each day I would go to the market, basket in hand, to pick out fresh vegetables for our daily meal. Vegetables were delivered to the market each morning at the crack of dawn. The kaleidoscope of color, sounds, aromas and dynamic drama of the marketplace was always an adventure.

FOR A SHORT PERIOD OF TIME, MATTHEW WORKED IN A SMALL CITY IN SOUTH INDIA, CHITTOR. They furnished us with a house and the luxury of a refrigerator. There was only one small hitch—the design of the small kitchen—where I was to spend most of my day. It was a veritable closet, just big enough to turn around in. The only window faced a brick wall, and it was just a small hole in the wall with thick bars running vertically. In the summer with the temperatures rising easily into the 100s, this tiny cave was merciless. I had a gas propane stove with two burners, a few shelves for storing pots and pans, a tiny cement slab to cut vegetables, and a concrete hole on the counter attached to a pipe, which was called a sink. I spent every day there making the same meal—curried vegetables, dhal, homemade yogurt, and our staple—either whole-wheat chapatis or rice. Although at times it was grueling work, the country and its people endeared themselves to us. And although the diet sounds monotonous, we never grew tired of it.

We had some papaya trees on the property. With a long bamboo stick we would pry a few ripe fruits free and attempt to catch them in midair. After quite a few splattered fruits, we became adapt at this sport. Cutting them up, we would sprinkle lemon juice and a pinch of cayenne pepper on them for an evening refreshment. After a blistering day in the kitchen, sitting outside under the wafting palms, surrounded by cooler tropical evening breeze, was a healing balm.

Spending a few years in Tiruvannamalai, South India—at the base of the Arunachala mountain, the kitchen was more spacious. A family of monkeys would wait until the cooking began, cling to the open window, observing. If for some reason I was not vigilant enough to secure the front door, they would sneak in and help themselves to whatever was available. Many fruits and breads found their way into monkey hands.

PAN-FRIED GREEN BEANS

Serves 4 to 6

GMENSY

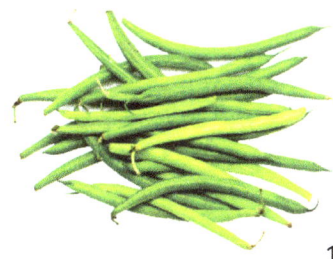

This has become a lovely standard recipe. If you have to prepare food really quickly, this is a great dish to build a meal around.

2 to 3 T avocado oil
½ t black mustard seeds
½ t cumin seeds
1 to 3 red chilis, dried, depending on how hot you like your food
1 t ginger, freshly grated
½ t turmeric
1 t coriander powder
1 t salt
Pinch of sugar or jaggery
4 C French cut green beans, frozen work very well
¼ C unsweetened coconut, finely grated (available in an Asian grocery)

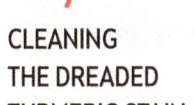

CLEANING THE DREADED TURMERIC STAIN

Dab it with straight 3% Hydrogen Peroxide. Dabbing, not rubbing, is the secret.

1. HEAT oil and add mustard seeds until they pop.
2. ADD cumin seeds and red chilis until brown.
3. ADD ginger, spices, salt, sugar, and green beans.
4. COVER pan and let stir fry about 10 minutes, stirring occasionally.
5. UNCOVER and add coconut, cook another 10 minutes until green beans are cooked and yet still slightly crispy, not mushy.

 SIDEBAR   THE MIRACLE OF TURMERIC

When you read the list of benefits turmeric provides, you will start using it abundantly! The question is what does it not do? As member of the ginger (zingiberaceae) family, it is native of Asia. The part of the plant used is the fleshy orange rhizome (underground stem). For centuries it has been used as a natural dye (as anyone knows who has cooked with turmeric.) While internally it helps conditions such as fever, allergies, jaundice, and liver ailments, it also aids digestion, helps fight infection and guards against heart attacks. Turmeric is known for its cleansing and purifying agent, inhibiting toxin accumulation, and supporting liver and gall bladder function by stimulating the flow of bile. Externally, it is used for reducing inflammation and swelling due to sprains, cuts, and bruises. The crucial chemical found in turmeric is curcumin. Its health benefits include reducing Alzheimer's-related inflammation of brain tissue.

East Indian Cooking

EGGPLANT CURRY

Serves 4 to 6

G M E N S Y

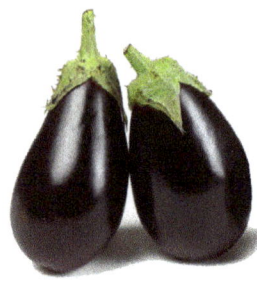

2 eggplants, 2 tomatoes (roast in 350 Degrees oven for 30 to 40 minutes and scoop out cooked pulp. Remove eggplant and tomato skins and slightly mash together).
1 T tamarind paste (you can use 2 T lemon juice to replace tamarind)
1 onion, chopped
2 T avocado oil
1 t black mustard seeds
1 t cumin seeds
2 cinnamon sticks
½ to 1 t cayenne powder
2 t coriander powder
1 t salt or to taste
¼ C cilantro, chopped small

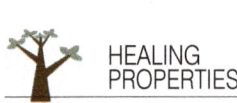

Eggplant
- Helps to protect the lipids in brain cell membranes
- Antiviral
- Lessens free-radical damage in joints
- Helps with the absorption of iron
- Helps to prevent cellular damage that may promote cancer

1. BLEND the tamarind paste, onion, and garlic in a blender with ½ C water.
2. ADD oil to pan and roast mustard seeds until they pop, then add cumin seeds and cinnamon sticks and roast until they brown.
3. ADD the eggplant/tomato pulp, cayenne powder, coriander powder, salt and tamarind paste mixture.
4. COOK on medium heat for another 5 to 10 minutes until it comes together as a thick curry, remove cinnamon sticks before serving.

 SIDEBAR   A BIT OF CORIANDER HISTORY

The word coriander can be used to describe the entire plant: leaves, stems, seeds, and all, but when speaking of coriander, most people refer to the spice produced from the seeds of the plant. The leaves of the plant are more commonly referred to as cilantro (the Spanish word for coriander), and due to its strong aroma, it can be an acquired taste. The seeds often combined with lemon in Middle Eastern cuisine. Little is known about the origins of the coriander plant, although it is generally thought to be native to the Mediterranean and parts of southwestern Europe. Experts believe its usage dates back to at least 5,000 BC. References to coriander can be found in Sanskrit writings, and the seeds were discovered in Egyptian tombs. Coriander is even mentioned in the Old Testament. In Exodus, chapter 16, verse 31: "And the house of Israel called the name there of Manna: and it was like coriander seeds, white; and the taste of it was like wafers made with honey."

TOFU OR PANEER AND ZUCCHINI RED CURRY

Serves 4 to 6

GMENY

This takes separate pots to ensemble, but it's worth the effort. This is a wonderful recipe and once you try it, you'll want to make it a staple. You can buy packaged paneer in Indian grocery stores or simply make your own.

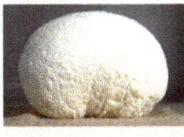

MAKING PANEER

6 C milk
2 to 3 T vinegar or lemon juice

Preparation:
Heat the milk in a big pot on medium-to-low heat for about 10 to 15 minutes, then add vinegar or lemon juice until milk solids begin to float on top. You may need to add more acid, depending on the milk. Remove solids and put in a cheese cloth lined colander. Let sit for about 1 hour, bind tightly and squeeze out the rest of the water to create a solid block of paneer.

Stir-fry Vegetables
1 T avocado oil
1 red onion, chopped fine
1 red pepper, chopped fine
5 zucchinis, medium, peeled and cut into 1-inch cubes
¾ t salt

Coconut Sauce
2 T fresh ginger, minced
½ t turmeric, 1 t coriander powder, 1 t cumin powder, and ½ to 1 t cayenne
½ t salt
1 C cherry tomatoes, cut in half
1 can light coconut milk

Topping
Splash of lemon juice
¼ C cilantro, chopped fine

Pan-Fried Tofu or Paneer
2 T avocado oil
1 pound extra firm tofu or 2 C paneer, cut into 1-inch cubes
¾ t kosher salt
Corn starch

Stir fry
1. SAUTÉ onions and peppers in oil until almost tender.
2. ADD zucchini and salt, cover and sauté until tender, about 10 minutes.

Pan-Fried Tofu or Paneer
3. SPRINKLE tofu or paneer chunks with salt, dredge in corn starch and aggressively remove excess, sauté batches in oil until lightly brown.
4. SAUTÉ spices and salt to pan you used to fry paneer, cook for 1 minute then add tomatoes and fry an additional 2 minutes. Add coconut milk. Process sauce in a blender until smooth.

Combine
5. ADD fried tofu or paneer, coconut sauce, stir-fried veggies; cook together until slightly thickened (about 5 to 10 minutes).
6. TOP with cilantro and a splash of lemon juice.

COCONUT CAULIFLOWER AND POTATO CURRY

Serves 4 to 6

GMENSY

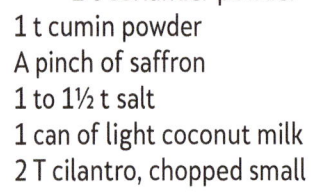
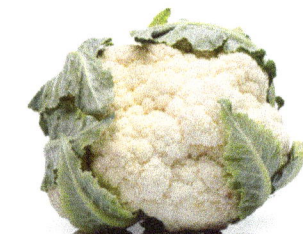

2 baking potatoes
1 cauliflower, cut into florets
2 T coconut oil
½ t black mustard seeds
1 to 2 green chilis, de-seeded or 1 to 2 dried red chilis
2 tomatoes, de-seeded and chopped
½ t turmeric powder
1 t coriander powder
1 t cumin powder
A pinch of saffron
1 to 1½ t salt
1 can of light coconut milk
2 T cilantro, chopped small

> This can easily become an all-time favorite and staple. Serve over rice or let the sauce cook uncovered until it is a bit reduced and serve it with chapatis or any flat bread.

1. BAKE potatoes about 1½ hours until very soft; peel and chop into 1" chunks. I often bake the potatoes in advance and cool.
2. STEAM cauliflower until almost cooked; it should remain a bit crisp.
3. HEAT oil in a large pot, then add mustard seeds until they pop.
4. ADD chilis, brown; be careful not to burn them.
5. ADD tomatoes, spices, and salt and stir until well mixed and the tomatoes begin to break apart.
6. ADD coconut milk, chopped potatoes, and steamed cauliflower. Continue to cook on low-medium heat, uncovered, for about 10 minutes until all the flavors merge.
7. TOP with cilantro.

 SIDEBAR   **ABOUT SAFFRON**

Saffron goes back to ancient Egypt and Rome where it was used as a dye, in perfumes, and as a drug, as well as for culinary purposes. It reached China in the 7th century and spread through Europe in the Middle Ages. The majority of today's saffron is imported from Iran (Southern Khorason) and Spain, which are recognized for producing the best quality, but it can also be found in Egypt, Kashmir, Morocco, and Turkey.

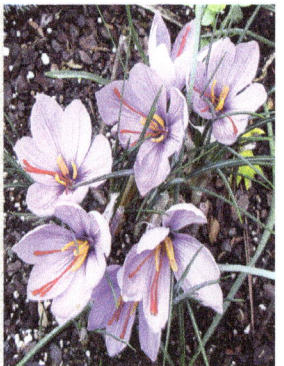

AN INDIAN MEAL

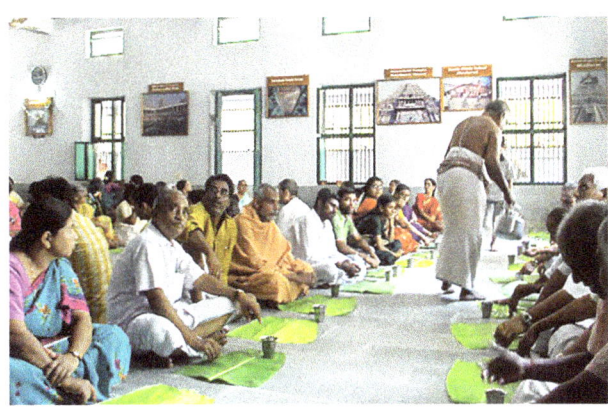

The dining hall in Sri Ramanasramam, Tiruvannamalai, India.

THE ART OF INDIAN COOKING has been handed down through many generations and the various, colorful spices are both aromatic and medicinal. Chilis, though quite powerful, are also one of the best sources of vitamin C, and ginger and cumin are excellent for digestion.

I vividly remember the first time I ate a South Indian meal. It was in 1973 on our first visit to India. We sat in long rows on the stone floor of the dining hall in Sri Ramanasramam. We sat in long rows on the stone floor of a dining hall. Banana leaf plates were spread before us and soon buckets of steaming rice and lentils were laden on each plate. The South Indian vegetarian diet goes back for centuries. It is a balanced diet combining the protein of beans, vitamins and minerals of vegetables, and the digestive properties of yogurt.

From the beginning, Indian cooking made a deep and lasting impression upon me. When I began creating my own meals, I made a visit to the ever-fascinating local vegetable market. I also acquired a wonderful array of stainless-steel utensils, which are used for both cooking and eating. My only purchase splurge was a pressure cooker, which was essential for certain dishes. I used a few stainless-steel inserts, placed on top of each other to cook multiple items at the same time.

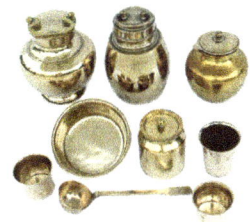

For those who have not ventured into Indian cooking, you need not acquire all the special spices mentioned in these recipes. I have tried to make them simple and, wherever possible, indicate when a spice is optional. Learning to cook with spices and herbs can literally change your palate and your life. Cooking with spices doesn't mean it has to be (hot) spicy; it just means you are daring enough to bring a new flavor to your meals.

East Indian Cooking

SIDEBAR   SAGE LESSONS IN THE KITCHEN

It was during our time in India, while we were staying in Sri Ramanasramam, where I imbibed the love of feeding others and cooking with great care and mindfulness. The many stories of how Ramana Maharshi prepared food is both inspiring and instructive. Up and about at 3 a.m., he would begin cutting vegetables and helping the other cooks in the kitchen. He always made sure whoever came to the Ashram should be fed and was insistent that nothing was wasted. Even stray mustard seeds or grains of rice were carefully placed back into their tins. He did not waste any parts of vegetables that others often ignored and was a master of adaptation, suggesting additions to enhance a dish.

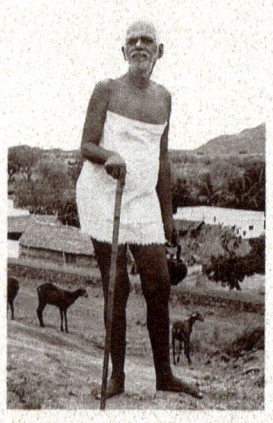

There is a lovely poem/song Ramana wrote about making poppadums, a complicated process of making thin fried lentil wafers. The song follows the story of when his mother wanted to make some for him; when she tried to enlist his help he told her: "you make your's and I will make mine" He knew she used to like to sing Tamil folk songs, so he composed one on this occasion. *An excerpt from the song*:

With an inward turned pestle of mind, pound away 'I-I'
Unrelenting at its stubborn out-going disobedience
Then with the rolling pin of Shanti (peace), roll out on the platter of evenness
The *Appalams* and see for yourself!

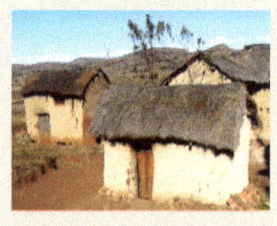

Indian Hospitality
During our first visit to India we also stayed in a remote village in North India, the state of Bihar. The only way to get into the village was a single file dirt walking path. While our luggage was hauled on the heads of villagers, we ventured on the muddy, deep puddled path during the infamous 1973 monsoon season. It was quite an adventurous trek to the center of this village. After a few days of sleeping on a typical wooden bed (charpoy) and becoming a part of the rhythm of village life (we felt we were living a few centuries ago), we were invited to visit a family who lived in a small hut about half a mile from where we were staying. When we arrived, a blanket was spread on the hard mud floor, in their tiny one room hut. The hosts sat across from us with beaming faces. We were the first Westerners they had ever seen. They were considered the poorest of the poor, but with great excitement and the utmost hospitality they handed each of us two cardamom seeds and a cupful of fresh well water. Their inner wealth was a graciousness which I found truly remarkable.

UPMA

Serves 6 to 8

MESY

This dish is customarily served as a light breakfast or an afternoon snack. It is very simple and quick to prepare. Have all the vegetables (cut up quite small) and spices ready before you turn on the stove, since the process goes quite quickly once you begin.

2 C semolina or Cream of Wheat cereal
1 T ghee or margarine
2 T coconut oil
½ t black mustard seeds
1 t urad dhal (optional, available from Indian or Asian markets)
5 to 6 curry leaves (optional)
Pinch asafetida (optional)
1 onion, large, chopped small
1 green chili, de-seeded or 1 dried red chili
1-inch fresh ginger, minced or chopped fine
½ C fresh raw cashews or peanuts, chopped
1 carrot, 1 potato, chopped very small
4 C water
½ lemon, squeezed for juice
1 T salt
¾ C peas, fresh or frozen
2 T fresh cilantro, rinsed and chopped small

1. ROAST semolina slowly with ghee or margarine on a very low heat, until it is light brown. This can be done ahead of time.
2. HEAT coconut oil and add mustard seeds until they pop. Then add urad dhal and curry leaves. Keep an eye on the urad dhal so it doesn't brown too much, add asafetida, and fry a few seconds.
3. ADD the onions, green or red chili, and ginger. Stir fry until onion is translucent; then add nuts and fry until golden brown.
4. ADD vegetables (except peas), fry 5 minutes. Add water, lemon juice, and salt. Boil, uncovered, and cook 7 to 10 minutes, until vegetables are tender. Add peas.
5. LOWER heat and very slowly begin to add the roasted cereal, stirring at the same time. It will begin to thicken very quickly. When the mixture is fully incorporated, put a lid on and reduce heat to the lowest possible setting, let sit for about 5 minutes. Top with cilantro.

HINT

UPMA CUTLETS

If you have any Upma left over or you want to cook it ahead of time and serve it later, here's a good idea.

Spread the warm Upma on an 11" x 7" greased baking pan. Let cool and then cut into squares. Pan fry with a little ghee or margarine to brown. Serve warm as a cutlet. You can accompany it with any chutney. (See Chutney Chapter on Page 246.)

POTATO AND GREEN PEPPER VEGETABLES

Serves 4 to 6

GMENSY

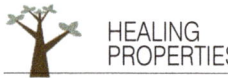
HEALING PROPERTIES

Green Peppers
- Contains vitamin B6 and folic acid
- Rich in vitamin A, protects against emphysema
- Rich in vitamin C, helps degenerative arthritis

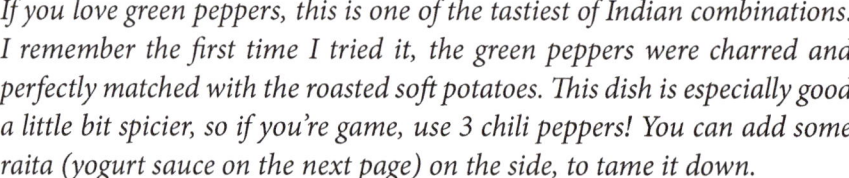

If you love green peppers, this is one of the tastiest of Indian combinations. I remember the first time I tried it, the green peppers were charred and perfectly matched with the roasted soft potatoes. This dish is especially good a little bit spicier, so if you're game, use 3 chili peppers! You can add some raita (yogurt sauce on the next page) on the side, to tame it down.

3 T avocado oil
½ t black mustard seeds
½ t cumin seeds
1 to 3 red chili peppers, dried
1½ inch ginger, minced or chopped small
7 curry leaves (optional)
½ t turmeric, 1 t coriander powder, and 1 t cumin powder (combined) or
    1½ T commercial curry powder or 1½ T curry paste
1½ t salt
4 medium potatoes, chopped
3 green peppers (Roast in oven until the skins are charred and place in a bowl with a lid. Let it sit covered for five minutes. Then remove the membrane, skin and seeds and slice into long strips.)

1. HEAT 3 T oil and add the mustard seeds. Let them pop.
2. ADD cumin seeds and chili peppers. Fry another minute or more.
3. ADD ginger and curry leaves, spices or curry paste, and salt.
4. ADD chopped potato, reduce heat, and put a lid on the pan. Roast slowly for about 10 to 15 minutes. Stir occasionally, checking to make sure potatoes are not sticking to the bottom of the pan. Cook until tender, not mushy.
5. ADD roasted green peppers to cooked potatoes, simmer on low-to-medium heat, with the lid on. Fry an additional 5 minutes, stirring occasionally to prevent vegetables from sticking to the pan.
6. REMOVE from heat. Do not overcook or the potatoes will break apart.

TURMERIC AND GINGER PICKLE

This is a healthy and simple addition to any Indian meal. Buy fresh turmeric root (specialty store or online) and ginger root. Peel and cut into very small, julienne pieces. Add lemon juice and salt. Marinate for a day or so and store in the refrigerator.

VEGETABLE YOGURT SAUCE – RAITA

Serves 4 to 6   G M E N S Y

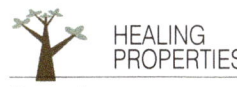

Cucumber
- Contains silica, an essential component of healthy connective tissue
- Helps prevent water retention
- High in fiber

2 C plain low-fat yogurt or alternative yogurt
½ C cucumber, de-seeded, peeled, chopped small
½ C tomatoes, de-seeded, chopped small
¼ t salt
1 t fine brown sugar or jaggery (Indian sugar)
½ t coriander powder
¼ t cayenne pepper
¼ t paprika
½ t ground ginger or 1 inch fresh, minced

Garnish
½ t oil
¼ t black mustard seeds
¼ t cumin seeds
¼ t urad dhal
¼ C cilantro, chopped small

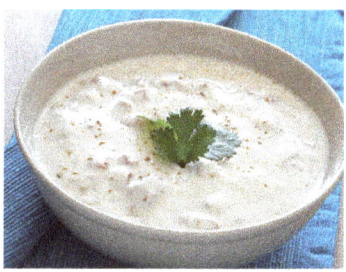

1. COMBINE the first 9 ingredients in a bowl, mix well.
2. HEAT oil in a small pan. Add the mustard seeds until they pop, then add the cumin seeds and urad dhal. Carefully "brown" the dhal, making sure not to burn it.
3. ADD the oil and spices to yogurt and top with cilantro.

 SIDEBAR   ABOUT CILANTRO (CORIANDER LEAVES)

People have used cilantro for thousands of years. It has been found in ancient Egyptian tombs dating back 3,000 years. The Hebrews of biblical times originally used cilantro (at some point parsley became the substitute) as the bitter herb in the Passover meal. The Roman soldiers under the reign of Julius Caesar took coriander with them, using it as a meat preservative and to flavor food. Cilantro was introduced into the Americas around 1670, one of the first herbs grown by the colonists, because this herb was believed to have a variety of medicinal uses, such as alleviating abdominal pain.

Fresh cilantro has a peculiar effect on people: they often dislike it or end up being totally addicted to it—so don't give up on it too quickly. Although the flavor of fresh cilantro is quite reminiscent of the crushed coriander seeds, we are more familiar with, it is much stronger and pungent, so a little goes a long way.

FRIED OKRA

Serves 4 to 6

GMENSY

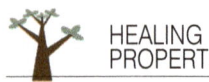
HEALING PROPERTIES

Okra
- Contains silica, an essential component of healthy connective tissue
- Helps prevent water retention
- High fiber and extra fluid

Rich in magnesium and potassium, okra is known in the Southern states as gumbo and in India as lady's finger. Do not put a lid on the pan when cooking it, or it will gum up. Okra pieces should be crisp on the outside, tender on the inside. Fried okra also goes great with chapatis (see page 197), yogurt and poppadum.

3 t avocado oil
½ t cumin seeds, ¼ to ½ t cayenne pepper, ½ t turmeric, ½ t coriander powder
½ to ¾ t salt
¼ C cilantro, chopped fine
1 lb. okra, fresh

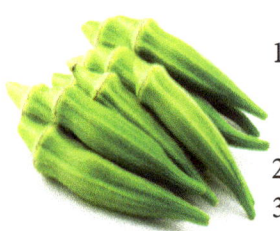

1. RINSE okra, then dry each piece. (Any excess water will make okra slimy. I have used frozen okra with satisfactory results; you have to cook it a little longer, uncovered, until all the water evaporates.)
2. CHOP okra into small rounds (remove hard tops)
3. HEAT oil, add cumin seeds, roast until brown, add the spices and salt.
4. ADD the chopped okra.
5. FRY on medium-high heat, uncovered, stirring often.
6. COOK until okra is crispy and slightly charred.
7. TOP with cilantro

 SIDEBAR   POPPADUM

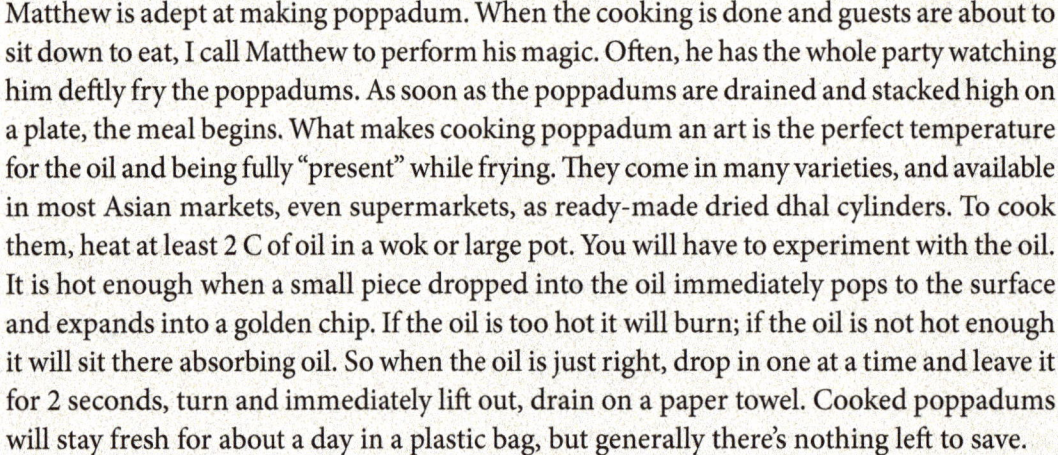

Matthew is adept at making poppadum. When the cooking is done and guests are about to sit down to eat, I call Matthew to perform his magic. Often, he has the whole party watching him deftly fry the poppadums. As soon as the poppadums are drained and stacked high on a plate, the meal begins. What makes cooking poppadum an art is the perfect temperature for the oil and being fully "present" while frying. They come in many varieties, and available in most Asian markets, even supermarkets, as ready-made dried dhal cylinders. To cook them, heat at least 2 C of oil in a wok or large pot. You will have to experiment with the oil. It is hot enough when a small piece dropped into the oil immediately pops to the surface and expands into a golden chip. If the oil is too hot it will burn; if the oil is not hot enough it will sit there absorbing oil. So when the oil is just right, drop in one at a time and leave it for 2 seconds, turn and immediately lift out, drain on a paper towel. Cooked poppadums will stay fresh for about a day in a plastic bag, but generally there's nothing left to save.

SOUTH INDIAN SPECIALTIES

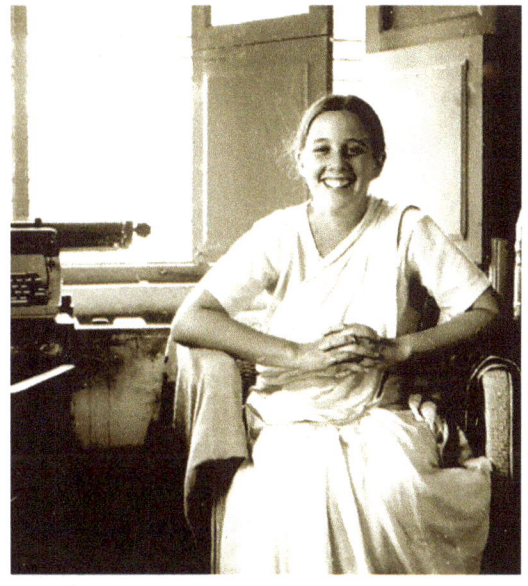

In the one room Indian cottage at Sri Ramanasramam, where we cooked, slept, wrote and designed publications.

MY FIRST ATTEMPT AT DOSA (A THIN, CRISP RICE PANCAKE) WAS A DISASTER. Not one came off the pan, without breaking or crumbling. A friend was passing by my Indian cottage, and I put my head out of the door and yelled, "Help!" She deftly lifted the pancake off the griddle on her first attempt. Such is the merit of experience and knowledge. It took years to figure out this relatively simple procedure.

Idlis are steamed, sourdough rice cakes that are served for breakfast throughout South India. In the morning, large cakes are served with a dot of ghee and either chili powder or brown sugar. They are highly digestible. A special idli maker, which can be purchased in Asian markets, makes it easy.

If you don't have an idli maker, you can improvise with cupcake shells (in stacks of three) or an egg poacher. Idlis work well as an appetizer, you can also get creative and introduce spinach and tomato puree for a lovely green and red variation.

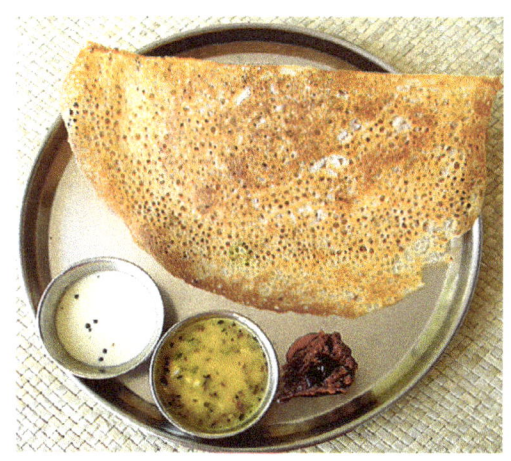

East Indian Cooking

DOSA

Makes 15 to 20 Dosas

Dosa can be served with potato stuffing, chutney, or sambar.

1½ C long grain white rice
⅔ C urad dhal, 1 t salt
Oil for frying

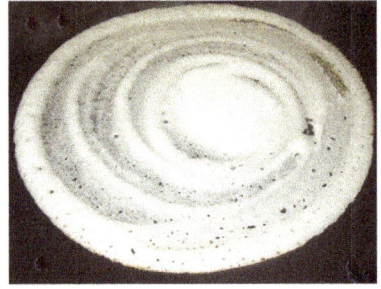

Both idli and dosa are made from the same slightly fermented batter. The quantity of rice to urad dhal (purchased in specialty Asian stores) do differ. Measure and rinse both the rice and dhal. Soak each in a separate container (in at least 3 C of water) overnight. The next day, using a heavy-duty blender, begin processing (about 1 C of rice at a time) with a bit of the water (the same water you soaked the rice in) until the rice becomes a course meal. Continue doing this until all the rice is blended.

Then repeat the process with the urad dhal. The dhal should be light and fluffy. Combine the batter, it should resemble a somewhat thick pancake batter. (You can always add more water at the end of the process.)

Stir gently with the palm of your hand. I have been told by a reliable source that the magic of rising the batter comes from mixing it with your hands. Set aside in a warm place. This is the most important part of the whole process. If you live in South Florida, a warm place may be your garage. If you live in Madison, Wisconsin and you are making dosa or idlis in January, the warmest place perhaps could be on top of a hot water heater with lots of blankets on top of the bowl or in a gas oven with a pilot light. If these are not available, I have found that turning the oven on for about 30 seconds heats the oven up enough to remain warm for a few hours. Every few hours repeat the process of turning on the oven for 30 seconds. Do be careful—I have learned the hard way. I turned on my oven for its 30-second interval when the phone rang, I then forgot all about it until I found a strange smell wafting through the kitchen. I had baked the entire batch of batter!

The batter is ready anywhere from 8 to 14 hours. The batter should double in size, with tiny bubbles on the top. It should also be fermented and give off a slight sour/sweet smell. This enhances its flavor, nutritional value, and digestive property. Add salt and more water, if necessary, at this point, so that the batter is a thin pancake consistency for dosa and slightly thicker for an idli batter. Now you are ready to cook the *dosa*. Have a plate handy to put each cooked dosa on. You can keep them warm by transferring each cooked dosa to a cookie sheet lined with aluminum foil, and putting it into a warm oven, or on a food warmer.

1. PRE-HEAT a cast iron griddle. This is very important.
2. PREPARE a dish of oil. Cut a small onion or potato in half. Spear it (on the top) with a fork and use to spread the oil on the pan. With the onion/potato brush, put a thin layer of oil on the hot griddle.
3. POUR a ladle (use a slightly rounded bottom type) of batter in the center of the pan. Immediately place the bottom of the ladle in the center of the batter and begin to spread it outward in a continuous motion until the dosa batter reaches the edges of pan and is very thin, almost transparent on the hot pan and has a lot of air bubbles all around, similar to a crepe but even thinner.
4. DRIZZLE a little oil over the surface and around the edge of the dosa. Cook for about 2 minutes until it begins to crisp and looks golden. Ease a spatula around the edge to loosen the dosa and flip it over carefully.
5. COOK about 30 to 45 seconds on the second side. The first dosa, like a regular pancake, may have to be sacrificed until the pan is well-seasoned and is at the perfect temperature.

MASALA DOSA

4 to 5 potatoes, chopped into medium/large chunks
2 T avocado oil
½ t black mustard seeds and ½ t turmeric
½ inch piece of fresh ginger, minced
1 to 2 green chilis
1 onion, sliced thin
1½ t salt and 1 t lemon juice
¼ C cilantro, chopped fine
½ t ghee, butter, or margarine for inside of dosa

1. BOIL potatoes until tender, but not falling apart.
2. ADD mustard seeds to oil, when they pop add turmeric, ginger, and green chilis and fry a few moments.
3. ADD onions and cook until translucent.
4. FRY cooked potatoes, salt, and lemon juice with onion mixture for a few minutes. Mash potatoes slightly.
5. ADD 2 T of potato mixture to the center of each dosa.
6. TOP with ghee, butter, or margarine and fold in half.

IDLI

Makes 18 to 24 Idlis

GMENSY

Follow the dosa recipe to soak, grind, and rise the batter. When the batter is ready and it has doubled in size with tiny bubbles on the top, add the salt and baking powder. Gently mix it together, adding more water, if necessary, until the batter resembles a pancake batter.

1 C long grain white rice
½ C urad dhal, with the black skin removed
1 t salt
¼ t baking soda, add just before you cook idlis
Melted ghee or oil for brushing on idli plate (available at Asian markets), cupcake shells, or cake pan.

Preparing Idlis

1. PREPARE the special idli plate by spreading a thin film of ghee or oil inside each cup, place a few spoonful's of batter almost to the top.
2. HEAT 1 inch of water until it comes to a rousing boil, in a pot large enough to hold the idli plate, cupcake shell, or cake pan.
3. LOWER the idli plate into pot of boiling water (the plate usually has 3 to 4 tiers that makes 9 to 12 idlis at a time).
4. STEAM for about 12 to 15 minutes. Insert a toothpick into an idli in about 12 minutes to see if it comes out clean. When they are done, remove from idli plate. Be careful, the steam can easily burn you.
5. REMOVE the idlis. When you begin the next batch, grease once again and add more water to the pot. Begin the cooking process again.
6. REHEAT by steaming idlis for about 5 minutes. Cover with a napkin.

Idli Upma

1 T oil
½ t mustard seeds
1 t urad dal
A few curry leaves
1 onion, chopped
1 green chili, chopped
½ t turmeric
Pinch asafetida
5 to 6 idlis, crumbled
1 t salt
¼ C cilantro

HEAT oil; add mustard seeds, dhal and curry leaves. Sauté onion and chili, then add idlis, salt, and cilantro.

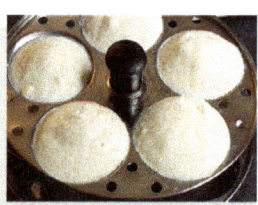

HOMEMADE IDLI MAKERS

- **Cupcake Shells:** If you are using the cupcake shells use a double boiler, vegetable steamer or prop them up with an inserted steamer or rack so that they are not touching the water.
- **Cake Pan:** In a 12" fry pan heat 2" of water and bring to a boil. Place one round 8" cake pan on the bottom with the flat side up. Grease a second 8" cake pan and fill with batter. Place on top of flat cake pan. Cover fry pan and cook idilis on medium heat for 10 to 12 minutes. Turn off heat and a let sit another 10 minutes. Remove from cake pan and cut into pieces.

TIFFIN

IN INDIA, THE INTENSITY OF THE HEAT MAKES AN AFTERNOON NAP ALMOST A NECESSITY. Between the hours of noon and 3:00 p.m., even if you are not in the habit of napping, the heat slows you to the point that a rest is pretty basic to survival. This period of rest and inactivity is followed by a rousing afternoon hot drink at 4 p.m. In South India, you are often given two stainless-steel cups to pour the boiling liquid back and forth, until it is finally cool enough to put one cup to your lips. (With practice, your hands can move further and further apart and still pour from one cup to the other—I have seen adepts in this pouring art form reach a distance of three feet; it is only limited by the length of your hand!)

Tiffin, or snacks, is a time-honored European tradition that stowed away on one of England's merchant ships during the days of the British Raj. When it jumped ship in India, tiffin stayed on and continues to be part of the fabric of Indian life.

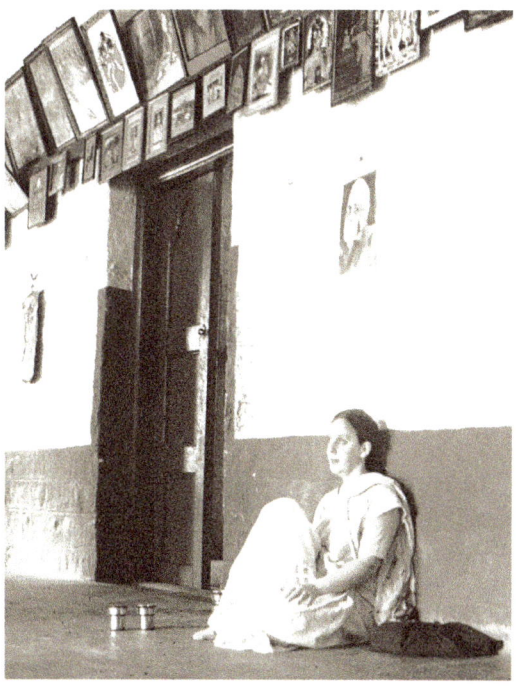

Coffee time, in the dining hall, at the hermitage of Ramana Maharshi.

DAHI VADA

Makes 18 to 24 Vadas

FRYING VADAS

Immerse fried and drained batch in a bowl of salted water, this removes excess oil, and allows vadas to soak up the yogurt.

After placing the vada in water, gently squeeze out excess water without breaking the vada and then place in yogurt. Though the whole process seems like a juggling act, once you get a momentum going, it is quite easy.

Put on soothing music and plan to meditate on cooking, draining, and squeezing vadas for at least one hour. Yes, it's worth all the effort.

This is not a low-fat snack by any means, but an occasional treat. These crisp fried dhal doughnuts are immersed in fresh plain yogurt (dahi).

1 C urad dhal, skin removed
¼ t fenugreek seeds
2 green chilis, de-seeded
½ t fresh ginger, grated
½ t peppercorns
1½ t salt
¼ t baking soda
3 C plain low-fat yogurt, ½ t salt added
¼ C cilantro, fresh, chopped
½ t ghee or avocado oil and ½ t black mustard seeds

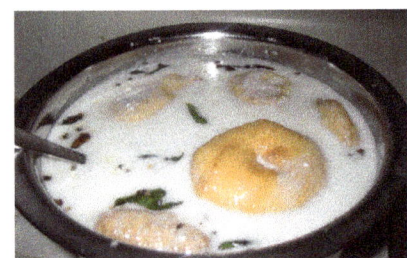

1. SOAK dhal and fenugreek in plenty of water for at least 6 to 8 hours.
2. GRIND the chilis, ginger and peppercorns in a blender until coarsely ground, transfer to a bowl.
3. BLEND the soaked and drained dhal/fenugreek with approximately ½ C of water until it is a light and fluffy batter.
4. ADD the dhal mixture to the bowl of ground spices; blend together with your hand to make the batter light and buoyant.
5. ADD water to make it the right consistency, which should resemble a slightly thick batter, like a quick bread.
6. ADD salt and baking soda just before you begin frying.
7. HEAT a wok or deep fry pan with about two to three inches of oil. Bring it to a frying temperature (about 350 Degrees). Gently lower a tablespoon of batter into the hot oil. If it begins to cook too fast, lower the heat. About five to six vadas should cook, brown and become crispy in about three minutes.
8. DRAIN on paper towels, immerse in salted water (see Hint).
9. PREPARE a separate bowl of yogurt which has been whisked and creamed. Add ½ t salt and chopped cilantro to the yogurt.
10. HEAT ghee or oil, add mustard seeds until they pop.
11. ADD popped mustard seeds to the yogurt/vada mixture.
12. CHILL vadas in the yogurt sauce for an hour before serving. (Chilling them overnight is even better.)

PAKORA: VEGETABLE FRITTERS

Makes 18 to 25 Fritters

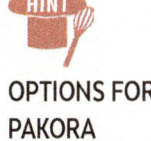

OPTIONS FOR PAKORA

Spinach; eggplant, sliced thin; bell peppers, chopped or sliced; cauliflower florets; green beans, whole; frozen peas; onions, chopped small or sliced thin; jalapeño peppers, chopped small or sliced thin; zucchini flowers, a delicacy; potatoes, sliced very thin; sweet potato, sliced very thin.

Pakora, fried vegetable fritters made from chickpea flour, is a very simple preparation and can be improvised using almost any vegetable. Chickpea flour happens to be a healthy and interesting alternative for those who are wheat sensitive.

2 to 2¼ C chickpea flour
1 to 2 T rice flour, add for crispiness (optional)
1 to 1½ C water
½ t whole cumin seeds
¼ to ½ t cayenne pepper or 1 freshly chopped Indian green chili, de-seeded, chopped fine
½ t turmeric
½ t fresh ginger, minced
1 t coriander powder
1 t salt
¼ to ½ C cilantro, chopped
½ t baking soda (optional)

1. MIX all ingredients together except for baking soda.
2. ADJUST the water to form a semi-thick, crepe-like batter.
3. ADD whatever vegetables you are using to the batter.
4. ADD baking soda just before frying.
5. HEAT oil to frying temperature and add tablespoons of vegetable batter and fry until golden. Drain pakoras on a paper towel.
6. PREHEAT oven to 150 degrees. As each batch comes out of the oil, and is drained well, add to a baking dish waiting in a preheated oven. This will keep the pakoras hot and crispy until the entire batter is fried.

CHANA DHOKLA

Makes 10 to 14 Pieces

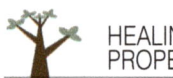

HEALING PROPERTIES

Garbanzo Beans
- Excellent source of fiber
- Significant amount of folate and magnesium
- Protein powerhouse

Dhokla Seasoning

1 t avocado oil
1 t cumin seeds
1 t mustard seeds
Pinch of *hing*

Add all ingredients to heated oil. After mustard seeds pop add ¼ C water and remove from heat.

Steamed chickpea soft bread is a traditional North Indian tiffin (snack), often served with chutney or yogurt sauce. This is my friend Chetna's recipe.

2 C chickpea flour
1½ C water
1 t salt and ¾ t turmeric
1 t baking soda
2 t lemon juice
2 t brown sugar
2 t avocado oil
1 T jalapeño or more to taste, de-seeded, finely minced
1 T ginger, finely minced (optional)
Pinch of *hing* (asafetida, available in Asian markets)

1. MIX all ingredients together.
2. POUR the batter into 2 eight-inch greased cake pans.
3. STEAM in a large pot 8 to 9 minutes, make sure the cake pan is raised up from the bottom of the pot (see Hint on page 240).

Topping
¼ C cilantro, finely chopped
1 T coconut, unsweetened, finely shredded

Garnish:
1. COOL in the pan.
2. CUT the dhokla into 2 inch squares and sprinkle evenly with Dhokla Seasoning (see left column).
3. TOP with coriander and coconut.

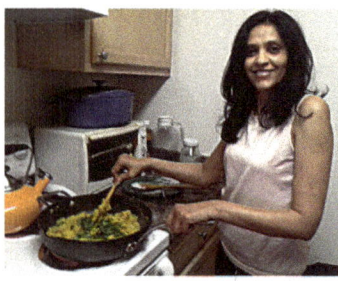

Chetna in her kitchen

DHOKLA OPTIONS

Using the same dhokla ingredients, add additional water to the batter; then add finely chopped onions and make a crepe or an egg-free omelet. If you are making an omelet, use any filling you would for an omelet, such as cooked mushrooms, tomatoes, spinach, etc.

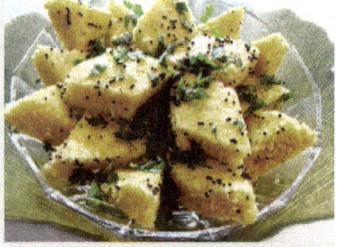

A Culinary Journey

CRISPY CHICKPEA COOKIE BREAD

Makes 8 to 10 Cookies | Preheat Oven to 350 Degrees | Bake: 20 to 24 Minutes   G M E N S Y

 **HEALING PROPERTIES**

Black Pepper
- Stimulates the taste buds, increasing hydrochloric acid secretion which improves digestion
- Diuretic, promotes sweating
- Antioxidant and antibacterial effects
- Outer layer of peppercorn stimulates the breakdown of fat cells

This is delicious for breakfast or may be used in place of bread with a generous pat of butter. It is a gluten-free and vegan, a cross between a savory biscuit and black pepper scone.

2½ C chickpea flour
½ C olive oil
1½ t salt
1 t black pepper, freshly ground
1 t oregano, dried
½ t thyme, dried
1 t ginger, freshly minced
2 T brown sugar
¼ C sesame seeds, toasted
1 t baking soda
1 to 3 T water, as needed

1. COMBINE all the above together. Add more water if it is too dry to shape, don't over handle them, as you would making biscuits.
2. SHAPE into 1 inch round balls, flatten to ¼".
3. PLACE on baking sheet.
4. BAKE until golden, let the cookie sit on the baking pan until completely cool.

 SIDEBAR   PEPPER

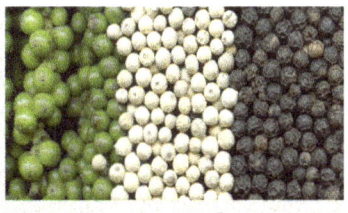

Black pepper is a seasoning produced from the fermented, dried, unripe red berries of the plant *Piper nigrum*. (The same fruit, when unripe and green, can be dried, or preserved in brine or vinegar, to make green peppercorns; or when ripe, dried and dehusked to make white peppercorns.) In fact, it is said that during a war with Rome, "Alaric the Visigoth" demanded a ransom of gold, silver, and pepper.

Native to India, pepper has played a very important role throughout history and has been a prized spice since ancient times. Since ancient Greece, pepper has held such high prestige that it was once used as currency and a sacred offering. It is one of the most common spices in European cuisine. It was critical during the Middle Ages to conceal the taste of partially rotten meat. Pepper became an important spice that catalyzed much of the spice trade. The pungent potency of black pepper is due to the chemical *piperine*.

CHUTNEY

JUST A TOUCH OF CHUTNEY adds an engaging and spirited addition to any meal. The consistency of chutney can be compared to an Indian-style pesto, without the Parmesan cheese. Chutney enlivens and enhances any dish with its subtle play of supporting flavors—sweet, spicy, and sour. It is a good companion for many Indian preparations, and it can accompany a simple meal of rice and vegetables. An interesting way to try chutney is to mix it with plain rice and ghee (clarified butter) and then shape it into balls. For an extra special treat immerse the rice balls in a pakora batter (see page 243) and deep fry. Yum! In most Indian households, fresh chutneys are made daily in stone mortars. The mortars are large, smooth stones with a hole scooped out at the center. An equally heavy pestle is used to grind the ingredients together into a paste.

After some time in India, I finally purchased one, because the ancient process looked so effortless, I loved watching cooks wielding stone upon stone. However, I found it quite challenging to do. It seemed to require a skill that must have been handed down from generations, or perhaps implanted in one's DNA.

I fondly remember the day our stone mortar arrived at the front door of our little cottage in India; it felt as if a century had slipped away. The first chutney we made, by the art of vigorously grinding, was by far the best we had ever eaten; but cleaning the mortar was another matter. You can't carry this large stone to the sink. Buckets of water, and a deft scooping motion of one's palm to remove the water, seemed to go on endlessly. Not having the resources to ship back this enormously heavy stone mortar, I discovered an ordinary blender does the work almost as well. I finally found a heavy-duty blender works wonderfully well grinding spices and making these pastes.

A stone spice grinder remains on my counter for a quick spice pounding, its heady, earthy aroma lingers for hours in the kitchen.

COCONUT CHUTNEY

Makes 1 Cup

GMENSY

This is a favorite recipe of ours. When buying a fresh coconut, shake it and make sure it's filled with plenty of water. Peel the hard, dark crust off the coconut; it will take some time. It is done slowly with a sharp knife or grater; peeling coconut will either improve or try your patience. If you have any extra coconut pieces you can secure them in a plastic bag for freezing. If frozen, thaw completely; these defrosted coconut pieces work quite well for chutney. Fresh chutney will keep well for 2 to 3 days in the refrigerator, but is best if served immediately. If it becomes too thick you can add a bit more water, then adjust salt and chilis to taste.

1 C fresh coconut, peeled and chopped into small pieces (you could also use unsweetened desiccated coconut in a pinch)
¼ C fresh ginger, grated or cut into small pieces
¼ C cilantro
1 t salt
¼ C roasted split chana dhal (a specialty item available in Asian markets)
¼ C lemon juice, fresh
1 to 2 green chilis, de-seeded and roasted, or ¼ (slightly spicy) to 1 t cayenne pepper (extra spicy)
¼ C water (you can use coconut milk for a richer flavor)

1. BLEND together very well, adding a little bit of water or coconut milk as you blend, until it is a soupy consistency.
2. ADJUST salt.
3. ADD garnish seasoning to chutney.

Garnish Seasoning

½ t ghee or oil
½ t black mustard seeds
½ t urad dhal
Pinch of *hing*

1. HEAT oil, add mustard seeds until they pop, add urad dhal until golden.
2. ADD *hing* at the end.

 SIDEBAR   THE MANY FACES OF COCONUT

Coconut juice or coconut water is the liquid inside a coconut. • Coconut milk is produced by steeping grated coconut in hot water then straining it. • Coconut cream is coconut milk cooked down until it thickens, or grated coconut steeped in hot milk instead of water. • One fresh coconut yields about 2 cups chopped. • Shredded coconut: 1 pound equals about 5 to 6 cups. • The easiest way to open a coconut is to pierce the 3 "eyes" with a nail or an ice pick and drain the liquid. Bake the shell at 350 Degrees for about 10 minutes. Then put it on a firm surface and tap it with a hammer in several places to crack it.

MINT OR CORIANDER CHUTNEY

Makes 1½ Cups

G M E N S Y

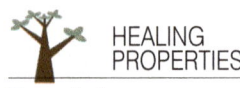 **HEALING PROPERTIES**

Tamarind
- As ointment good for inflammation, or rheumatism
- Restores sensations from paralysis and sunstroke

This chutney keeps well for about 1 week in the refrigerator. Because this chutney is so tasty, it usually doesn't last that long! Mint is about the easiest herb to grow yourself. It grows like a weed so it is best to plant it in a large container and let it spread out, otherwise it will take over the entire garden. The more you pick, the more it grows.

1½ C mint and ½ C cilantro fresh, or any combination of both
2 T tamarind paste (made into a paste) or ⅛ C lemon juice
¼ C coconut, freshly grated or unsweetened desiccated coconut, toasted
2" piece fresh ginger, grated or cut into very small pieces
1 t brown sugar
1 to 2 green chili, de-seeded and roasted, or ¼ (slightly spicy) to 1 t cayenne pepper (extra spicy)
1 t salt
4 T water

1. CUT green chili, discarding the seeds. Use them sparingly as they are quire powerful.
2. BLEND all ingredients very well, adding a little bit of water, as needed.
3. ADJUST salt.
4. ADD seasoning to chutney (see page 247).

 SIDEBAR   TAMARIND

Stately tamarind trees line many Indian villages. Its long and dusty pods (known as the Indian date) have a fruit-like, sour flavor. A little goes a long way. Tamarind pulp has more sugar and fruit acid per volume than any other fruit; it is also one of the main ingredients in Worcestershire sauce.

For some reason few plants seem to survive growing beneath a tamarind tree and there is an Indian superstition that it is harmful to sleep under it. It may be because of the corrosive effect that fallen leaves have on fabrics in damp weather. Many Asian countries venerate the tamarind tree as sacred. To Burmese the tree represents the dwelling-place of the rain god, and some hold the belief that the tree raises the temperature in its immediate vicinity. In Malaysia, a little tamarind and coconut milk is placed in the mouth of an infant at birth, and the bark and fruit are given to elephants to make them wise.

TOMATO CHUTNEY

Makes 2 Cups   GMENSY

USING BLACK MUSTARD SEEDS

Popping black mustard seeds is an art in itself. They will bounce everywhere so it is best to put a lid on the top of the pan, but leave the lid ajar, as they can burn in an instant.

This very simple chutney can be prepared at a moment's notice and it's one of my all-time favorites. In India, I often made it to accompany morning idil's.

2 T avocado or coconut oil
1 t black mustard seeds
1 t curry leaf powder (see Hint below)
2 small red onions or shallots chopped into strips
1 T ginger, grated
4 large tomatoes, chopped

1 t coriander powder
1 t salt
½ t brown sugar
¼ C cilantro, chopped
1 C yogurt, or alternative

1. HEAT oil, add mustard seeds and let them pop, add curry leaf powder.
2. SAUTÉ onions, ginger, and coriander, for about 5 minutes.
3. ADD tomatoes along with sugar and salt.
4. SAUTÉ for about 7 minutes, until tomatoes are soft.
5. ADD cilantro and let cool.
6. FOLD yogurt into cooled tomato mixture.
7. REFRIGERATE at least a half an hour before serving.

CURRY LEAF POWDER   Makes 1 Cup

Curry leaves can be sautéed in oil with mustard seeds and often with asafetida (*hing*). Strip the leaves from their stalk before frying, tear or slightly crush them between your fingers to release their essential oils. Some people don't like the mouthfeel of cooked curry leaves in a dish and go to great pains to pick them out while they eat and place them on the side of their plate. If this is the case you could make Curry Leaf Powder, here is the recipe:

4 C curry leaves   2 T coriander seeds   ½ t methi seeds   2 T urad dal   2 T dried coconut
2 T cumin seeds   1 to 2 red chilis, dried   ½ t coconut oil   2 T chana dal, dried   ½ t salt

1. DRY roast curry leaves over medium heat, remove from pan and let cool.
2. DRY roast cumin, coriander, chili, and methi seeds until fragrant, remove from pan and let cool.
3. HEAT oil in the same pan and sauté urad and chana dal until brown and aromatic, remove from pan, add coconut and roast for 2 minutes. Allow everything to cool completely.
4. BLEND all ingredients with salt until finely ground.
5. STORE in an airtight container. It will last up to 2 months.

RICE

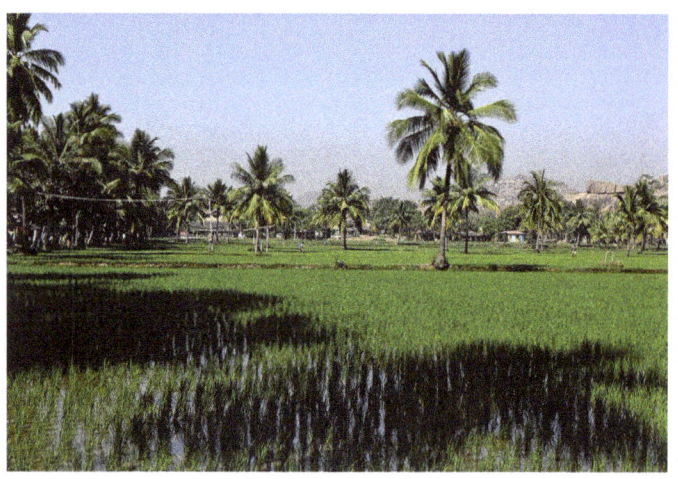

RIDING THROUGH THE SOUTH INDIA LANDSCAPE, PADDY (RICE) FIELDS stretch out like a green tapestry upon the flat land. It is a scene that is serene and vibrant, one that remains imprinted in my heart. In India, we witnessed the essential role rice plays in the lives of the people. In fact, almost three-fourths of the world's population depend on rice as their staple food. In the West people often prefer whole grain brown rice. Organic basmati white rice provides a light change of pace and works well with Indian food. Although in current times rice is being replaced by other high fiber grains, because it is a high carbohydrate, rice in moderation can also be a good source of fiber.

One day, as we were about to embark on a long train journey from Chennai to Delhi, a special friend, Saraswati, prepared three unique rice dishes for the trip. In her sparse Chennai kitchen, she made a large batch of rice, fried lots of spices and mixed various ingredients for each specific dish. Generations of South Indians carried these rice packets with them on their various travels; the spices in the rice helped make these meals last the many days of one's journey, without refrigeration.

As a guest in an Indian home, we were not allowed to resume our journey without being given these preparations, each wrapped in a single serving leaf package, for our three-day train trip. In this chapter are adaptations of these three rice dishes. They are also perfect for a picnic.

Here are a few instructions on preparing organic basmati long-grain rice:

1. There is a slight possibility that the rice may contain foreign matter such as small stones, stems, and bits of unhulled rice grains. It is best to pour out the amount of rice you are going to use on a flat surface and remove any of the foreign matter.
2. Before cooking the rice, fill the cooking pot with water. Stir the rice briskly—a film of starch and perhaps some husks may rise to the surface. Pour this off and repeat until the water is clear.
3. Use a heavy-bottom pot with a well-fitting cover for proper rice cooking. The general rule is 1 cup of rice to slightly less than 2 cups of water. Each cup of dry rice will yield approximately 3 cups of cooked rice. Add the rice and water to the pot, bring the rice to a vigorous boil. This will not take very long, so don't leave it unattended. When the rice has come to a boil, immediately turn the heat down very low so that it maintains a gentle simmer, with a tight-fitting lid on. For white rice check on it in about 15 minutes and see if all the water has been absorbed. If not, let it continue to cook another 5 minutes until it is done. Do not stir the rice while it is cooking. You can easily substitute brown rice in any of the following recipes. The water is the same, but the cooking time is about 40 to 45 minutes, after you have lowered the heat.

TYPES OF RICE

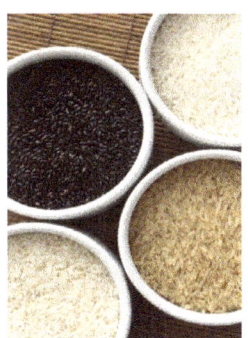

Arborio Rice is an Italian white rice grown in the Piedmont and Lombardy regions of Italy and also in California. It is a short, plump grain, and when cooked, it has a creamy texture while the inner grain remains firm. Arborio absorbs more liquid than other rice, requiring additional liquid to be added throughout the cooking process. It is used primarily in the Italian dish, risotto. Arborio is often considered the pasta of Northern Italy.

Suggested Use: Arborio rice is used primarily in risotto dishes. Add seasonal flavors, herbs, and vegetables.

Basmati Rice is a nutty flavored, aromatic rice grown in India and Pakistan around the Himalayan foothills, as well as in Iran. It is known for its delicate fragrance. The grains of this rice cook up separate and fluffy.

Suggested Use: Use basmati rice in any dish with a fragrant flavor, such as Indian curries and stews.

Brown Basmati Rice is a thin, long grain that is light tan in color. Brown basmati still retains the bran coating, which gives the rice a higher fiber

COOKING RICE IDEAS

Add a few drops of lemon juice to your pot of boiling rice, this will keep the grains from sticking together.

Add brewed green tea, coconut milk, or veggie broth to the pot instead of water.

Add fresh herbs to the pot while cooking rice: basil leaves, thyme sprigs, and bay leaves and take them out once the rice is cooked.

content and a stronger aroma than white basmati. This rice has a nutty, earthy flavor and cooks up to a firm, separate and fluffy texture.

Suggested Use: Brown basmati is an all-purpose rice, traditionally served with South Asian curries and coconut milk dishes. The rich, nutty flavor is delicious in lentil dishes or in casseroles. It makes a tasty base for stir fry and adds flavor and texture to soups.

Botan Rice is also known as sushi rice because this is the type of sticky rice used in sushi. Botan rice is a small, round, ivory colored grain with a mildly sweet flavor. Botan rice becomes sticky as it cooks and holds together well. Botan rice is a glutinous rice which also works well in Asian desserts.

Suggested Use: Botan rice is most commonly used as sushi rice, which includes a combination of rice, vinegar, and sugar. Botan rice can also be used as dessert rice in puddings and custard molds. In some countries, glutinous rice is also cooked with coconut milk and sugar for sweet dishes.

Short Grain Brown Rice is a small, almost round grain of rice that contains a higher starch content than long or medium grain rice. Short grain brown rice tends to be moister, causing the grains to stick together. It is also known as pearled rice or glutinous rice (though it does not contain gluten). This type of rice is easy to handle with chopsticks and is preferred in Eastern cuisine. This rice cooks up like the Italian arborio rice. They are similar in shape and texture. The short grain brown rice retains a high fiber bran coating giving it a nuttier flavor.

Suggested Use: Short grain brown rice is great in creamy dishes and stuffing. Use as a substitute for arborio or mochi rice. You can also use to make confections, crackers, rice balls, rice cakes and rice molds. Its starchy consistency makes it ideal for rice puddings.

Himalayan Red Rice has been grown in South Central Asia for many centuries. The rice paddies located in the foothills of the Himalayan Mountains produce the most aromatic red rice. Himalayan red rice is also grown in France. Similar in shape to brown rice but with a deep rosy color, red rice contains more of the natural bran than white rice. For this reason it requires a longer cooking time and has a nuttier more complex flavor than processed white rice.

Suggested Use: The firm and hearty texture of red rice is perfect for rice salads and rice pilaf dishes. The full shape and rosy color make it a wonderful choice for meals showcasing rice. It goes

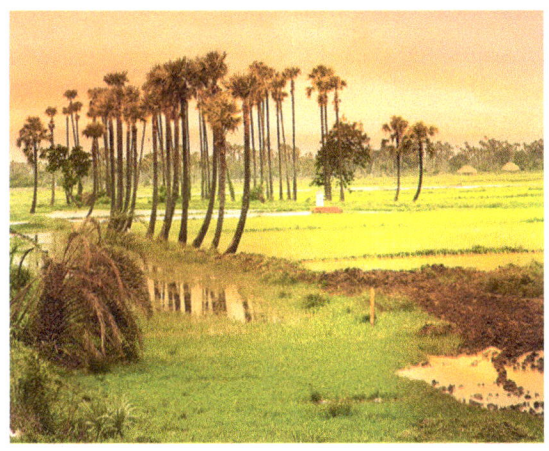

remarkably well with steamed vegetables, tofu and tempeh dishes. You can combine red rice with white rice for textural and visual interest.

Jasmine Rice is fragrant and aromatic, with a very soft and delicate flavor. It has been prized for centuries in Thailand for its silky texture and sweet nutty flavor. Jasmine rice cooks up separate and fluffy and gives off a delicate fragrance reminiscent of jasmine tea. Although originally grown in Thailand, jasmine rice is now cultivated in India and the United States. It has a similar flavor and texture to basmati rice.

Suggested Use: Excellent served with spicy dishes, its mild aromatic qualities help to balance hot foods.

Mochi Rice is a hulled, short grain, glutinous white rice. Its flavor is mild and slightly sweet. This rice has a very high starch content, which makes mochi extremely sticky. A traditional rice of Japan, mochi is most frequently used to make rice cakes. To make the cakes, cooked rice is pounded until it becomes sticky enough to hold together. It's then shaped into balls or cakes, wrapped with seaweed, or filled with little pieces of tofu. Mochiko flour is made from this rice and used to make crackers and rice noodles.

Suggested Use: Mochi is often used to make confections, crackers, rice balls, rice cakes and rice molds. Its sweet flavor and starchy consistency make it a good choice for making sushi. Due to its sweet, starchy nature, it also makes a wonderful rice pudding. It is also good to use in veggie patties as a binding ingredient.

Wild Rice (Zizania Aquatica) is not really a rice; it is a seed from an aquatic grass. Wild rice was important to the survival of many tribes in the upper Midwest. The harsh winters of Minnesota made hunting and fishing difficult and wild rice was often the subsistence food for entire tribes. Wild rice is very dark brown to black in color; each grain can be as long as one inch.

Suggested Use: The high price of wild rice usually makes it a featured part of a menu. The rice has a chewy, nutty flavor and combines well with other long grain rice. Wild rice and wild mushrooms are also a great combination in soups or pilafs.

FRAGRANT VEGETABLE RICE

Serves 5 to 7

GMENSY

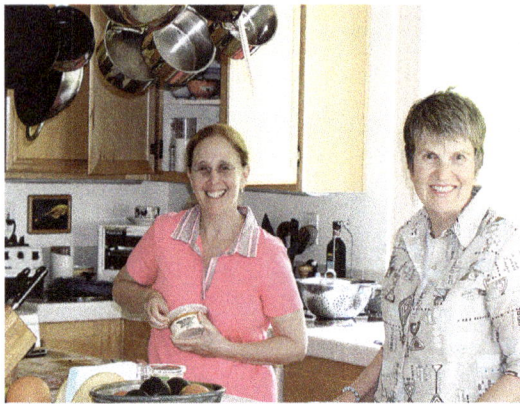

I love sharing the kitchen with friends. Often my friend Joan Loomis would arrive early to help in food prep for special dinner gatherings.

1½ C organic basmati rice, cook—yields about 4 to 5½ cups of cooked rice, cool
3 T ghee, vegetable, or coconut oil
½ t black mustard seeds
2 onions, chopped small
1 T fresh ginger, grated
1 garlic clove, crushed
¼ C cashews
½ C fresh or frozen coconut, grated or unsweetened dry coconut
1½ t salt
1 t garam masala spice mixture (page 112)
2 carrots, sliced thin
½ small cauliflower, cut into small 1-inch florets
½ C frozen green peas
2 T cilantro, cut small and splash of lemon juice

1. HEAT ghee or oil, in a large heavy bottom pot or cast-iron wok.
2. ADD mustard seeds and let them pop.
3. ADD onions, cook until translucent, then add ginger, garlic, and cashews. When the cashews are golden, add coconut, spices, salt and all vegetables, except peas.
4. STIR FRY vegetables on medium-to-low heat, until tender. Check and stir often to make sure they do not burn. When vegetables are tender, stir in frozen peas and let soften. Add the cooled cooked rice, cilantro, and lemon juice. Taste; adjust salt.
5. COMBINE well.

Coconut Rice Balls

Coconut rice balls is a variation for this recipe. It makes a great hor d'oeuvre. With ghee or oil on your hands roll vegetable rice tightly into small balls and refrigerate for half an hour to firm up. Then roll the balls into unsweetened, dry coconut. Bake in a 350 degree oven for 7 minutes. Make sure the coconut does not burn. Serve with chutney or Indian pickle.

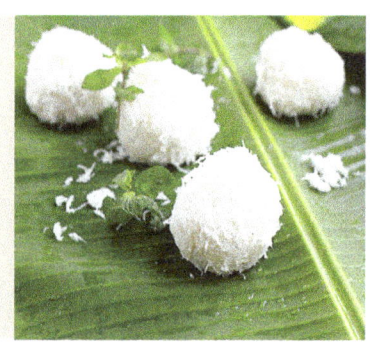

A Culinary Journey

SOOTHING YOGURT RICE

Serves 4 to 6   GENSY

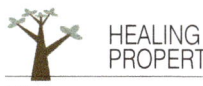
HEALING PROPERTIES

Mint
- Helps relax and smooth the muscles surrounding the intestine
- Helps with stomach spasm
- May inhibit growth of certain fungus

This is a very simple but satisfying rice dish, especially in the summer. It goes well with lemon pickle and fried poppadum dhal wafers.

2 T vegetable oil,
½ t mustard seeds and ½ t split urad dhal
½ t salt
6 curry leaves (optional)
1 green chili, de-seeded, finely chopped
1 t ginger, freshly grated
3 C cooked organic basmati rice
1½ C fresh low or nonfat yogurt or alternative
6 to 7 mint leaves, fresh, ripped

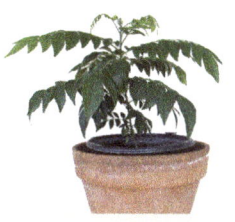

In warmer climates you can easily grow your own curry leaf tree.

1. HEAT oil and add mustard seeds until they pop, then add urad dhal. Remove the pot from the heat so the dhal does not burn. You want the urad dhal to be a golden brown, which takes a few moments.
2. ADD the following to the pot of roasted spices: curry leaves, chili, and ginger; fry a few additional moments. Then remove from pot and grind in a mortar and pestle or blender, adding a few tablespoons of water, to make it into a paste.
3. ADD yogurt, salt, and spice mixture to the cooled rice.
4. SPRINKLE top with mint leaves.
5. REFRIGERATE if you are not serving immediately.

 SIDEBAR   THE HISTORY OF MINT

There are about 25 different species of mints; the two main varieties are: peppermint which has a strong, bold flavor and spearmint, a little more cool and subtle. Mint, an ancient herb, is known for its culinary, medicinal, and aromatic properties. From Europe to India to the Middle East, mint has been used as an herb to clear the air. It has also come to symbolize hospitality in many cultures. In ancient Greece, mint leaves were rubbed on dining tables to welcome guests, while in the Middle East, the host still traditionally offers mint tea to guests upon their arrival. Mint has played an important role in the American tradition as well. While the Native Americans were using mint even before the arrival of the European settlers, the early colonists brought this prized herb with them from the Old World, long honored for therapeutic properties and used to make a hot beverage.

LEMON RICE

Serves 4 to 6

GMESY

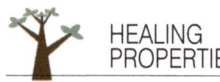 **HEALING PROPERTIES**

Asafetida
- Used to eliminate waste from the intestinal tract; especially good at clearing out toxins and impacted waste
- Added to lentils and beans to make them more digestible, reduces gas and relieves flatulence, abdominal pains, and digestive disorders
- Helps to prevent constipation

This lovely hued very lemony rice has a sweet/tangy aroma. You have to add enough salt since the lemon takes over and mutes the salt as the rice cools.

1 C organic basmati rice, cooked (yields 3 cups of rice)
3 T avocado oil
½ t black mustard seeds, 1 t split urad dhal (optional) and 6 to 7 curry leaves
1 to 2 fresh hot green chilis, finely chopped
1 t fresh ginger root, finely chopped
Pinch of asafetida (*hing*)
1 onion, chopped very small
¼ C whole raw cashews or peanuts
½ t turmeric powder and a few strands of saffron
1½ t salt
½ t turbinado brown sugar
Juice of 2 lemons or ¼ C
1 T lemon zest
¼ C cilantro, chopped

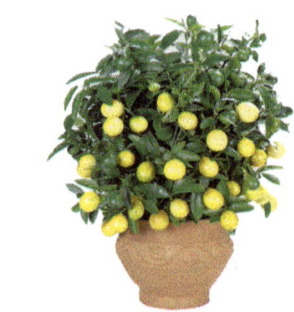

Grow your own miniature lemon bush.

1. HEAT oil in a heavy-duty pot, add mustard seeds until they pop.
2. ADD urad dhal and curry leaves. As soon as the dhal browns, which takes about 30 seconds, add the chili, ginger, and asafetida.
3. FRY a few moments, add the onions, and cook until translucent. Then add the nuts, let them turn a golden color.
4. STIR in turmeric, saffron, and salt.
5. ADD cooked rice, lemon juice and zest; stir in very well, taste and adjust salt, if needed.
6. TOP with cilantro.

 ASAFETIDA (HING)

Asafetida is a brownish, bitter, resinous material obtained from the roots of several plants of the *genus ferula* in the parsley family. It is extremely helpful in digestion. Available as a powder, this resin is very strongly scented and must be used with care. It is absolutely necessary to fry this powder very quickly in hot oil. The two reasons to heat the asafetida are: the resin dissolves in the hot oil and gets better dispersed in the food, and the high temperature changes the sulfuric taste to a much more pleasant one.

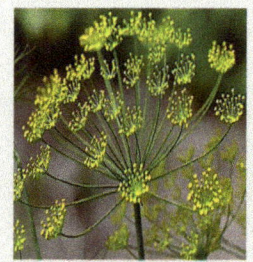

DHAL DAY

FOR A PERIOD OF SIX MONTHS, EVERY FRIDAY WAS "*DHAL* DAY." *Dhal* is the Indian term for legumes—the dried beans that come in many different sizes, colors, and shapes. Legumes form the protein powerhouse of Indian vegetarian cuisine.

How did "*dhal* day" begin? Chetna, a close friend, began working with us one day a week, and of course stayed for lunch, since whoever finds their way to the Inner Directions office rarely leaves without a meal. So our Friday lunches began to take on a distinctly Indian atmosphere, with *dhal* holding center court.

Each Thursday, I began to contemplate which *dhal* I'd be making the following Friday morning. My favorite was split mung, a quick-cooking, easily digestible *dhal* that incorporates the various flavors of the vegetable it comes into contact with. Split mung surrenders to the vegetable without losing its own distinction. Other *dhals,* I experimented with were whole-mung—a more robust and nuttier flavored *dhal* good for winter months. Additionally, there are brown and red lentils, which are the more dominant flavored *dhals*. These combine well with tomatoes and cumin seeds. Split pea is the most common *dhal*, very similar to our own split pea soup but with a unique Indian flare. Freshly roasted and ground cumin seeds and dried chili peppers give this *dhal* a special quality—a North Indian staple. Whenever I eat this *dhal* I find myself reminded of traveling on an Indian train in the early 1970s. It was on

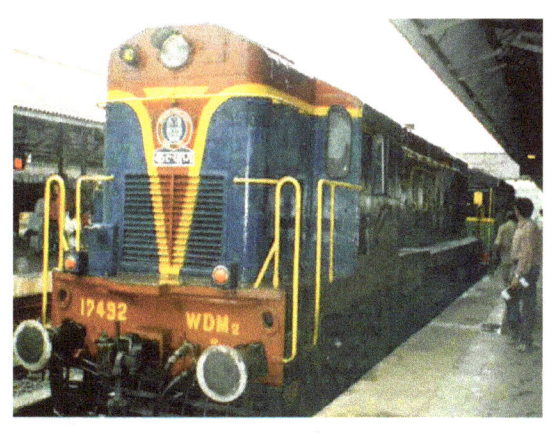

East Indian Cooking

COOKING TIPS FOR DHAL AND BEANS

Dhal contains a wide range of amino acids.

Hints

- If you are soaking whole bean dhal, drain water and replace with fresh water before cooking, a few times.
- After bringing beans to a boil, skim the top.
- Add fresh, minced ginger and turmeric to the pot while cooking.
- Add salt at the end of the cooking process, otherwise the beans will not soften.
- Split dhals don't need to be soaked.
- Add a pinch of asafetida fried quickly in hot oil when finishing the beans to aid digestion.

that train that we were given a stainless- steel tiffin carrier with our meal in different steel bowls that fit, one into the other. The food included the best split-pea *dhal* we'd ever tasted. We ate this thick *dhal* with whole wheat chapatis and rice as the train chugged along at snail speed through the vibrant green paddy fields of the Indus Valley. The other split-pea *dhal* I still remember fondly is the one served at the Ramakrishna Monastery in Kolkata. This *dhal* was truly sublime—its bright turmeric yellow color and fresh from the cow ghee flavor was very simple and

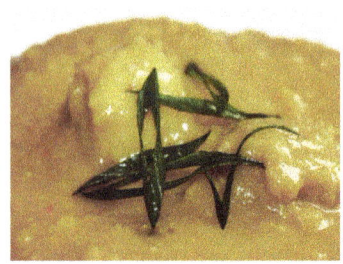

distinctive, an elegant dish. It was served with a unique puffy rice which still had a bit of husk attached to it (special to the state of Bengal), along with a few whole, boiled and salted, straight from the field, baby potatoes. We ate this particular meal every day for the entire week we stayed there.

Sambar, the South Indian dish that consists of *toor dhal*, is another favorite. This *dhal* is a bit more challenging to digest for sensitive stomachs. And, although not technically a *dhal*, chickpeas married with tomatoes and a hint of cinnamon make a wonderfully rich stew, with a similar texture to dhal.

Once *dhal* is made, you simply have to cook up some rice, add a side vegetable, lemon pickle (see recipe below), a dish of yogurt or *raita*, and you've got a complete meal.

Easy Lemon Pickle
Makes 1 (12 oz.) or 2 (6 oz.) mason ball jars

1. BOIL 3 C of water, put 2 large or 3 small whole lemons into pot, cover and let sit off the heat for 10 minutes. Remove from water, dry, and cut each lemon into 10 to 12 (large) or 8 (small) pieces, remove seeds, add juice of 1 lemon (½ C).
2. PAN ROAST and pulverize into powder: ½ t red chili flakes and 1 t fenugreek seeds. Mix with 2 T salt, ½ t turmeric, 1 t cumin powder, 2 T brown sugar.
3. HEAT 3 T cold pressed sesame or avocado oil, add 1 t black mustard seeds, 6 curry leaves (optional) and a generous pinch of asafetida. Let mustard seeds splutter, add to lemons and juice, mix thoroughly.
4. PLACE in sterilized jars and store in refrigerator, lasts up to 1 month.

SAVORY SPLIT MUNG DHAL WITH SPINACH

Serves 6 to 8

This is a favorite dhal recipe, filled with wonderful, healing spices; the aroma of spices permeates the kitchen while this dish is being made. Shown to me by a friend visiting from India, it's become a staple, because it is such a simple and complete meal in itself. I received more comments about this dhal than any other recipes printed in the Inner Directions Journal*. I once gave a fun-filled cooking lesson to my friends Nan and Peter, who often requested this dhal, which I would share with them when I made a potful. If you want a smoky, less potent chili you can use Aleppo.*

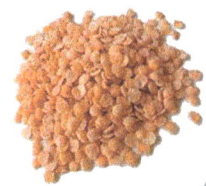

2 to 3 T avocado, ghee, or coconut oil
½ t cumin seeds and ½ t brown mustard seeds
Pinch of *hing* (asafetida)
1½" piece of ginger, skin removed, grated
1 garlic clove, smashed and chopped very small [optional]
½ t turmeric powder
1 t coriander powder
¼ t cardamom powder
¼ to 1 t cayenne or Aleppo pepper, depending how hot you like it
2 onions, sliced thin
2 plum tomatoes, chopped or ½ (8 oz.) can canned roasted diced tomatoes
3 C fresh spinach, roughly chopped or 1½ C frozen
1 C split mung dhal, orange, rinsed well and drained
4 to 5 C water and 1 (14 oz.) can light coconut milk
1½ to 2 t salt
½ C cilantro, chopped small and splash of lemon juice

1. HEAT oil in large soup pot (I often use a heavy-duty Dutch oven).
2. ADD cumin and mustard seeds, fry until they pop, add the rest of the spices, and stir fry for 1 minute.
3. STIR FRY ginger and garlic for one minute
4. SAUTÉ onion until translucent, then add tomatoes and fry until soft.
5. ADD dhal, and 4 cups of water, bring to a boil. Skim foam from top and lower heat to a simmer. Cook for 15 to 20 minutes.
6. ADD spinach and cook another 30 minutes on low heat.
7. ADD coconut milk and salt and additional water if necessary. Dhal should be thick like a creamed soup. You can blend slightly or mash with a potato masher. Top with cilantro and lemon juice.

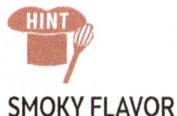

SMOKY FLAVOR

To add a smoky flavor to any dhal, simply add a few drops of liquid smoke at the end of cooking, a little goes a long way. This ingredient simply contains water and natural hickory smoke.

SPLIT PEA DHAL

Serves 5 to 6

GMENSY

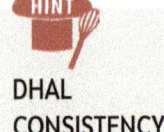

DHAL CONSISTENCY

To eat this dhal with chapatis: (See page 197). Make a thicker dhal, reducing water to 4½ C, mash slightly at the end.

To eat with rice: Add the full 6 C and cook dhal until tender, but not mushy.

This is a traditional North Indian recipe. Special Indian green chili gives this dhal an authentic taste, but if you don't have it on hand, dried red pepper flakes, or jalapeños, work just as well. If you want a smoky, less potent chili you can use Aleppo pepper.

1 T coconut or avocado oil and 2 T ghee, butter, or margarine
½ t cumin seeds
½ t black mustard seeds
¾ t turmeric powder, 1 t coriander powder, 1 t cumin powder
1 to 2 green chilis, de-seeded, chopped small or 1 t dried red pepper flakes
1" ginger piece; skin removed, grated
1 onion, chopped very small
1½ C green or yellow split peas (rinse well)
4 to 6 C water and 2 T lemon juice
1½ t salt

1. HEAT oil and ghee, butter, or margarine in a large soup pot.
2. ADD cumin and mustard seeds, fry until they pop. Add green chili or red pepper flakes. Let brown slightly.
3. ADD turmeric, coriander, and cumin powder.
4. STIR FRY ginger for 1 minute.
5. SAUTÉ onion until translucent.
6. ADD split peas, water, and lemon.
7. SIMMER on low-medium heat, skim top foam, cook approximately 30 minutes. Peas should be intact, soft, but not be completely dissolved, add salt at the end.

SIDEBAR GREEN CHILIS

Fresh green Indian chilis are usually long and thin and can be found in the produce area of an Indian grocery store or through a mail order supplier. When selecting fresh chilis make sure they are firm, smooth, and glossy with no signs of splitting. Refrigerate them in a plastic bag for up to 3 days. When handling fresh chilis, it is best to protect your hands with rubber gloves and avoid touching your face or eyes. They are hard to come by, so I usually buy plenty and simply freeze the balance in an airtight container for later use.

A Culinary Journey

HEARTY CHICKPEA CURRY

Serves 6 to 8

GMENSY

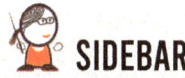 **SIDEBAR**

THE HISTORY OF CHICKPEAS

Chickpeas are the most widely consumed legume in the world. They originated in the Middle East as a reliable source of protein.

The first record of when garbanzos were eaten is about 7,000 years ago.

They seemed to grow wild for about two thousand years, and were first cultivated around 3,000 BC, in the Mediterranean basin and then spread to India and Ethiopia.

When using dried beans, soak overnight. An Instant Pot is ideal, the beans cook quickly and absorb the intense flavor. In a Dutch oven bring to a boil and then cook on medium heat. I have used canned chickpeas as well. (If you are using canned chickpeas, rinse twice, and drain really well, the cooking time is reduced to 15 minutes.)

2 T avocado oil
½ t cumin seeds
½ t black mustard seeds
2 onions, chopped
4 tomatoes, large, chopped, or 1 (14 oz.) can fire roasted tomatoes
½ t turmeric powder
1 t garam masala (see page 132)
½ t cardamom powder
2 bay leaves and 2 cinnamon sticks
½ to 2 t cayenne pepper, depending how hot you like it
1 t brown sugar or jaggery
2" ginger piece, skin removed, grated
2 C dried chickpeas, soak overnight, drained and rinse twice with fresh water
Add Enough water (in Instant Pot) to go half way up to the top of chickpeas, ½" over the top of chickpeas (for Dutch oven)
2 t salt and ½ C cilantro, chopped small

1. HEAT oil in Instant Pot (use Sauté setting) or in a heavy-duty Dutch oven.
2. ADD cumin and mustard seeds, fry until cumin seeds brown and mustard seeds pop.
3. STIR FRY ginger for 1 minute and sauté onions until translucent
4. MARINATE tomatoes, turmeric, garam masala, cardamom, bay leaves, cinnamon sticks, and cayenne powder in ½ C water for 15 minutes.
5. ADD tomato mixture to spices in pot and cook for a few minutes until thickened.
6. ADD chickpeas and water to the Instant Pot cook (on Stew Setting) for 30 minutes or in the Dutch oven cook for about 1½ hours, until chickpeas are very soft, add salt at the end.
7. REMOVE bay leaves and cinnamon sticks and adjust salt to taste.
8. TOP with cilantro

MUMBAI KITCHEN

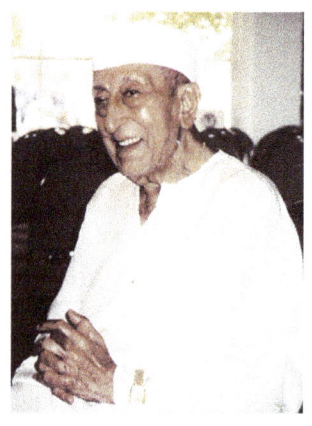

FOR ONE WEEK IN JUNE 1999, WE HOSTED AN INDIAN TEACHER, SRI RANJIT MAHARAJ in our home. We were very blessed by his visit as he passed away about a year and a half later. We had never met him but knew it would be a very special visit. He arrived with three dedicated people to assist him: Naleen, Laurance, and Ujjwala. Each had their specific duties, but Ujjwala cooked for everyone! This skilled team graciously allowed us to join them in the kitchen for the week. And much was going on in the kitchen. The kitchen crew chopped cilantro, grated ginger, and stirred pots of vegetables, all under the watchful eyes of Ujjwala. She is a mother of three and works as a teacher in a school for the deaf in Mumbai (Bombay). Always smiling, Ujjwala taught us the true meaning of selfless service. In a practical way there was much to learn by being in the kitchen with her, from various ways to utilize spices in dry and wet combinations to balancing the delicate blend of condiments with vegetables and legumes. The main lesson of the week we learned from Ujju was: "Laugh and be free. If we must cook, let it be a joy. Cook from joy—let your hands be infused with love."

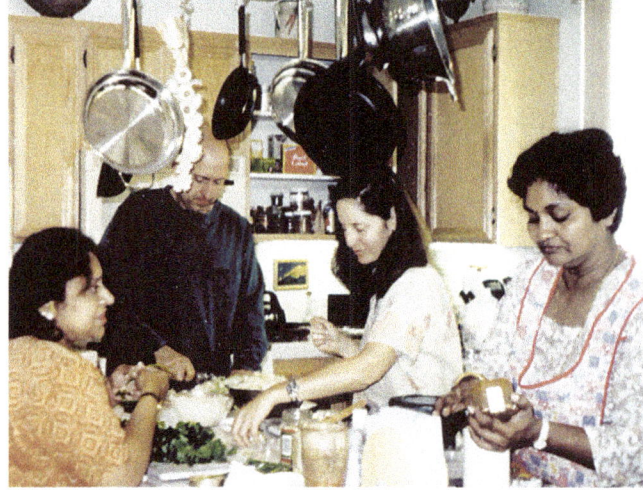

When you're in the kitchen with Ujju (far right) you should wear an apron; turmeric is a natural dye.

A Culinary Journey

STIR-FRIED GOURD OR ZUCCHINI

Serves 6 to 8

GMENSY

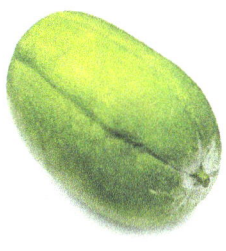

There are so many gourd varieties. In our travels throughout India, we ate a variety of them, depending on the season and region we were visiting. Because there are so many different curries, both dry and wet, we never got tired of them. Ujju's version is a simple but satisfying way to eat any summer squash.

3 T avocado oil
1 t black mustard seeds
Generous pinch asafetida (*hing*)
7 C zucchini or Indian gourd, skin left on, cut into cubes
¾ t turmeric
1½ to 2 t salt
1 t turbinado or jaggery sugar
Splash of lemon juice
2 T cilantro, chopped

Ginger/Chili Paste

1 to 2 green chilis, de-seeded and chopped
1" piece of ginger, chopped very small

GRIND together with a little water to make a thick paste.

1. HEAT oil in large frying pan, add mustard seeds, let them pop, then add asafetida.
2. STIR in cut vegetables and top with turmeric and salt.
3. FRY on a medium heat, keep lid on pan between stirring often. You want them to steam in their own juice, yet not burn.
4. ADD ginger/chili paste (see recipe on side), remove lid, continue frying until veggies are tender.
5. ADD sugar and lemon at the end of cooking.
6. TOP with cilantro.

 SIDEBAR   MUSTARD SEEDS

Both the Biblical and Buddhist stories of the mustard seed are favorites of mine, as are the mustard seeds themselves. Indian cooking generally uses the brown or black mustard seeds, rather than the yellow ones most commonly used for mustard. They need to be tempered by frying them with a little oil and waiting for them to pop, to release their distinctive essence.

Mustard, like black pepper, is one of the most widely used spices in the United States. It is not known when it was first used as a condiment, but the Romans blended these small seeds with "must" to make a sauce. "Mustard" is an ancient name, stemming from the Latin word *mustem ardens*. *Mustem* means "must" (fermenting grape juice that has not yet become wine), and *ardens* means "burning," alluding to the pungent hotness of the seeds.

UJJU'S HEAVENLY TOMATO SOUP

Serves 6 to 8   GMENSY

This is a delightful soup to top any rice dish. Serve simply with plain rice or alone as a fiery soup. This recipe needs the green chilis to give it its unique flavor. You can substitute three Indian green chilis for one jalapeño, but make sure to remove the seeds and white membranes.

2 T avocado oil
3 to 4 onions, medium, chopped small
¾ t turmeric
1 t coriander powder and 1 t cumin powder
1½ t salt and 1 t sugar
8 to 10 very ripe tomatoes, chopped
1 can light coconut milk
2 T cilantro, chopped

Blend together with a small amount of water:
1½" piece of ginger, cut into small pieces
1 to 3 Indian green chilis (de-seed or add seeds to make it as hot as you wish. Ujju used 3 and boy was it hot!)

1. HEAT oil and sauté onions until translucent.
2. ADD spices, salt, sugar, and tomatoes and cook on medium heat for about 10 minutes until tomatoes are fully cooked.
3. ADD coconut milk, blended ginger and green chilis, heat for another few minutes, adjust salt if needed.
4. COOL slightly and blend until smooth, add cilantro at the end.
5. REHEAT to serve, but don't bring to a boil.

Chopping Cilantro

1. Immerse in cold water for a few minutes to remove debris, then drain well on a paper towel.

2. Remove any discolored leaves and long stems.

3. Finely chop cilantro you are using.

4. Wrap unused cilantro in a paper towel and place in a plastic bag. Store in the refrigerator for a few days.

 SIDEBAR   LIGHT COCONUT MILK

I love using light coconut milk since it imparts the same unique flavor as regular coconut milk without the excess fat. After opening a can and using a small portion, I save the remainder in the refrigerator for other uses. Recently, I discovered that freezing the remainder in ice cube trays and transferring the cubes to a plastic bag or container allows me to use a small portion at a time. Make sure to label and date the plastic bag or months later you'll have no idea what the cubes contain.

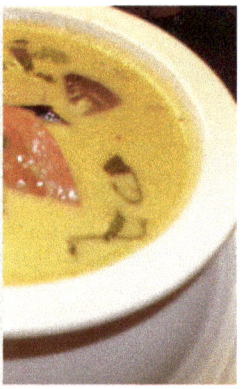

BOMBAY BAIGAN BHARTA (EGGPLANT CURRY)

Serves 6 to 8

GMENSY

ADDITIONAL ITEMS FOR EGGPLANT CURRY

You have an option of adding ½ C cashew nuts or green peas when frying onions to add an additional level of flavor.

Roasted Eggplant and Chilis
3 small eggplants, charred or roasted
1 to 2 Indian green chilis, de-seeded.

Tomato Mixture
3 T avocado oil
Pinch asafetida and 6 to 7 curry leaves (optional)
3 onions, chopped very small
3 tomatoes, chopped small

Spices
½ t turmeric, 1½ t coriander powder, and 1½ t cumin powder
1 t garam masala powder (see page 132)
1½ t salt and 1 T brown sugar or jaggery
½ C cilantro, chopped small

Blended Spices*
1 to 2 garlic cloves, peeled and chopped
1½" piece of ginger, remove skin and chopped small

BLEND together with a small amount of water to make a paste.

1. CHAR eggplants and green chilis by placing directly onto gas range and rotating until soft inside and black outside. You can also roast them in the oven; turn often to ensure even cooking. Remove skins and chop into pieces. Remove excessive seeds from eggplant and chilis.
2. FRY asafetida and curry leaves in oil for a few minutes, then add onions. Sauté until translucent, then add tomatoes.
3. COOK tomato mixture until all liquid is evaporated.
4. MIX spices, salt, and blended spices* with roasted eggplant and chilis.
5. ADD eggplant mixture to tomato mixture and cook together on medium heat, covered, for about 10 minutes.
6. ADD sugar at the end, top with cilantro.

 SIDEBAR   JAGGERY

Jaggery is an unrefined crude brown sugar obtained from the sap of the East Indian jaggery palm. It is produced by boiling the sap of the palm (similar to maple sugar production) and is popular in India and Southeast Asia as a sweetener and an ingredient in curries, especially vegetarian curries. Jaggery tastes somewhat like a combination of dark brown sugar and molasses and can be used interchangeably with brown sugar. Sold as solid cakes, it is also known as "palm sugar."

EGGPLANT MASALA (SPICE) RICE BALLS

Serves 8 to 10

GMENSY

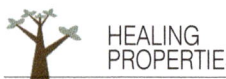

Bay Leaves
- Soothing for the stomach, relieve abdominal cramps
- Help strengthen and tone digestive organs

Definition of ma·sa·la

Any of a number of spice mixtures ground into a paste or powder for use in Indian cooking.

¼ C coconut oil
9 bay leaves and 6 to 7 curry leaves (optional; available in specialty store)
1 t cumin seeds
½ C raw cashews, chopped
2 onions, chopped small
3 C basmati white rice (uncooked)

Dry Ingredients (dry roast spices until fragrant and then grind spices in a coffee grinder or mortar and pestle)
20 cardamom seeds (remove from shell), ½ t peppercorn, 2 cinnamon sticks, 2 T cumin seeds, 1 T coriander seeds and 2 bay leaves, ½ C coconut (finely shredded, not sweetened)

Wet Masala (grind in blender)
2 C cilantro
2 to 3 green chilis
1 to 2 garlic cloves
1½" piece of ginger, grated
½ C water
1 eggplant (remove skin) chop, boil and drain

Additional Ingredients
5½ C water
2 T salt
½ C cilantro, chopped small

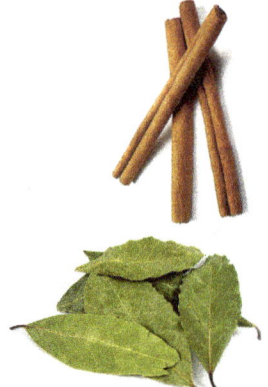

1. HEAT oil in a large, heavy bottom pot; add bay leaves, cumin, curry leaves, cashews, and onions. Cook until onions are translucent.
2. ADD rice and stir fry a few moments.
3. ADD dry spice ingredients, blended wet masala, water and salt to rice mixture. Mix well then bring to a boil. Lower flame and simmer about 15 to 20 minutes until rice is completely cooked. Watch carefully since it can easily burn on the bottom of the pot.
4. TOP with cilantro.
5. COOL rice mixture, knead together, adding oil to your hands for shaping.
6. SHAPE into one-inch round balls, then flatten.
7. BAKE at 350 Degrees for 10 to 20 minutes, until golden.

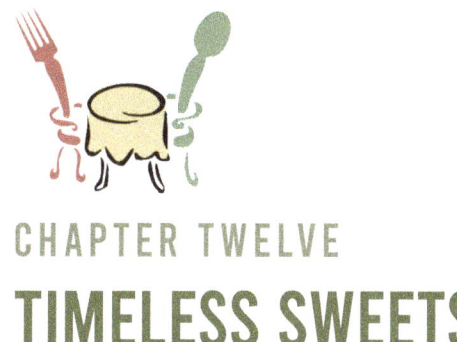

CHAPTER TWELVE
TIMELESS SWEETS

PIES
CAKES, COOKIES AND BARS
CREAMY CREATIONS
INDIAN DESSERTS

PIES

Gluten-Free Flour Recipe for Baking

This combination can stored it in a container in the refrigerator. To use: measure the amount you need for your recipe and subtract ½ cup, then add ¼ C almond meal and ¼ C oat flour.

See page 288 and 310 for gluten-free binding agents that need to be added to this mix.

3 C brown rice flour
1 C potato starch
½ C white rice flour
½ C tapioca flour

EVERY SUMMER, BEGINNING AT AGE SEVEN TO ELEVEN, my family vacationed in a bungalow colony in upstate New York called, "Salon's Lodge." Mr. and Mrs. Salon were quite old by the time my family started spending summers in the old, run-down cottages that surrounded their land. The land had a number of ancient apple trees, whose apple variety names were long forgotten. The land also skirted a small forest with wild berries that grew like weeds, and a hand-dug pond where we were sure monsters lived.

Many of my aunt's and multiple cousins, including Grandma Molly, spent the entire summer with us. While the dad's worked all week and visited on the weekends, the mom's and grandma's days revolved around cooking and baking, especially Grandma Molly. So, before we could do anything fun for the day, we had to check with Grandma about which pie she would be making, berry or apple. Berry picking often carried the possible risk of poison ivy or oak, so we had to negotiate the woods carefully. Apple picking sometimes required a ladder, so it was deemed more fun. After picking the apples we delivered them to Grandma Molly who carried them to the communal kitchen tucked into her well-worn apron. We knew by afternoon the warm pie would be sending its lovely fragrance throughout the front yard.

Following in Grandma Molly's footsteps I often make pies. I bake them according to what is in season, blueberry in midsummer, apple and pumpkin in the fall, and pecan in winter. Pies first became a part of my life in Nova Scotia. There was an old, dormant apple orchard on the property and somehow the trees survived decades of neglect. The varieties were small, tangy, and funnily shaped, perfect for pies and sauces. Having a fresh pie cooling on the kitchen counter is about as close to heaven as you can get. These recipes are pretty basic, with a few healthy twists.

TRADITIONAL PIE CRUSTS

Preheat Oven to 350 Degrees | Bake: 10 to 12 Minutes

MENSY

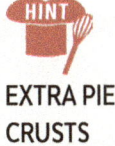

EXTRA PIE CRUSTS

Pie crusts were always a challenge until I created the fool-proof recipe; it is a flaky, non-temperamental recipe. I like to make extra crusts at the same time, I place each one in a tin foil pie plate, double wrap in plastic bags, and store in the freezer, so whenever I feel inclined to bake a pie the crust is already waiting.

FOOL-PROOF PIE CRUST (DOUBLE CRUST)

You can always half this recipe for a one crust pie. This can also be done in a food processor, using the pulse setting.

2¼ C unbleached white pastry flour
½ C whole wheat pastry flour
¾ C + 2 T butter or margarine, cubed and chilled
1 t salt
1 t vinegar
½ C ice water

1. MIX flours (sifted together) salt, butter or margarine with your hands, until it resembles pea-shaped balls.
2. MIX vinegar and very cold water.
3. COMBINE wet mixture (beginning with ⅓ C) to dry mixture, adding extra tablespoons (as needed), so dough just comes together.
4. PLACE rough dough on top of cling wrap, pull up the sides up, until it forms a round, split into two sections and wrap each separately.
5. CHILL in refrigerator at least 30 minutes or more before rolling out.

WHOLE GRAIN PIE CRUST (SINGLE CRUST)

1 C whole wheat pastry flour and ½ C oat flour (sift together)
½ t salt
8 T butter or margarine, chilled
3 to 5 T ice water

1. ADD flours and salt to butter or margarine, until the mixture resembles peas. Add just enough chilled water for mixture to come together.
2. MOLD into one ball; cover with wax paper or parchment paper and chill at least 30 minutes or more before rolling out.

 PIE CRUSTS TIDBITS

• Work with cold ingredients and utensils. • To measure flour: lightly fluff up then dip a cup into the flour and sweep off excess with knife. • Before rolling out chilled dough, remove from fridge and let sit for 10 minutes. • Work quickly before the dough softens. • Roll from the center out. • Lift and move dough in a circle, adding the minimum amount of flour to the board to make sure it doesn't stick. • Re-roll scraps by stacking on top of each other, side by side, if narrow. Roll between sheets of wax paper to avoid having to add excess flour, or on a Silpat (see the appendix).

Timeless Sweets

WHEAT-FREE CRUSTS

Preheat Oven to 350 Degrees

GMENSY

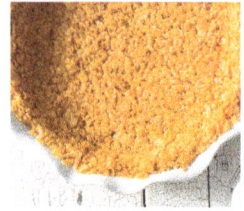

SWEET CORNFLAKE PIECRUST (SINGLE CRUST)
A sweet, gluten-free crust, which works for many dessert pies.

4 C corn flake cereal, enough to make 1¼ C crushed
1 T maple syrup and 1 T agave syrup
2 T margarine or butter, melted

1. PULVERIZE corn flakes until they are fine crumbs.
2. MIX melted margarine or butter with syrups, add to crumbs.
3. PAT into an 8" or 9" pie pan, bake for 5 minutes.
4. CHILL thoroughly.
5. ADD filling to chilled crust.

Fluting Crust

You use two hands to "flute" the edge of the crust, by pushing your thumb from one hand in between the thumb and index finger of the opposite hand.

You can also use one hand to "flute" the edge of the crust between your thumb and the side of your index finger. Either method will work.

SAVORY OATMEAL CRUST (SINGLE CRUST)

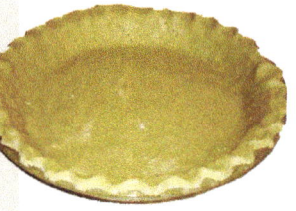

1 C gluten-free flour blend and ½ C rolled oats, whirled in blender until fine
½ t xanthan gum (omit if your gluten-free blend already contains it)
½ t salt
6 T margarine, butter or coconut oil, or any combination of the three, cube and chill
3 to 5 T ice water

1. COMBINE flour, oats, xanthan gum, and salt in a bowl.
2. ADD chilled margarine, butter, or coconut oil, mixing it in with a fork, until it resembles fine crumbs.
3. ADD just enough ice water to forms a ball, cover and chill.
4. ROLL into a 9" round, adding flour as needed, fold in half and place in pie plate, tine bottom and flute crust.
5. BAKE for 10 minutes, until almost golden, chill before filling.

MORE WHEAT-FREE CRUSTS

Preheat Oven 350 Degrees | Bake: 5 to 7 Minutes   GMENSY

HEALING PROPERTIES

Amaranath
- Packed with manganese
- High in phosphorus, a mineral that is important for bone health.
- Rich in iron, which helps your body produce blood
- Good source of health-promoting antioxidants

GRAHAM-CRACKER LIKE PIECRUST (SINGLE CRUST)

This crust is suitable for pumpkin pie, fruit pie or cheesecake. It is a sweet, almost graham-cracker tasting crust.

4 T margarine or butter, chilled
¾ C amaranth flour (this flour and date sugar gives it a graham-crackery taste)
¼ C arrowroot flour (also called arrowroot powder)
¼ C tapioca flour
¼ C almond meal/flour
½ salt
½ C date sugar
3 to 5 T ice water

1. CHILL margarine or butter, cut into small cubes.
2. MIX all dry ingredients together.
3. ADD just enough water to hold it together.
4. PRESS into a pie plate.
5. BAKE until almost golden.
6. COOL crust before filling.

GMSY

 SIDEBAR   AMARANTH HISTORY

Before the Spanish conquest in 1519, amaranth was associated with human sacrifice. Aztec women made a mixture of ground amaranth seed, honey, or human blood, shaping this mixture into idols that were eaten ceremoniously. This practice appalled the conquistadors who reasoned that eliminating the amaranth would eliminate the sacrifices. The grain was then forbidden and consequently fell into obscurity for hundreds of years. If the cultivation of amaranth had not continued in a few remote areas of the Andes and Mexico, it might have become extinct.

ALMOND CRUST (SINGLE CRUST)

Dry Ingredients
2 C almond meal
¼ t salt and ¼ t baking soda
2 T maple or brown sugar
3 T margarine or butter
1 egg

1. MIX dry ingredients together.
2. BLEND margarine or butter with the egg, add to dry ingredients until it is finely and uniformly distributed.
3. PRESS the crumble into a pie plate.
4. BAKE until almost golden, checking often, as it can burn quickly.

Timeless Sweets

BLUEBERRY CRUMBLE PIE

Makes 1 Pie | Preheat Oven to 350 Degrees | Bake: 40 to 45 Minutes   G M E N S Y

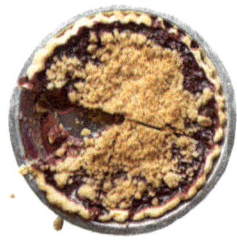

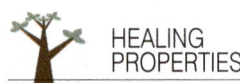
HEALING PROPERTIES

Blueberry
- Packed with antioxidant phytonutrients, helps to neutralize free radical damage.
- May improve nighttime vision
- Helps to protect the brain from oxidative stress and age-related conditions, such as Alzheimer's
- Helps relieve both diarrhea and constipation, with its soluble and insoluble fiber
- Contains tannins that can reduce inflammation

Growing up in Northern New Jersey I remember blueberries ushering in each summer season. A vivid memory is one of picking blueberries in the forest behind "Salon's Lodge" (in the Catskill Mountains) and the woods near my house in Glen Rock, New Jersey, before they turned it into a large housing development. I picked just enough for a fresh blueberry pie. Even now, the smell of cooked blueberries takes me back to the amazing wonder and freedom of childhood summer vacations. This blueberry pie uses less sugar, plenty of lemon and a slight hint of coconut. The crumb topping is golden and crumbly, has a warm buttery flavor, and it's oh so easy to make. When baking I place my berry pie on a cookie sheet, since it can bubbly up quite a bit.

Blueberry Mixture

4 C blueberries (approximately 2-pint cartons)
½ C brown, maple, or date sugar
2 T corn starch and ½ t cinnamon
2 t lemon juice and 1 t lemon zest

Crumb Topping

½ C brown sugar
½ C whole wheat flour or ¾ C gluten-free flour blend (½ C if you omit oats)
½ C margarine or butter, softened
¼ C rolled oats
¼ C finely shredded unsweetened coconut and pinch of salt

1. COMBINE blueberry mixture in a bowl and let sit for 15 minutes. Pour into a prepared pie crust.
2. BLEND the sugar, flour, butter or margarine, oats, coconut, and salt together.
3. SPRINKLE crumb topping evenly over pie filling.
4. ADD aluminum foil to the edges; remove after baking 30 minutes.
5. BAKE until juices bubble thickly, and crumb top is golden.

 HINT — STORING BROWN SUGAR

Store brown sugar in an airtight plastic container. To soften brown sugar that has gone hard, just add a slice of fresh bread or a slice of apple to the container for a few hours. When the sugar is soft, remove the bread or apple slice.

MOM'S APPLE PIE

Makes 1 Pie | Preheat Oven to 350 Degrees | Bake: 50 to 60 Minutes

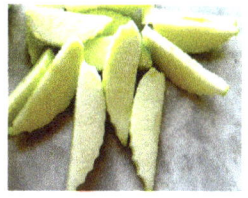

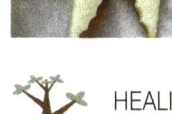

This was one of my mom's favorite recipes, which we had in the early fall. I would walk over to Herald's Farm (a small roadside stand that is long gone) and get some apples that had just arrived from upstate New York apple farms. Mom often used a few different varieties of apples to give her pies a tart/sweet taste but turned to "Granny Smith" for the largest proportion of apples. She was always quite generous in her use of spices. The fragrant juices that flowed from her pie were a deep auburn color.

Apples
- Contain insoluble and soluble fiber and natural pectin (found primarily in the skin) that grab toxins like heavy metals, lead, and mercury
- Contains dynamic antioxidants
- Inhibits growth of liver and colon cancer cells, according to several studies

7 large apples, cored, peeled, and sliced, don't slice too small
½ C brown sugar
1 T cinnamon, ¼ t nutmeg, ¼ t allspice, ¾ t ginger powder, ½ t cardamom
½ t salt
3 T flour or corn starch
1 T lemon juice and 1 T lemon zest
2 T margarine or butter, cold

1. COMBINE the sliced apples, sugar, spices, and flour together, add the lemon juice and zest until it's mixed well, and fill a prepared pie crust.
2. TOP with margarine or butter bits, chopped very small.
3. PLACE top crust over the apples and prick with a fork to release the steam; then sprinkle top with a cinnamon/sugar mixture.
4. BAKE until top is golden.

SIX GREAT APPLE PIE VARIETIES

Any good cooking apple usually works, though knowing apple varieties is helpful because some apples contain more liquid and may need extra thickening ingredients to ensure that the pie isn't soggy.
Golden Delicious: Pale gold, freckled skin. Sweet, crisp, and mellow. HINT: Cut down the sugar in pies and sauces made from these apples.
Granny Smith: Bright green with a pink blush. Tart and crisp. HINT: Holds it shape and blends nicely with sweeter apples.
Macintosh: Light to deep red with green blush. Sweet with a tart-tang, very juicy. HINT: Tender flesh cooks down quickly; might need extra thickener in pie.
Rome: Bright red. Slightly tart, firm. HINT: Holds it shape during baking.
Cortland: Deep red/pale yellow blush. Sweet with a hint of tartness. HINT: Juicy, use extra thickener.
Jonagold: Creamy yellow flesh/blush stripe. Honey-sweet, hint of tartness, juicy and crisp at same time.

CREAMY PECAN PIE

Makes 1 Pie | Preheat Oven to 350 Degrees | Bake: 40 Minutes   G M S Y

Pecans are natively grown in central California, so whenever we travel from the south to the north, we end up stopping at a pecan stand. Pecans, like all nuts, don't last very long in the pantry, so if you have an abundance of them, it's a good idea to refrigerate or freeze them. This recipe is a slightly lighter version of the traditional pecan pie.

2 eggs, large and 3 egg whites
½ C maple syrup and ½ C light corn syrup (or 1 C agave or brown rice syrup)
⅓ C dark brown sugar and ½ t salt
1 C pecans, chopped (an additional 10 whole pecans for top)
1½ t vanilla extract

HINT

CUTTING PIE

When cutting a sticky pie, coat your knife with a thin layer of oil. It will slice clear through.

1. BEAT all the eggs and next four ingredients, with a whisk or mixer until very well-blended.
2. STIR in the chopped pecans and vanilla extract.
3. POUR into a prepared crust.
4. TOP with 10 whole pecans.
5. BAKE for 20 minutes, then cover with foil.
6. BAKE an additional 20 minutes, until custard is set.

 SIDEBAR   THE ART AND HISTORY OF THE PIE

Originally, individual pies were filled with meats and vegetables cooked together inside a solid ridge of pastry (called *pasty*), hand crimped along the top. The pasty allowed a miner or traveler to grasp the pastry of the pie for eating and then discard the crust to avoid germs and contamination from dirty hands. Early Irish Catholic priests also prepared them to carry as they walked about the countryside preaching. When the Irish people migrated to northern England they took the art of pie-making with them. Soon every miner in northern England took pies down into the mine for noon lunch. English sailors took pie-making as far as the shores of Russia (known as *piraski* or *pierogies*). Then the Pilgrims brought their favorite family pie recipes with them to America. The colonists adapted their pie ingredients and techniques to what was available in the New World. At first, they baked pies with berries and fruits pointed out to them by the Native Americans. Colonial women used round shallow pans, instead of pasties, to stretch the ingredients.

HOLIDAY PUMPKIN PIE

Makes 1 Pie | Preheat Oven to 350 Degrees | Bake: 50 to 60 Minutes   GMENSY

LIGHTER VERSION TO REPLACE EGG YOLKS IN RECIPE

- 2 envelopes unflavored gelatin and 2 T water
- fat-free evaporated milk
- 3 egg whites

Sprinkle gelatin over water, let stand 5 to 10 minutes. Bring 1 C milk just to a boil, stir into gelatin. Stir in ¼ C egg whites to temper eggs, then add rest of the egg whites. Follow baking instructions for the rest of the pie.

I once tried to make pumpkin pie with a rather large pumpkin from our Nova Scotian garden. It just didn't work; it actually tasted bitter. There are so many wonderful varieties of organic canned pumpkin pulp available that making this pie is almost as simple as opening the pumpkin can. It goes really well with a dense, whole grain crust. This pie can easily be made without eggs, by using soft tofu to bind it.

1 (15 oz.) can of pumpkin pulp
½ C date, maple, or brown sugar
¼ C maple syrup, agave, or combination of the two
2 eggs* or ½ C soft tofu blended with 1 T oil
1 (12 oz.) can evaporated milk or 1 C vanilla soy, macadamia, almond, coconut, or rice milk
1 t vanilla extract
1 t cinnamon, ground, 1 t ginger, ground
　¼ t nutmeg, ground, ½ t cloves, ground,
　½ t cardamom, ground
½ t salt

1. MIX pumpkin pulp with sugar and syrup.
2. BLEND eggs or tofu mixture, milk, vanilla, spices, and salt together, add to pumpkin mix and viciously blend well.
3. POUR into a prepared pie crust.
4. BAKE 425 degrees for 10 minutes, reduce oven to 325 degrees for 45 to 50 minutes, until the center of the pie is set.

*You can also separate the eggs, add the yokes to the batter, make a meringue from the egg whites and fold into the batter at the end.

 NIFTY HOMEMADE SPICE CABINET

This is a simple and innovative way to make a spice cabinet utilizing your existing spice jars. Purchase sticky-back Velcro strips. Stick the grab part on the bottom of your over-the-counter cabinets. Stick 1-inch pieces onto the tops of spice jars so the jars hang down in full view. Grab and loosen spice bottle when you are ready to use. When a jar is empty, save the old cap and switch it to the new jar. You can buy double sticky velcro by the yard at a fabric store.

Timeless Sweets

INTENSE CHOCOLATE TART

Makes 1 Pie | Preheat Oven to 325 Degrees | Bake: 40 to 45 Minutes   GMNSY

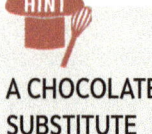

A CHOCOLATE SUBSTITUTE

Carob has been used as a food for over 5,000 years. Both the seeds and pods are edible; the ground seeds are used as a substitute for cocoa. Carob powder is also used as a food stabilizer and a darkening agent. You can substitute carob powder and chips equally to chocolate.

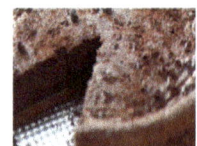

This is a holiday treat, a pie I have made for many Passover seders. It's very rich and satisfying, a little goes a long way. Since there is no added flour, substituting a gluten-free tart shell makes this a great alternative dessert.

5 oz. unsalted margarine or butter
5½ oz. semisweet chocolate or carob chips
8 T unsweetened cocoa or carob powder, sifted and ½ t salt
4 eggs or 2 eggs and 3 egg whites (made into meringue)
7 ounces turbinado or sugar cane (non-refined brown), processed until fine
3 T maple or agave syrup
3 T sour cream or vegan alternative
10-inch flan or tart shell; prebake, cool before filling

1. PLACE the butter, chocolate, cocoa powder (or carob) and salt in a bowl over a pan of simmering water and allow to melt slowly, stirring occasionally, until well-mixed, cool slightly.
2. BEAT the eggs and sugar together until light and creamy; then add the maple syrup and sour cream.
3. STIR chocolate mixture into egg and sugar mixture (fold in meringue if you are using it). Then pour into a prepared tart shell.
4. BAKE until a crust forms on top, check at 40 minutes.
5. REMOVE tart from the oven and allow to cool on a rack for at least 45 minutes. The skin will crack, and filling will shrink slightly.

 **SIDEBAR**   THE HISTORY OF CHOCOLATE

In 1519, Spanish Conquistadore Hernando Cortez led an expedition into the depths of Mexico to capture gold and silver treasures from the Aztec. The Emperor Montezuma, along with his subjects, welcomed these strange-looking visitors, served them a cold, bitter popular drink called cacahuati. From the Aztecs, the Spaniards learned about the drink's mystical connections—from the juice of the seeds of the cacao tree. Montezuma himself attributed strength and energy to the drink. However, it was too bitter, so he added sugar to make it more pleasant. Cortez decided to introduce this drink into the Spanish Court, calling it chocolat. It became an instant success, served piping hot. Soon Spanish ships were bringing regular supplies of cacao beans to satisfy the demand that spread across Europe.

CAKES, COOKIES, AND BARS

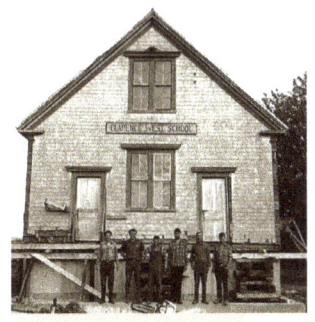

Sharing Cookies
I honed my baking skills when Matthew (far left) and local workers were hard at work relocating and renovating the original one room schoolhouse back onto the Nova Scotia property, transforming it into a meditation hall. I took them treats and drinks to give them a break. It gave me the opportunity to try new variations on many classic cookie and bar recipes.

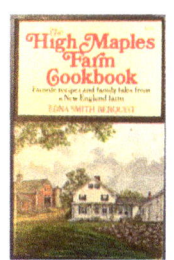

I STARTED BAKING COOKIES IN NOVA SCOTIA. We had so much homemade butter, local farm honey, and maple syrup on hand that I had to find ways to use them up. Developing cookie recipes on cold, snowy days was great fun.

My first inspiration for cookies came from a book. When we lived in rural Canada, a bookmobile would come by the house once a week. In the middle of the week, even during a snow storm, a large beep in front of the house announced its presence. It was there that I discovered the *High Maples Farm Cookbook*. It included wonderful stories about a Vermont family who for generations operated a maple farm. The book had many recipes for cookies using maple syrup as a foundation. I also tried to bring a more wholesome edge to the cookies by adding seeds, nuts, raisins, and whole grain flours. Often, they became mini meals in themselves. Recently, Matthew found a copy of the book online and now, after decades, I have it in my library.

On the farm rhubarb and raspberries are perennials we waited for each year. Rhubarb came first, even before the spring frost left the ground. Raspberries waited for the warmth of summer, so teaming them with rhubarb for bars and treats (see page 280) are the perfect way to use them.

For many years we didn't eat eggs, so it was a challenge to create recipes without them. When Matthew was not able to eat chocolate, carob substituted quite well. Then glutinous flours were out, so I worked on flour alternatives by using gluten-free flour blends and a combination of almond and coconut flour. Many combinations can be substituted in these recipes. If nuts are a problem, you can also use garfava flour, a combination of garbanzo and fava beans. As you can see, these recipes are adaptable to the extreme.

ORGANIC PINEAPPLE-CARROT CELEBRATION CAKE

Makes 1 Cake | Preheat Oven to 350 Degrees | Bake: 35 to 40 Minutes

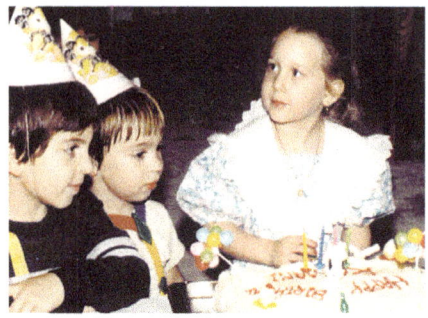

Ramani's 5th birthday traditional carrot cake

When my daughter Ramani was little, I always baked a special birthday cake, something healthy and festive. I don't think she ever really understood about the healthy part, but it was always a big hit with the moms. It can easily be made with all organic ingredients.

Wet Ingredients
1 C organic apple sauce, no sugar added
½ C avocado oil
¼ C maple or agave syrup
2 eggs
1½ T vanilla paste, or extract
1 T lemon zest

Dry Ingredients
1 C whole wheat pastry flour, sifted and 1½ C unbleached white flour or use 2½ white flour for a lighter cake
1 T baking powder and 1½ t baking soda
1½ C brown, date, or maple sugar
½ t salt
1½ T cinnamon, ¾ t ginger powder, ½ t cardamom powder

Stir-in Ingredients
2 C finely grated organic carrots (4 to 5 small to medium carrots)
1 (16 oz.) can crushed pineapple, drain (reserve ½ C for layers and 1 T for icing)
½ C walnuts, lightly toasted and chopped very small (optional)

1. MIX wet and dry ingredients together, in separate bowls.
2. COMBINE the two bowls into one; mix until smooth.
3. STIR in carrots, pineapple, and walnuts.
4. DIVIDE batter into three prepared round pans that have been lightly greased, with cut wax paper circles for the bottom of the pans.
5. BAKE until cake tester comes out clean. Cool for 5 minutes in pan; remove cake and cool completely before icing.
6. SPREAD ¼ of the frosting on first layer, top with ¼ C crushed and very well drained pineapple, duplicate frosting, and pineapple on second layer. Finish by frosting top and down the sides of cake. (You can also make this a naked cake and not frost the sides of the cake.)

Cream Cheese Icing

8 oz. softened, low fat cream cheese or vegan alternative
½ C margarine or butter
1 t vanilla extract
¼ t salt
1 T crushed pineapple
4 C powdered sugar

Mix first 5 ingredients together until smooth, add sugar and blend until creamy. Adjust sugar if too loose.

HOLIDAY BISCOTTI

Makes 12 to 16 Biscotti | Preheat Oven to 325 Degrees | Bake: 32 to 40 Minutes   M N S Y

VARIATIONS

1. Macadamia nuts and dried cherries (chopped into small pieces)

2. Coconut and dried pineapple

CHOCOLATE EDGE

You can also dip the long bottom edge in chocolate. Heat 1 C semisweet chocolate chips and 1 T coconut oil over a double boiler for 1 minute, until soft, stir well. Place in a shallow pan and dip the long side of the biscotti into the chocolate and place back on the wire rack to cool and harden.

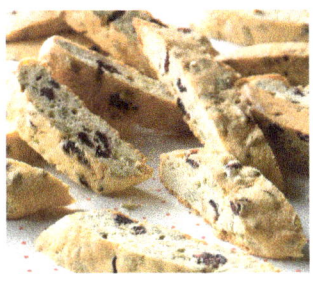

This is one of my very favorite treats for dipping, it's both crisp and light and not too sweet. I also love to give this out for holiday treats!

Wet Ingredients
2 large eggs, room temperature
½ C olive oil
1 C turbinado sugar
1 T vanilla extract
1 t orange zest (save juice for hydrating dried fruit)

Dry Ingredients
2 C unbleached organic all-purpose flour, sifted
1½ t baking powder
¾ t cardamom powder and ½ t cinnamon
½ t salt

Stir-in Ingredients
1 C salted toasted pumpkin seeds (any seed or nut will do)
½ C dried cranberries (or any dried fruit) hydrate in orange juice, drain well

1. BLEND the first five wet ingredients.
2. WHISK flour, baking powder, cardamom, and salt in a separate bowl.
3. ADD wet to dry ingredients, mix until just moistened (dough will definitely be very sticky). Stir in seeds or nuts and dried fruit.
4. DIVIDE mixture in half. With slightly wet hands shape each portion into flat rectangles, about 8" long and 1" thick, place on parchment paper and then onto a baking sheet. Bake for 25 to 30 minutes, until the center of the logs are baked and edges are just beginning to brown.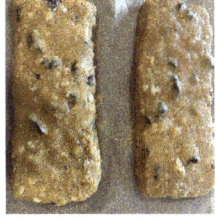
5. REMOVE logs to wire racks and cool 15 minutes. Transfer to a cutting board. Using a serrated knife, cut diagonally into ¾" slices. Return to baking sheets, cut side down.
6. BAKE about 7 to 10 minutes on first side and then turn them over and bake another 10 minutes, until lightly browned.
7. REMOVE from pans to wire racks to cool. Store in airtight container.

RHUBARB-RASPBERRY COBBLER

Makes 1 Cobbler | Preheat Oven to 400 Degrees | Bake: 20 to 25 Minutes   MENSY

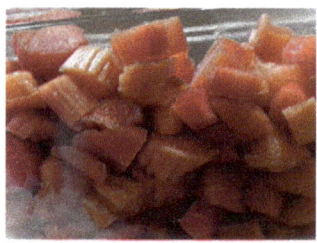

Fruit Ingredients
½ C water, 1½ t corn starch, ¾ C turbinado sugar
2 C rhubarb stalks, chopped in cubes
1 vanilla bean, split or 1½ T vanilla extract
1 C raspberries
1 T lemon zest

TURBINADO SUGAR

- Partially refined sugar retaining some of the molasses, with a caramel flavor.
- Sometimes called raw sugar—a term implying that it's minimally processed.

Cobbler Ingredients
1 C organic white pastry flour, ¾ C dark brown sugar, ½ salt, and ½ t cinnamon
4 T butter or margarine, cut-into pieces
1 egg and ¼ C almond milk or ½ C almond milk

1. GREASE sides and bottom of an 8" baking dish.
2. PLACE the water, corn starch, sugar, vanilla bean and rhubarb in a saucepan and bring to simmer, stirring constantly, cook for 5 minutes. Remove from the heat, stir in raspberries and zest, cool completely.
3. COBBLER TOPPING: Combine flour, sugar, salt and cinnamon, cut in butter, until it resembles peas, add the liquids until just combined.
4. SPREAD the cooled fruit mixture on the bottom of the baking dish, spoon the cobbler topping evenly over the fruit.
5. BAKE until golden brown on the top.
6. REMOVE from oven and let cool 10 minutes before serving.

 SIDEBAR   HISTORY OF COBBLERS

The pie was developed from a Roman concept in the 2nd Century B.C. of sealing meat inside a flour and oil paste as it cooked. Cobblers were an early adaptation of the pie and go by a multitude of names: tart, torte, pandowdy, grunt, slump, buckle, crisp, croustade, bird's nest or crow's nest pudding. Yet, they are simply variations based on cooking seasonal fruits and berries, fresh ingredients that are available in your locale, and topped with some sort of topping. Early American settlers improvised, when they first arrived, they bought their favorite recipes with them, but not finding the ingredients they needed they invented new dishes with unique names. Early colonists were so fond of these juicy dishes that they sometimes served them as a main course, for breakfast, or even as a first course in the larger meal. It was not until the late 19th century that they primarily became desserts.

RASPBERRY-PECAN BARS

Makes 16 Bars | Preheat Oven to 325 Degrees | Bake: 60 Minutes

BAKING SODA & POWDER

Baking Soda
Sodium bicarbonate. When mixed with an acid, like sour cream, molasses, or lemon juice, gases are released. You should then bake immediately.

Baking Powder
Comprises baking soda and an acid, usually cream of tartar.

Double-acting Baking Powder
Made of baking soda, sodium aluminum sulfate, calcium acid phosphate, and corn starch. It reacts at first when it contacts the liquid and a second time when it's heated. Therefore, you can mix the ingredients ahead of time and wait to bake it.

Dry Ingredients
½ C whole wheat pastry flour, 1¼ C unbleached white flour, and ¼ C coconut flour or 1½ C gluten-free flour blend and ½ C coconut flour (you can omit gluten-free substitute)
½ t baking soda and ½ t baking powder
½ t salt
1 t cinnamon
½ t cardamom powder

Wet Ingredients
½ C coconut oil
½ C brown sugar, firmly packed
¼ C maple or agave syrup
1 egg and 2 egg whites (or ¼ C soy, almond, or rice milk with 1 t corn starch mixed in)
1 T vanilla
¾ C pecans, chopped small (roasted for 5 minutes in a 325-degree oven)

Filling
⅔ C raspberry jam (an all-fruit jam is best)
1 T lemon juice

1. GREASE an 11" x 7" x 2" baking pan with margarine or butter.
2. SIFT dry ingredients together.
3. BEAT coconut oil until creamy; add sugar and syrup and beat again until light and fluffy.
4. ADD eggs (or alternative mixture) and vanilla and beat until well mixed, stir in pecans (reserving 3 T for top).
5. STIR wet into dry ingredients to make top and bottom dough.
6. STIR jam and lemon juice together in a saucepan and heat slightly to make a spreading consistency, cool.
7. PRESS half the dough (about 1½ C) evenly on the bottom of the pan.
8. SPREAD the jam filling on top without disturbing the bottom layer.
9. CRUMBLE the remaining (sticky) dough evenly on top. Sprinkle with reserved pecans.
10. BAKE until golden brown.
11. COOL on wire rack and cut into squares.

OATMEAL-DATE SQUARES

Makes 16 Bars | Preheat Oven to 300 Degrees | Bake: 30 to 40 Minutes   GMESY

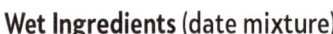

When we first visited Nova Scotia to look for a house to buy, we stayed at a local bed and breakfast owned by Mr. and Mrs. Greenlaw. They took us into their home and hearts. Once we moved there, we remained friends. Often on Sundays, we would "visit," as it was called. We'd sit in the flower wallpapered front sitting room, talk about simple matters—the weather, crops, and cows, while eating Mrs. Greenlaw's oatmeal-date squares and other "fancy cakes," accompanied by milky tea. Some squares were made with her homemade strawberry jam and literally melted in your mouth, but the favorite of all were her date squares, which I have updated, utilizing dates from local California desert towns.

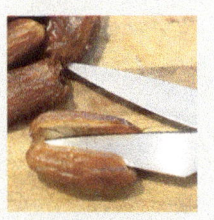

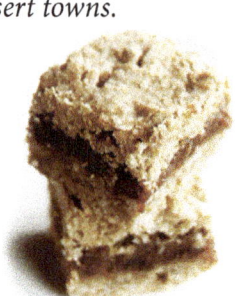

CUTTING DATES

Put dates and other sticky fruits in the freezer for about an hour before cutting.

Using oiled cooking shears to cut them makes it easier—no sticky fingers.

Wet Ingredients (date mixture)
3 C dates, cut into pieces
¼ C turbinado sugar and ¼ C maple or agave syrup
¾ C water
1 T corn starch
1 T lemon juice and 1 t lemon zest

Dry Ingredients (crumb topping)
1½ C rolled oats
1¼ C whole wheat pastry flour or gluten-free flour blend, sifted
¾ t salt
½ C brown sugar and ¼ C date, or maple sugar
2 T corn starch
1 t baking soda
½ C margarine or butter, chilled
½ C walnuts, chopped small

1. GREASE an 11" x 7" baking pan with margarine or butter.
2. COOK dates, sugar, syrup, water, corn starch, lemon juice and zest on low heat until mixture is thick, about 10 minutes and cool mixture.
3. COMBINE dry ingredients together, cut in margarine or butter, stir in nuts, mix until a wet crumb mixture is formed.
4. SPREAD ¾ C of the crumb mixture on the bottom of the pan. Top with date mixture carefully so you don't disturb the bottom layer and add the rest of the crumb mixture on top and pat down.
5. BAKE and cool, then cut into squares.

HEALTHY DARK CHOCOLATE MOCHA BROWNIES

Makes 16 Bars | Preheat Oven to 325 Degrees | Bake: 35 to 40 Minutes   G M N S Y

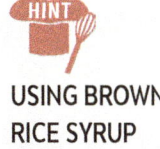

USING BROWN RICE SYRUP

Brown rice syrup is a liquid sweetener with the consistency of honey. It has a unique caramel-like flavor that can be used to enhance a recipe, but its flavor will not interfere if used sparingly.

It's made by combining barley malt and brown rice and cooking the mixture until all the starch is converted to sugar. It is then strained and cooked down to a syrup that is only 20 percent as sweet as sugar.

These bars marry the wonderful combination of chocolate and coffee, in a less sweet and low-fat but intensely flavorful and moist bar. Adding coffee enhances the richness of chocolate.

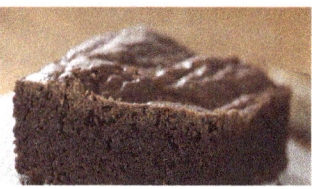

Dry Ingredients
½ C unbleached white flour and ¼ C whole wheat pastry flour, sifted
    ¾ C gluten-free flour blend (you can omit gluten-free substitute)
¾ C unsweetened organic cocoa or carob powder
¾ t salt
¼ t cinnamon
¾ C organic brown sugar

Wet Ingredients
¼ C avocado or olive oil
¼ C applesauce
¼ C brown rice syrup
¼ C maple or agave syrup
2 eggs and 3 egg whites
1¼ t vanilla extract
½ C dark chocolate or carob chips, reserve ¼ C and melt the remaining ¼ C
    over a double boiler.
¼ C dark brewed coffee (decaf is fine), if you have a milder coffee, you can
    boil it down for about 5 to 10 minutes to concentrate, then cool.
OPTIONAL: ½ C pecans, toasted and chopped very small

1. GREASE 9" x 13" baking pan.
2. STIR dry ingredients together.
3. WHISK wet ingredients together until light and fluffy; stir in melted chocolate and coffee.
4. STIR dry ingredients into wet ingredients.
5. MIX in reserved chips and toasted pecans (if you are using them).
6. SPOON into prepared baking pan.
7. BAKE until cake tester comes out clean, don't overbake.
8. COOL on wire rack and then cut into squares.

Timeless Sweets

AUNT BEA'S POPPY SEED MOON COOKIES

Makes 30 to 35 Cookies | Preheat Oven to 325 Degrees | Bake: 15 to 20 Minutes   M S Y

CHECKING DOUBLE ACTIVE BAKING POWDER FOR FRESHNESS

To check and see if the baking powder in your pantry is still active, stir 1 t into one-third cup hot water. There should be immediate vigorous bubbling. If there is no bubbling or the bubbling is sporadic, the baking powder is past its prime, better to discard.

These poppy cookies have been made by my mother's family for generations. I'm not quite sure where the name "moon" came from, but that's what we always called them. My mother finally pinned down Aunt Bea and got her to measure the ingredients while she made them, to preserve this very simple and delicate recipe. I adapted the recipe to make them healthier without sacrificing their original flavor. These cookies are usually made in large batches, you could easily cut the recipe in half. I love how Aunt Bea shaped the cookies with an ordinary juice glass. I've included a slimmed down alternative by reducing the number of egg yolks.

Dry Ingredients
1¾ C whole wheat pastry flour, sifted
2 C unbleached white pastry flour, sifted
¼ C corn starch
¾ C turbinado sugar, blend in a food processor to make it finer
½ C poppy seeds

Wet Ingredients
2 eggs and 4 egg whites or 3 eggs
¼ C maple or agave syrup
2 T vanilla paste or extract
2 t baking powder
¾ C avocado oil

1. MIX dry and wet ingredients in separate bowls, then combine to form a dough, don't over handle.
2. CUT into four parts and wrap with plastic, chill at least one hour.
3. SPRINKLE a bread board with confectionery sugar and roll out to a ½" thickness, cut into rounds with a glass or 3" biscuit cutter.
4. BAKE until slightly brown edges. Don't overbake.

 **SIDEBAR   POPPY SEEDS**

Poppy seeds were introduced to India and Persia by Alexander the Great. In Ayurveda they are used as a sedative or an aphrodisiac. They relieve anxiety and prevent diarrhea. They are also sometimes used in a paste to thicken gravy in Indian and Middle Eastern dishes.

PEANUT BUTTER/NUT CHIP COOKIE

Makes 18 Cookies | Preheat Oven to 350 Degrees | Bake: 10 to 15 Minutes   GMESY

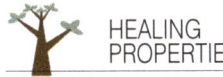
HEALING PROPERTIES

Nut Butters
- 8 grams of protein for every 2 tablespoons
- Good source of folic acid
- Contains significant fiber and vitamin E

I have worked on this recipe for years. My goal for these cookies has been to make something that produces a rather traditional, yet healthy cookie.

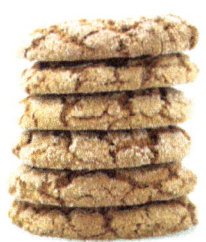

Wet Ingredients
½ C margarine or butter, softened
½ C low-fat peanut butter, almond, macadamia, or cashew butter
½ C organic granulated brown sugar (reserve 2 T for rolling)
½ C maple or agave syrup
1 egg, 2 egg whites or substitute with vegan meringue (see page 308)
1 T vanilla extract

Dry Ingredients
1 C whole wheat pastry flour, sifted and ½ C unbleached white flour or
    1¼ C light gluten-free flour blend, sifted
1 t baking soda (add an additional ½ t if you are not using egg or omit if you are baking soda sensitive)
½ t salt
½ C chocolate or carob chips
½ C walnuts, chopped very small

1. MIX dry and wet ingredients, in separate bowls, then combine both to form a dough.
2. CHILL in a covered bowl until cold (overnight is fine).
3. SHAPE into small balls (1 inch) and roll in reserved sugar (if the dough is a little sticky, use a small scoop and add some sugar to your palm).
4. PLACE on cookie sheet and press down slightly with a fork in both directions to make a crisscross design (sugar the fork before you press the cookie down). Be careful not to burn.

COOKIE IDEAS

Shaping Cookies: Use a small ice cream scoop to make uniform cookies.

Baking Cookies in Summer: Cookies are like sponges absorbing moisture from the atmosphere. On hot, humid days they can turn from crispy-crunchy, to soft and limp, within hours. Fortunately, the cooler months are when we feel most motivated to bake. If you do bake in the heat of the summer and find your cookies spreading too much or turning soggy, try adding 2 egg yolks instead of one egg. The fat content of egg yolks keeps the dough tender while its emulsifying action keeps it moist after baking.

MINI CHOCOLATE CHIP COCONUT COOKIES

Makes 38 cookies | Preheat Oven to 375 Degrees | Bake: 11 to 14 Minutes   GMSY

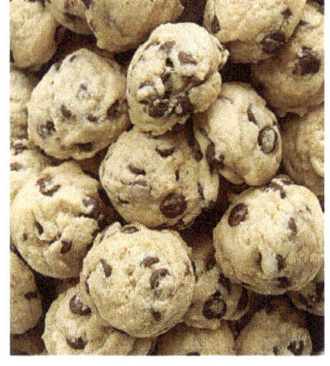

Here's a classic mini cookie recipe that utilizes what I have on hand in my pantry, at any given time. It has a hint of coconut flavor, though if you don't want excess coconut flavor, simply leave out the shredded coconut. I also tried to make them just a little bit healthier with the addition of nuts and/or seeds. The secret is in the soft dough, but they do need to chill for about an hour to be able to handle them better.

To form the cookie, use a small ice cream scoop and don't flatten. I usually put this dough in the refrigerator, tightly wrapped, for at least an hour and up to a week to harden. You can also bake one cookie at a time, for out of the oven loveliness and the smell of freshly made cookies wafting through your home.

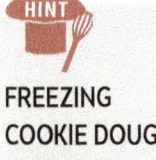

FREEZING COOKIE DOUGH AND BAKED COOKIES

You can always bake one sheet pan of cookies and freeze the balance for another time. Or bake them all and freeze half the batch, double bag or place in an airtight container.

Wet Ingredients
½ C coconut oil and ¾ C turbinado brown or coconut sugar
1 egg
1 t vanilla extract

Dry Ingredients
¾ C unbleached white flour/ ¼ C oats/ ¼ C whole wheat pastry flour (or any combination of flours, you could also use 1¼ C gluten-free flour blend
½ t salt
½ t baking powder

Extra Ingredients
¼ C bittersweet chocolate mini chips or chunks
¼ C any nuts or seeds, chopped (I often use walnuts or pumpkin seeds)
¼ C coconut shredded (optional)

1. MELT coconut oil and add sugar, mix really well. Blend in egg and vanilla, until it's fully incorporated.
2. WHISK the flour, salt, and baking powder, add to melted oil/sugar mixture and stir to combine. Stir in chips, nuts, and coconut. Chill the dough for at least an hour.
3. SCOOP cookies and spread them out to allow for expansion.
4. BAKE for about 11 to 14 minutes, just until the edges are golden. Don't overbake.
5. STORE at room temperature for about 3 to 4 days or freeze a batch.

OATMEAL/WALNUT-RAISIN COOKIES

Makes 18 to 24 Cookies | Preheat Oven to 350 Degrees | Bake: 10 to 15 Minutes   M E S Y

In 1971, we started a yoga class in the local Quaker Meeting House and called it Awareness Unlimited. We did a few yoga postures, sang (accompanied on the guitar by our friend), read from books, and ate. Everyone brought something to share after each class. One lady always brought her oatmeal-walnut-raisin cookies, which she called, "the healthy ones." After weeks of eating these wonderful cookies, I asked for the recipe. Though I don't remember her name, through all the years and travels, I still have the original index card she gave me. It is now splattered and well-worn, and the cookies are still the best I have ever found. I've adapted the original recipe to make it lower in fat and a bit less sweet.

EGG REPLACEMENT FOR BAKING

For each egg add an extra 1 t baking soda and use:
- ¼ C water and 2 T egg replacement powder (Ener-G Foods)
- 1½ T flaxseed meal blended in ¼ C water until smooth.
- ¼ C soft tofu and 1 T oil.
- ¼ C apple sauce or prune puree.

Wet Ingredients
½ C margarine or butter, softened and 2 T avocado oil
½ C organic brown sugar
½ C maple or ⅓ C agave syrup and 1 t vanilla
2 eggs and 2 egg whites or egg substitute (see Hint)
2 T vanilla extract or scrape seeds from one vanilla pod

Dry Ingredients
1 C whole wheat pastry flour, sifted
1 C old-fashioned toasted* rolled oats, whirled in blender until chopped fine
¾ t salt
1 T baking soda (if you a baking soda sensitive, you can omit if you use eggs or make a meringue from the egg whites)
½ t nutmeg, freshly grated and 1 t cinnamon
½ C raisins and ½ C walnuts (chopped small)

1. MIX dry and wet ingredients together, in separate bowls, then combine to form a dough.
2. CHILL 30 minutes, then roll into a log, wrap in plastic wrap, and refrigerate a few hours or better overnight.
3. CUT chilled log into ¼" slices and place on a cookie sheet.
4. BAKE making sure not to burn.

TOASTING OATMEAL FOR COOKIES OR CAKES*

Sprinkle oatmeal over a cookie pan and heat in an oven on a very low heat for about 10 minutes.

Timeless Sweets

VEGAN MANGO/SORBET GLUTEN-FREE SANDWICH

Makes 24 to 28 Cookies | Preheat Oven to 350 Degrees | Bake: 25 to 30 Minutes   GMENSY

A great vegan dessert sandwich.

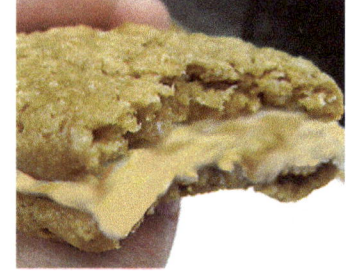

SORBET
2 C fresh mango, cut into pieces and frozen
1½ C almond, rice, or soy milk
3 T agave syrup

1. BLEND all ingredients until smooth. Pour onto cookie sheet about ½" in depth.
2. COVER and freeze for a least two hours until set.
3. CUT into rounds with the same cutter you use to make cookies.

SANDWICH COOKIES

Dry Ingredients
1½ C gluten-free flour blend with 1 t agar agar powder
½ C oats, ground fine (you can use gluten-free oats that are not processed on the same machines as wheat products or omit)
¾ t salt
½ t ginger powder
½ t cinnamon
¼ t cardamom powder

Wet Ingredients
½ C coconut oil
1 t vanilla extract
½ C agave syrup

1. PREHEAT Oven. Put parchment paper on a large baking sheet.
2. BLEND dry ingredients in a bowl.
3. COMBINE wet ingredients until creamy, then add dry ingredients to wet ingredients until well combined.
4. FORM into two disks, cover and put in refrigerator for at least 30 minutes.
5. ROLL each disk out to ¼" thickness and cut into large rounds
6. BAKE until golden, cool.
7. COMBINE two cookies with sorbet circle to form a sandwich.
8. FREEZE at least two hours before serving.

Binding Agents for Gluten-Free Recipes

You need binding agents in gluten-free recipes to counter the dryness, density, and heaviness of gluten-free flour. **Agar agar** is a natural, plant-based gelatin derived from seaweed. It's used as a stabilizer and thickening agent. **Xanthan gum** and **guar gum** are also substitutes, though agar agar, a natural gelatin, seems to be helpful for people who have digestive issues.

A little goes a long way, measure carefully as it can possibly make your baking product soggy.

GLUTEN-FREE CARDAMOM ROSE CUPCAKES

Makes 8 Cupcakes | Preheat Oven to 400 Degrees | Bake: 12 to 15 Minutes **G M S Y**

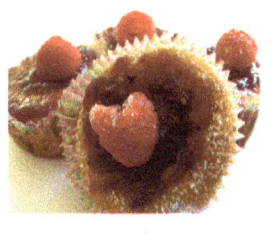

These are perfect for a Valentine's Day treat or any special occasion. Not only are they gluten-free but they're also low in sugar. Eggs are especially difficult to omit for this fluffy and light cupcake. You can use decorative cupcake holders to give it a festive look.

HINT: ALMOND FLOUR

Almond flour is high in protein and fiber and is rich and nutty.

Store almond flour in the refrigerator or freezer. Almond meal is coarser and not the same product as almond flour. It's not suitable for general baking but works well for pie crusts.

Wet Ingredients

3 eggs and 3 egg whites (whip 3 egg whites to hard-peaked meringue; beat 3 whole eggs; fold both gently together.)
6 T coconut oil, margarine, or butter, melted and cooled
⅓ C agave syrup
¼ C almond milk
¾ t rosewater and 1½ t vanilla

Dry Ingredients

1 t cardamom powder
½ t salt
3 T almond flour
4 T garfava flour and 2 T potato starch or 6 T coconut flour, sifted well
½ t xanthan gum
1½ t baking powder

1. BLEND wet into dry ingredients separately.
2. ADD wet ingredients to dry ingredients (it works best if you use a hand mixer or stir vigorously with a hand whisk).
3. FILL cupcake holder with ice cream scoop, to make them uniform. Make a little well on top of the batter with a spoon.
4. WARM 3 T all-fruit organic raspberry jam* until liquid, then cool.
5. SPREAD on thin layer on top of each cupcake and add one raspberry.
6. BAKE and then dust each cupcake with powdered sugar.

Low Sugar Strawberry or Raspberry Freezer Jam* | 4 (8 oz.) containers

3 lbs. organic berries, hulled & stems removed (6 C mashed)
1¾ C apple juice concentrate
¼ C agave syrup
1 package pectin

Mash the berries in a large bowl. In saucepan, bring apple concentrate, agave syrup and pectin to a boil for 1 minute. Add berries and stir for 1 minute. Cool and ladle into freezer containers. Place in the refrigerator overnight to let it set, then store in the freezer. Good up to 1 year in freezer, 3 weeks in refrigerator.

GLUTEN-FREE CHIP BLONDIES

Makes 16 bars | Preheat Oven to 350 Degrees | Bake: 20 to 28 Minutes   G M N S Y

BAKING WITH COCONUT FLOUR

Coconut flour has an extraordinarily high fiber content and absorbs more liquid than other gluten-free flour alternatives. It's nutty and mildly sweet with a light coconut flavor.

Baking ideas with coconut flour:
- Shift or blend well before measuring.
- Keep an eye on baking time as it bakes much faster than other flours.
- Keep in an airtight container in the refrigerator or freezer. But before using it in a recipe, allow it to return to room temperature.

This is one of Matthew's favorite desserts, he recently added baking soda and baking powder to his sensitivities to wheat, dairy, whole nuts, and chocolate. It is the essential ingredient for any quick breads, cookies, and cakes. In this recipe dates give it sweetness and keeps this bar moist and chewy, and the meringue helps lighten it up, without needing to add baking soda or baking powder.

Dry Ingredients
¾ C gluten-free flour blend or make your own combination:
2 T garfava flour
1 T tapioca starch
¼ C almond flour
½ C coconut flour
½ t xanthan gum
¾ t salt

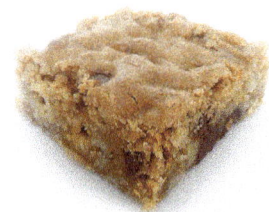

1. WHISK all above ingredients until well incorporated.

Wet Ingredients
½ C pitted dates (cover with warm water and let sit one hour; drain well)
⅓ C coconut oil, butter, or margarine, softened
¼ C agave nectar
1 t vanilla extract

Fold-in Ingredients
2 whole eggs or 1 whole egg and 2 egg whites or 4 egg whites (beat the egg whites into a meringue and fold into batter at the end)
1 C low-sugar butterscotch chips

1. PREHEAT oven and line an 8" x 8" baking pan with parchment paper and grease top of paper and sides of pan.
2. COMBINE wet ingredients in a blender, blend until smooth
3. ADD dry ingredients to wet ingredients
4. FOLD in meringue and chips and mix until incorporated into batter
5. POUR batter into baking pan.
6. BAKE checking often (it's better to underbake rather than overbake).
7. COOL on a rack and cut into 16 bars. They freeze very well when double wrapped.

CREAMY CREATIONS

Cashew Cheese Recipe

A good vegan alternative is Cashew Cheese:

2 C raw cashews
¼ C lemon juice
¼ C organic coconut oil
1½ t salt
¾ C cashew or almond milk

Soak cashews for at least 8 hours with enough water to cover them. Drain very well and blend with the rest of the ingredients, until smooth. Wrap cashew cheese in cheesecloth tightly and refrigerate overnight.

IN NOVA SCOTIA WE HAD TWO DELIGHTFUL COWS that produced a large bucket of warm milk early morning and late afternoon. The morning milk routine was to separate the milk into cream and curds (the curds ended up in the waiting mouth of our neighbor's lucky pig). We'd store the cream in the refrigerator for making butter. When we had enough cream stored up, we'd churn the butter in an original, turn of the century wooden churn and mold it into large squares from a lovely carved antique wooden butter mold that made a floral stamp on top. I also made ghee from the butter and used it in most Indian recipes (see page 298).

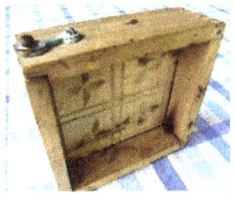
Decorative butter mold

In the late afternoon, milk was brought to pasteurized temperature, cooled, and refrigerated for daily use. Having so much milk meant that we had to be creative with ways to use it all.

Almost every day I made fresh yogurt, as well as making homemade cottage cheese and Indian paneer. In the summer we made ice cream using a hand-churned ice cream bucket, which used the salt and ice method. Now I use a more modern electric version, where the insert is frozen before the ice cream maker is plugged in. It's much easier!

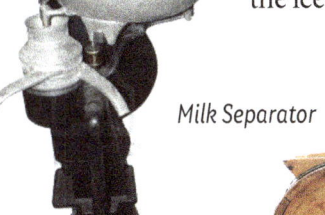
Milk Separator

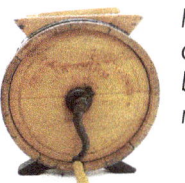
Hand churn butter maker

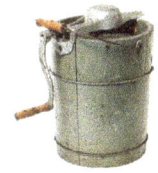
Hand churn ice cream maker

SPICY PUMPKIN CUSTARD

Makes 4 to 6 Pots | Preheat Oven to 350 Degrees | Bake: 45 to 50 Minutes   **G M N S Y**

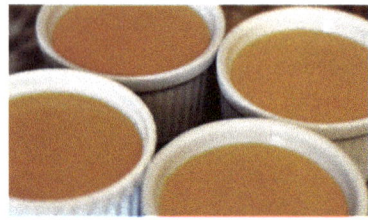

1½ C low-fat milk, soy, almond, or coconut milk
1½ C organic pumpkin puree, canned is fine
3 eggs
1 T vanilla extract
½ C agave syrup
1 T corn starch
1 T ground cinnamon
½ t ground cardamom
¼ t ground ginger
½ t ground nutmeg
½ t salt

USING COCONUT MILK OR COCONUT CREAM

Coconut Milk has the liquid consistency of cow's milk, it's made from simmering one-part shredded coconut in one-part water.

Coconut Cream is much thicker and richer, it's made from simmering four-parts shredded coconut in one-part water, making it a perfect milk substitute in various recipes that require heavy cream.

1. PREHEAT oven.
2. WHISK together milk, pumpkin puree, eggs, vanilla, and agave.
3. WHISK together the corn starch and spices. Slowly blend the corn starch and spices into the pumpkin mixture. Stir well until completely mixed.
4. POUR batter into lightly oiled ramekins. Use about ¾ C of pumpkin mix for each one. Place ramekins in a large baking dish and add enough hot water until it reaches halfway up the ramekins. Cover lightly with tin foil.
5. BAKE until set. Cool on rack and refrigerate for at least an hour.

CARDAMOM COCONUT WHIPPED CREAM

Makes ¾ Cup

1 (14 oz.) can whole fat coconut cream, chill
2 T maple or agave syrup
1 t vanilla extract
¼ t ground cardamom
Dash of salt

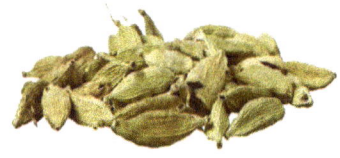

1. WHISK coconut cream in a bowl until well blended and place in the freezer for 20 minutes.
2. BEAT coconut cream with a mixer for 4 to 5 minutes until thick.
3. STIR in syrup, vanilla, cardamom and salt and place in freezer until firm, like a soft ice cream.

FRUITY YOGURT TART

Makes 1 Pie | Preheat Oven to 325 Degrees | Bake: 20 to 25 minutes   G M S Y

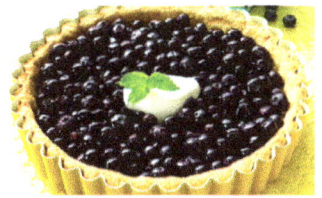

This is a wonderfully light and healthy holiday dessert, but you really have to love ginger to appreciate this fruity pie.

1 prepared tart crust (see page 160)
2-inch piece of ginger root (to make 2 T ginger juice)
2 eggs, 4 egg whites
¼ C brown sugar
¼ C agave syrup
1¼ C plain low or non-fat yogurt or cashew yogurt
1¼ T vanilla extract
½ t cardamom powder
¼ C whole wheat pastry flour (or 1 T almond flour and 3 T coconut flour, sifted)
¼ C almonds, slivered, roast until golden
½ C blueberries or any combination of berries (mix in 1 T brown sugar)

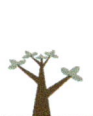 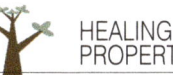 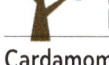

HEALING PROPERTIES

Cardamom
- Helps heal bronchial conditions and sore throats
- Eases stomach cramps
- Stimulates digestion
- Aids liver function, although too much cardamom may cause gallstones

1. PEEL ginger root and finely grate over a plate or bowl. Press grated ginger root through a sieve, tea strainer, or garlic press, to catch the liquid in a small bowl. Reserve liquid and discard the root.
2. BEAT eggs with sugar and agave for 2 to 3 minutes.
3. FOLD in yogurt, vanilla, cardamom, and ginger juice. Gradually add flour and combine.
4. ADD mixture to cooled tart shell.
5. BAKE until custard is done, don't overbake.
6. REMOVE from oven and spread with almonds and top with berries.
7. REFRIGERATE for 2 hours before serving.

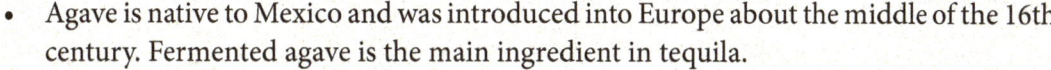

 **SIDEBAR**   **AGAVE FACTS**

- Agave is native to Mexico and was introduced into Europe about the middle of the 16th century. Fermented agave is the main ingredient in tequila.
- Some studies indicate that agave syrup may not raise your blood sugar in the same way sugar does as it's made up of 95% natural fructose.
- Agave is 40% sweeter than sugar, so you can adjust the amount without sacrificing the sweetness.

Timeless Sweets

EASY LOGANBERRY LIGHT ICE CREAM

Makes 8 to 10 Cups

GENSY

You can substitute any berry for logan but if you can get some, the taste is absolutely unique. This is a great, light recipe and its egg free, but not dairy free!

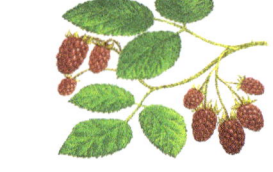

My father was born in Canada, and we still have relatives there.

Many summers when I was very young, we loaded up the car and drove to Crystal Beach, on Lake Erie, to be with our Canadian family. It was there that I discovered loganberry concentrate, which became the official summer drink.

1 (14 oz.) can fat-free sweetened condensed milk
3 C fat-free half-and-half
¼ t salt
1 T vanilla extract
½ C brown sugar
1½ C loganberries (frozen loganberries or concentrate are fine)

1. WHIRL loganberries with sugar in a blender until puréed. Set aside, or use 1 C loganberry concentrate.
2. PREPARE ice cream maker canister, making sure the insert is completely frozen before you begin.
3. COMBINE ingredients, except berries. Beat on medium-low to blend well, then mix in berry puree. Cool in refrigerator for a few hours.
4. POUR cooled ice cream mixture into frozen canister of ice cream maker and freeze according to the manufacturer's directions. A typical ice cream maker takes 20 minutes, until the ice cream thickens. Place in the freezer for a few hours before serving.

 SIDEBAR   HISTORY OF THE LOGANBERRY

The loganberry is a cross between a blackberry and a raspberry. It was accidentally created in 1883, in Santa Cruz, California, by an American lawyer and horticulturist, James Harvey Logan (1841–1928). In the 1880s, berry growers began to cross pollinate to obtain better commercial varieties. Logan was unsatisfied with the existing varieties of blackberries and tried to cross two varieties of blackberries to produce a superior variety. While attempting to cross two varieties of blackberries, Logan accidentally planted them next to an old variety of red raspberry, all of which flowered and fruited together. Logan gathered and planted the seed. The 50 seedlings produced plants similar to the blackberry parent but were larger and more vigorous. James was eventually honored when this new berry became known as the Loganberry and was introduced to Canada and Europe in the late 1800s.

STRAWBERRY OR RASPBERRY ICE CREAM

Makes 8 to 10 Cups

GMSY

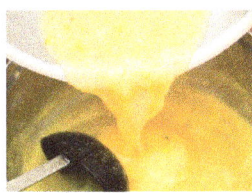

ICE CREAM BASICS

- Using brown sugar give this ice cream a caramelized flavor.
- Make sure the milk is not too hot when adding the egg yolks, the main goal is not to scramble them. If there are a few cooked pieces, straining it before cooling will remove them.
- Don't be impatient, make sure the custard is really cold before churning.

2½ C 2% milk or vanilla almond milk
3 large egg yolks
½ C organic fine brown sugar
3 T vanilla bean paste or vanilla extract
¼ C low-sugar strawberry or raspberry preserves

1. COOK milk or almond milk over a medium to low flame until just before it boils.
2. SEPARATE the egg yolks and beat in the sugar.
3. REMOVE milk from the stove, cool until warm. Add a little of the warm cream to the egg mixture to temper.
4. POUR the tempered egg mixture into the milk slowly and continue to dribble in the rest of the egg/sugar mixture, whisking thoroughly after each addition.
5. RETURN the custard to the stove. Over a medium to low heat stir until slightly thickened, about 7 to 10 minutes. Stir continuously. The custard should coat the back of a spoon, so that your finger leaves a clean line and doesn't bleed. Add vanilla and remove from heat.
6. POUR custard into a bowl and cover. Place in the refrigerator for a couple of hours, or overnight, so that it is completely chilled.
7. REMOVE ice cream mixture from the fridge and mix in the preserves.
8. PLACE in chilled (overnight) ice cream maker bowl.
9. CHURN according to directions of your ice cream maker.
10. REMOVE from the ice cream bowl and place in a tight-fitting freezer container. It stays fresh for at least 2 months.

 SIDEBAR   **ALL ABOUT USING VANILLA BEANS**

Vanilla is the number one flavor for baking and cooking. You can use it directly from the pod, though the more common way to use them is in an extract or as a vanilla paste.

Vanilla bean paste is similar to extract, though thicker; the consistency is like syrup, and you can substitute either 1:1 ratio, it's specialty is the lovely vanilla bean seed flecks, which tells us we are using real vanilla. You can also use a whole vanilla bean pod. Carefully cut the inside of the pod to scrape out the seeds. Each pod full of vanilla seeds, can be substituted for 3 t of paste or extract. Save the pod and put in your sugar bowl, for lovely vanilla sugar.

Timeless Sweets

INDIAN DESSERTS

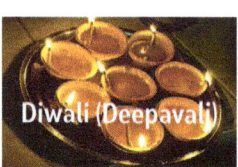

Diwali (Deepavali)

This five-day holiday in India and throughout Asia, includes:
- Lighting clay lamps filled with oil, signifying the triumph of good over evil.
- Cleaning house to make goddess Lakshmi feel welcome.
- Lighting firecrackers to drive away evil spirits.
- Wearing new clothes and sharing sweets and snacks with family members and friends.

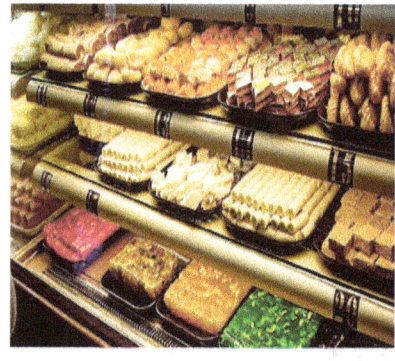

SWEETS IN THE INDIAN HOUSEHOLD, UNLIKE IN THE WEST are often reserved for special occasions. Families wait and savor these delights. Of course, they are loaded with sugar and butter, so they serve them as an occasional treat.

On one special occasion, we were staying with a family in Baroda (a large town in North India) to celebrate Diwali (see sidebar). The day before Diwali, the women in the household busied themselves boiling milk and sugar syrup for a variety of sweets. Dough was rolled thin and shaped into little triangles, deep fried, then immersed, while still hot, into a rose and cardamom syrup. Milk and coconut bars were arranged on platters, and heaps of semolina and raisin pudding were spooned into bowls. A sweet, spicy aroma permeated the entire household.

At the break of dawn, the sweets and other preparations were offered at the family shrine for blessings. Afterwards, the day brought an endless stream of visitors. Neighbors and friends stopped by to be offered sweets—whoever arrived at the door was an honored guest. We also went from door to door and were offered an array of magnificent sweet preparations, specialties from each family, handed down through the generations. Indeed, after such a day, one year is not too long to wait for next year's celebration.

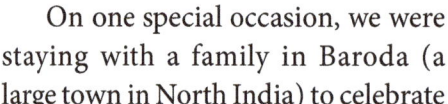

HALVA PUDDING

Serves 6 to 8 GMESY

SERVING HALVA

Halva is often served on special occasions. Just a spoonful at the end of an Indian meal is quite satisfying. It should be served as soon as possible, warm, when the halva cools down it hardens. You can re-purpose it by cutting into cubes and frying in 1 T ghee or margarine and ¼ t cardamom powder, until brown on all sides.

This is the most common sweet in India and the first one I learned to make. Toasting semolina (sugee) is the heart of the recipe. It should be toasted slowly, on a low flame, with a concentrated mind. The moment it is ready, the semolina turns a slight golden color and begins to emanate a sweet smell.

1 C semolina, Cream of Wheat, or Cream of Rice
½ C ghee, sweet butter, or margarine (reserve 1 T)
¼ C raw cashews and a few almonds
¼ C golden raisins
2 C water
½ C turbinado sugar or jaggery
¼ C maple or agave syrup
½ t cardamom, freshly ground
½ t rose water (available in Asian markets)
A few strands of saffron

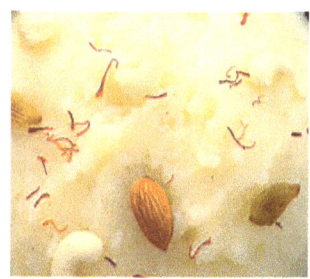

1. TOAST the semolina in ghee, butter, or margarine, in a heavy-duty fry pan on low heat. Stir often till the semolina is slightly golden, about 10 minutes.
2. SAUTÉ cashews and almonds in a separate pan with reserved 1 T ghee, butter, or margarine, until nuts are slightly roasted, and then add raisins until they are puffed—just a few minutes, add saffron.
3. BOIL water and add sugar, syrup, cardamom. Stir until dissolved. Then add sautéed raisins, nuts, rosewater, and saffron.
4. REDUCE heat and using one spoon to stir the water, very slowly begin pouring in the sautéed semolina. Stir constantly to prevent lumps from forming as it thickens. You know the halva is done when the raisins pull away from the pan. Ladle into a bowl and serve warm.

 SIDEBAR CARDAMOM

Cardamom is one of my favorite aromatic seasonings that showed up in Ayurvedic writings in the 4th B.C. The Vikings, who first discovered it on a trip to India, still enjoy cardamom in festival cakes. It was imported to Europe in 1214. Whole or ground, the unique flavor and aroma of cardamom defies the boundaries of normal sensory perceptions. It is compellingly strong, yet delicate; sweet, yet powerful, with a eucalyptus-like freshness. I buy the green pods and grind the fresh black seeds, a few teaspoons at a time, to have it handy for Chai Tea.

MATAJI'S CARROT BURFI (FUDGE)

Serves 8 to 10

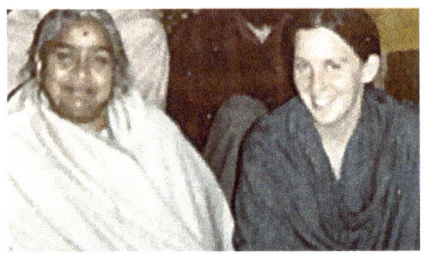

I first learned this traditional ghee-laden Indian dessert from Mataji (in the picture), an accomplished singer and protégé of Rabindranath Tagore. It was during my time in Nova Scotia when I had lots of homemade ghee, maple syrup, and home-grown carrots available.

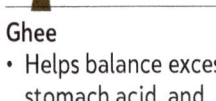 HEALING PROPERTIES

Ghee
- Helps balance excess stomach acid, and helps maintain/repair the mucus lining of the stomach
- Like aloe, prevents blisters and scarring if applied quickly to skin after a burn
- Helps promote all three aspects of mental functioning: learning, memory, and recall

3 T ghee or margarine
4 C carrots, very finely shredded
¾ C maple or agave syrup
½ t cardamom powder (you can grind the seeds, though discard gray seeds as they are too dry)
1 C milk powder (there are nondairy substitutes, see page 307)
2 T pistachios, chopped and slightly toasted

1. HEAT ghee or margarine in a heavy-duty pan. Add carrots and sauté a few minutes. Add syrup and cook for a few more minutes. Take the pan off the heat to cool slightly.
2. ADD cardamom to the carrots/syrup and, stirring constantly, slowly begin adding the milk powder.
3. COMBINE until smooth and return to low-medium heat. Stir, scraping the sides and bottom of the pan until the mixture draws away from the side. This should take about 3 minutes.
4. SPREAD hot mixture into a well buttered cake pan.
5. TOP with pistachios, cool and cut into squares or triangles.

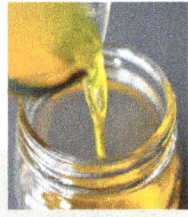

 HINT — MAKING GHEE

Ghee is an ingredient in many Indian sweet recipes. Here is an easy way to make it. In a heavy-duty pot, bring one pound of sweet butter to a gentle boil. Lower the heat so that the butter gently simmers. Simmer for about 20 minutes, until the fat gathers on the top and the ghee becomes a clear liquid (make sure to check it often, so the fat doesn't burn). Some fat will accumulate on the bottom, as well as float on the top. Let the ghee cool for ten minutes, with a spoon scrap off the top fat and then strain it through layered cheesecloth or a fine tea strainer into a clean and dry jar. It can remain fresh for many months, as long as no moisture gets in the jar, so no refrigeration is needed.

RICE PUDDING

Serves 6 to 8

GMESY

THE SPOON ON TOP OF THE MILK PAN TRICK

You can use the trick of placing a wooden spoon over the top of the pan, so the milk doesn't boil over easily. You still have to be vigilant in watching the milk as it rises and adjusting the heat.

Rice Pudding or Kheer, as it's called in India, is a quick, simple, and delightful dessert. All you need is a little rice and a few pantry ingredients, and you're done.

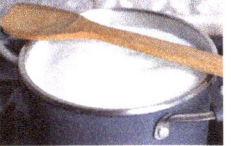

½ C basmati rice
1 T ghee or coconut oil and ½ t ground cardamom
4 C low or non-fat milk or 2 C milk and 2 C coconut milk
¼ C turbinado sugar and ¼ C jaggery (see page 265) or
    ½ C turbinado sugar
¼ C slivered almonds, chopped and slightly roasted
2 T raisins
1 t rosewater (depending how much rosewater flavor
    you prefer, you can start with ½ t)

1. SOAK rice in enough water to cover for at least 20 minutes and drain very well.
2. ADD ghee or coconut oil and cardamom to a heavy-duty pot, add rice and stir fry until aromatic.
3. ADD milk and bring to a boil, making sure not to let it boil over, stir often. Lower heat, and cook for about 10 to 12 minutes, until it begins to thicken, continue to stir so it doesn't stick to the bottom of the pan.
4. ADD sugar, almonds, and raisins. Continue cooking for an additional 5 minutes or until thickened and rice is tender. Add rosewater and chill.

 SIDEBAR   **ROSEWATER BEGINNINGS**

It was interesting to note that centuries ago, rosewater held a special place in Europe and the new colonies of America. It was made in what was called "the still-room," where the family's liqueurs and medicines were made and stored. Water that the petals were boiled in was used in puddings, cakes, and custards. In fact, a recipe in a 1755 English cookbook put rosewater in "waffles" and pumpkin pie. Early cookbooks warned that when grinding almonds, always add a little rosewater to keep them from oiling. But in the late 18th century, people slowly abandoned rosewater for the more versatile vanilla bean as their flavoring of choice.

TROPICAL FRUIT SALAD

Serves 6 to 8

GENSY

This is a refreshing and not-too-sweet dessert that is a light and a nutritious ending to any meal.

CUBING MANGOS

Stand the mango on end, slice along the sides of the large flat pit with a flexible knife, curving around the pit as you slice. You will have three sections: two larger, round sections and a flat center section. Score each section lengthwise into slices, then crosswise into chunks. Holding a rounded section by its edges, push at the curved bottom to turn the rind inside out. Cut chunks away from the rind and trim away rind from the flat center section and separate as much fruit as possible.

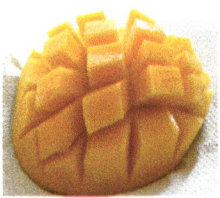

2 C mango, chopped small
2 bananas, chopped small
¼ C coconut, grated very fine (the finest dried coconut is from Indian markets.)
1 C oranges, de-veined and chopped small
2 C pineapple, chopped small
1 C red, green, or combination, grapes, halved lengthwise

1. MIX together in a large serving bowl.

Dressing

1 C ricotta cheese (see page 58 for vegan option)
¼ C orange or pineapple juice, left over from fresh fruit
¼ C honey or agave syrup
½ t cardamom powder
½ vanilla bean pod, scraped or 1 t vanilla extract

1. BLEND well until smooth.
2. TO SERVE: place fruit in separate bowls and top with dressing.

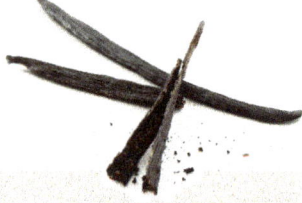

 SIDEBAR   DELIGHTFUL VANILLA

Vanilla is native to Mexico, where it is still grown commercially. Vanilla was used by the Aztecs and when Cortez brought chocolate back to Europe, he also brought vanilla bean pods. It was soon added to the cocoa concoction and the rest is history.

On our first trip to Hawaii, we spent time on the Big Island, and one of our excursions was to the Vanilla Bean Farm along the Hamakua Coast in the small hamlet of Paahulio. It was a long journey up a misty mountain overlooking the Pacific. The land has the soil, temperature, humidity, and climate to develop this incredible pod. As the first commercial growers of Vanilla in the U.S., they mentored in its birthplace, the rainforest of Micronesia, Mexico.

REFRESHING INDIAN MANGO SORBET

Serves 6 to 8

GMENSY

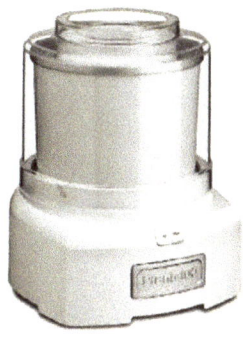

I make this sorbet a lot. It's a simple recipe with just enough added spices to give you a hint of an Indian dessert, and it's perfect after a hot curried dinner. It does require a ice cream/sorbet maker.

1 C water
1 (15 oz.) can mango pulp, Kerari, or Alphonso are the best. (You can buy this at an Indian or Mexican grocery or by mail order. Buy a few cans to have them on hand.) or 2 C fresh mangos, blended into a puree.
½ C brown sugar
½ t cardamom powder
Small capful of rosewater
½ t lemon zest
Fresh mint for garnish

1. FREEZE base of sorbet maker for at least 3 to 4 hours, overnight is best.
2. BOIL water and add the rest of the ingredients except mint.
3. STIR sugar/mango water mixture until sugar is completely dissolved. Put in refrigerator until very cold.
4. ADD cooled mango mixture to frozen base and turn on unit. Let it churn until slightly thickened, about 15 to 20 minutes.
5. TRANSFER to a freezer container. Before servind place ice cream scoop in hot water to help soften the sorbet for scooping.
6. TOP with fresh mint leaves.

 HOW TO TELL IF A MANGO IS RIPE

Ripe mangos usually have a sweet, full, fruity aroma emitting from the stem end. It is ready to eat when it's soft to the touch and yields to gentle pressure like a ripe peach. The ideal storage temperature for mangos is 55 degrees. They should last about 1 to 2 weeks. One of the best ways to ripen a mango to leave on the kitchen counter at room temperature. If you want to accelerate the process, place in a paper bag overnight (you can add an apple to the bag to create more natural ethylene gas).

TRADITIONAL ALMOND MILK (BADAM KHEER)

Serves 3 to 4   G M E S Y

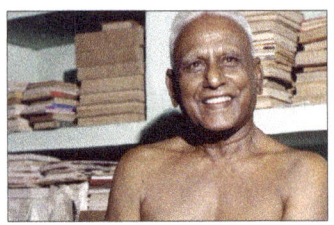

Balarama Reddy

We first had this dessert drink with a wonderful friend and mentor, Balarama Reddy, who we'd often meet in the Southern India city of Bangalore. We would go there to escape the heat, as it's famous for its moderate climate. Balarama would take us to the celebrated Mavalli Tiffin Rooms (MTR, as it is referred to, has been in business for over 80 years!). We would start with this thick, nutritious drink and then move on to numerous other tiffin specialties, until we were so full that all we could do was take a nap.

25 almonds (you can use blanched and skinned almonds, see page 29)
3 C milk or almond milk
½ C brown sugar, jaggery, or ⅓ C agave syrup
½ t cardamom powder
1 t rosewater and 5 to 7 strands saffron, soaked in warm milk or water

1. GRIND the almonds in a food processor. Add just a little milk to make it into a smooth paste.
2. BRING milk to a boil and reduce to 2½ cups (if you are using almond milk heat to almost a boil).
3. ADD almond paste, spices, and drained saffron.
4. SERVE chilled or warm; chilled is more traditional.

CHAI TEA

Serves 4   G M E N S Y

This is not traditionally thought of as a dessert, but it can be one and it's especially lovely served at the end of a meal. It's spicy and sweet and a great ginger-infused digestive.

Mataji taught me how to make this tea during our time together in Nova Scotia. We enjoyed many warm chai tea breaks by the bay window, overlooking twenty miles of the snow-filled Annapolis Valley.

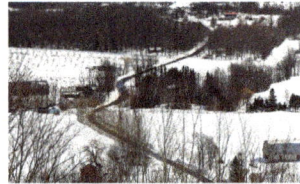

4 tea bags or 4 t loose, black tea
2 C low or nonfat milk, almond, or soy milk
2½ C water
1 T ginger, freshly grated

1 T cardamom powder
4 whole cloves
4 T turbinado sugar

1. HEAT milk and water in a heavy bottom pot until it comes to a boil.
2. ADD tea bags or loose tea and spices continue to simmer for 5 minutes until the milk/water turns a deep brown, strain before serving.

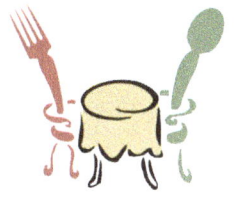

APPENDIX

STOCKING THE PANTRY

FOR EVERYTHING THERE IS A SEASONING

RESOURCES

THE ALLERGY CONNECTION

DEFINITION OF TERMS

INDEXES

STOCKING THE PANTRY

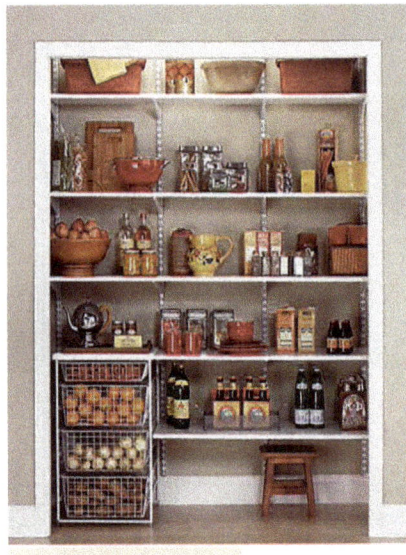

Cooking begins with the pantry, the heart of your kitchen. Organizing yourself before you begin to cook makes the actual preparation a joy and a time to unwind.

A PANTRY IS A WONDERFUL PLACE. It can be filled with remarkable scents from a wide variety of spices and condiments, plus reveal a spectrum of colors from different beans and grains. Best of all, it contains many of the essentials that go into the preparation of any meal. The first pantry I grew to appreciate was the one in our Nova Scotia farmhouse. It was where we separated the milk (from two cows), stored the summer bounty of jams and jellies, and kept 50-pound bags of lentils and brown rice that were purchased at bargain prices from a local food co-op. Whenever I entered the pantry, I felt a living pulse from the food on the shelves and the grains stored in tubs on the floor. A pantry need not be a separate room—it can be any area of your kitchen where you go to get ingredients for daily meals. Organizing your pantry is well worth the time and effort. You need not invest in expensive storage jars; large quart or gallon jars, the kind used in restaurants (often available in dollar stores) can make ideal containers.

Farmers markets are a great source for obtaining organic produce. In Southern California there is a Farmers Market in almost every town along the coast. Prices for certain organic foods, such as bananas, carrots, greens, and cauliflower are now often priced closely to their non-organic varieties.

Produce like strawberries and broccoli have thousands of places where chemical residues can hide and are hard to wash off. So, in at least a few instances, it's worth the trouble, and extra money, to buy them organically grown. If you live in a remote area, I've listed a few organic mail order suppliers and resources, later in this appendix.

POTS AND PANS

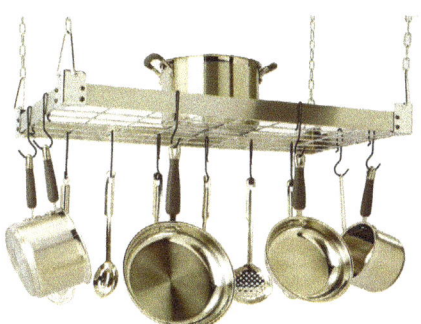

Utensils are uniquely important in food preparation. A high-quality set of stainless-steel pots and pans will last a lifetime. Years ago, I gave up all my nonstick cookware after reading research on the toxicity of Teflon pans. The problem with Teflon is that it leaches a combination of dangerous chemical substances into your food. In fact, canary and parrot owners have found that heating these pans to as little as 325 degrees can actually kill birds. There is also evidence that links these pans to neurological damage. There is also evidence that links these pans to neurological damage. Stainless-steel, heavy-duty cookware, like All Clad or similar brands are more expensive, but still a good, one-time investment. Though, they can be hard to clean. If you immediately fill the pan with hot water, add a few drops of lemon juice and bring it to a boil, it will make for less scrubbing. An interesting cleaning trick for stuck-on food is to use effervescent denture cleaner tablets mixed in warm water. Let the pot or pan soak for about 15 minutes, then it often cleans itself.

Another possible carcinogen can be found in inexpensive enamel casserole dishes, because the red, orange, or yellow glaze may contain cadmium. I've invested in a small collection of the French cookware, *Le-Creuset*. Each pan or dish has a cast-iron core sandwiched between hard enamel. You may find this brand in outlet stores. Some good comparable generic brands are now available. These pots cook food slowly and evenly, and cleanup is almost miraculous.

Two great items to have in your collection are a Dutch oven (perfect for stew, soups, and rice dishes) and a fry pan often referred to as "the green pan." I have two green pans, an 8" and 10." Their ceramic, non-stick formulation releases 60% fewer greenhouse gases than traditional Teflon non-stick technology. They should not be used at very high temperatures.

Cast iron has stood the test of time and actually does add iron to the foods that are cooked in them. You have to make sure you prepare the pan before its initially use, dry it immediately after rinsing it and oil it so it doesn't rust. A cast iron griddle and fry pan are great tools I have had on hand for over forty years. I have carted around my very first 10" cast iron skillet that I once used in the farmhouse kitchen. When I look for it in the back of my cabinet to make cornbread, it greets me like an old and trusted friend.

A stainless-steel pressure cooker and now an Instant Pot is a wonderful tool. A quick soup can be made in five minutes. Chickpea stew tastes more complex when it's made in a pressure cooker vessel. Once I had an accidental pressure blast that reached the ceiling of my kitchen, but in general, they are very safe and offer the benefit of locking in vitamins, minerals, and flavor. Instant Pots have now almost replaced the old pressure cookers, they are pressure cookers with specific settings and very safe pressure valves. I have grown to love mine and actually finally relented and gave up my original 35-year-old pressure cooker.

BAKING SUPPLIES

A Silpat (nonstick pad) is great to have for rolling out breads and baked goods. Not much sticks to it and you can use less flour when rolling out your dough. I prefer not to use it for baking as it may leach chemicals at high temperatures.

I use stainless-steel cookie sheets, bread and muffin tins lined with all-natural wax or parchment paper, just like Grandma used to do. *Chefs Select* makes 100% natural soy wax paper products that are petroleum free. These are clean, safe, non-toxic, and biodegradable. Use parchment paper rather than plastic lids or wraps, which can release dioxin into the food when heated in the microwave or conventional oven. Parchment is generally good up to 400 degrees.

You can get these products online at: www.chefsselect.com, or www.amazon.com.

PANTRY ITEMS AND ALTERNATIVES

Tofu: Tofu should be purchased weekly and kept in a tight-fitting container with the water changed daily. Firm tofu is best for frying and baking in main dishes. Soft or silken tofu is used in baking quick breads and desserts, and for blended soups.

Soy Sauce: Tamari and *shoyu* are wonderful, natural soy products, aged in kegs, using the centuries-old method of natural fermentation. They convert hard-to-digest soy proteins, starches, and fats into easily absorbed amino acids, simple sugars and fatty acids. *Shoyu* is made with whole soybeans, whole wheat, sea salt, and *koji*. Tamari can be made with or without wheat and contains less water, yielding a slightly thicker sauce.

TOP 5 HERBS

Basil
Basil may be the most fragrant and well-beloved herb of all. Widely used in Mediterranean, Italy, and Greece cooking.

Rosemary
A wild herb with robust aromatics and strong aroma, it should be used in small amounts or as sprigs and then removed.

Sage
Works wonderfully with vegetarian dishes, especially with pasta. A little goes a long way.

Oregano
What's an Italian dish without oregano? In the Mediterranean kitchen, this herb is often grown on the windowsill so it's always handy.

Cilantro
Native to the Mediterranean, cilantro is used all over the world. Every part of the cilantro plant is used.

Braggs Liquid Aminos is an alternative to soy sauce. It contains small amounts of the nonessential amino acids: alanine, arginine, aspartic acid, glutamic acid, glycine, histidine, isoleucine, and lysine.

Coconut Aminos is another substitute for soy sauce, gluten, and soy free! It's made from the sap of the coconut palm, but it doesn't taste like coconut: it's like a milder version of soy sauce that is less salty.

Miso: Miso is high in *umami*, the fifth basic taste described as "savoriness." It adds both denseness and intensity. A little miso goes a long way—it's about 8 to 14 percent salt, but most of its intense and complex flavor comes from fermentation rather than salt. A tablespoon of miso contains 680 mg of sodium (a tablespoon of table salt contains an astounding 6,589 mg of sodium).

When miso is to be heated, it's always best to add it at the end of the preparation. Miso can be found in small plastic containers in the refrigerated section at Asian markets, natural food stores, and well-stocked supermarkets. Look for naturally aged brands with no additives. It may be stored in the refrigerator for up to one year, but ideally should be used within 2 to 3 months, to take advantage of its optimal aroma.

Milk Alternatives: Milk can easily be replaced in any recipe with soy, almond, rice, or coconut milk alternatives. Soy is a bit thicker and richer and comes in a variety of styles: nonfat, low-fat, or vanilla. For people with IBS or sensitive stomachs, soy may be a bit harder to digest than rice or almond milk.

When a recipe calls for milk powder you can use rice, soy or potato alternatives. Milk-free powders are available in most health food stores; a good brand is *Dari Free Milk Powder.* You can also go to www.meyenberg.org for powdered goat's milk, www.naturesflavors.com for powdered soy milk, or www.vancesfoods.net for powdered potato milk.

When making dairy-free yogurt you will need a live, active culture. Check ingredients carefully, as milk-free starters may contain dairy ingredients. You can check with a few websites, such as: www.dairyconnection.com, www.giprohealth.com and www.healthy-traders.com. Another company you may want to check out is: www.gemcultures.com.

For severe milk allergies check products for casein, a milk protein often added to products labeled "dairy-free." Cream cheese, sour cream, and even Parmesan cheese are now available casein-free.

TOP 5 SPICES

Ginger
For centuries ginger was exclusively for the wealthy; its floral taste is woven into romantic legends.

Coriander
The potent and spicy coriander seed is from the cilantro plant. The ground seed is coriander powder.

Pepper
Black pepper is a tropical plant, which grows at the equator. The peppercorns are picked when they are under ripe and the color changes to black, as they dry.

Turmeric
Turmeric may be the most important spice of all. When dried and ground it becomes a wonderful orange hue. It's the essential ingredient in curry powder.

Paprika
With its gorgeous red coloring, all varieties of paprika are derived from *capsicum annum*, a sweet red pepper.

Eggs: If you do use eggs, organic pasture raised, or infertile are available almost everywhere, though a bit more expensive. *Ener-G* is an incredibly versatile and easy-to-use commercial dry egg replacer, available in most health food stores. While the instructions on the package say to mix Ener-G with two tablespoons of water, some recipes will need a bit more moisture when replacing eggs. When using Ener-G, a general rule of thumb is that one egg is equivalent to ¼ C of liquid, which means you need to compensate with more liquid, soy, rice, almond or coconut or cashew milk. Ener-G and other store-bought egg substitutes are relatively flavorless and work best in baked goods such as cookies, muffins and cakes and can also be used to bind ingredients together in a casserole or loaf dish.

You can also use mashed banana, prune puree, or applesauce as an egg replacer in baked goods, such as muffins, pancakes, or yeast-free quick breads, it adds the perfect amount of thick moisture, like eggs, but it won't help the dish rise or turn out light and fluffy, so you have to add a bit more baking powder or baking soda to make it rise.

Tofu can be a great egg substitute in dishes such as: quiche, frittata, or egg salad. The texture of crumbled regular tofu is similar to boiled or cooked eggs. Adding mustard or turmeric to the dish gives it an egg-like yellow hue. Silken tofu is also a good egg substitute in baked goods. To use: blend ¼ cup silken tofu with the liquid ingredients until smooth and creamy. While it won't alter the flavor of a recipe, using tofu as an egg substitute will make baked goods a bit heavier, so it works well in brownies and pancakes, but wouldn't work well in something like an angel food cake that needs to be light and fluffy. A general recipe for using tofu as an egg substitute, which also helps to lighten the recipe is: ¼ C soft tofu, 1 T oil, ½ t arrowroot powder, and 1 T baking powder. Blend until smooth with 1 T soy, rice, or almond milk.

There is a product called *Wonderslim* which is a fat and egg substitute made from dried plum concentrate, oat fiber and soy lecithin. It is available on Amazon. When baking you can substitute ¼ C of *Wonderslim* for each egg to replace the liquid portion of the recipe. Be aware that it is not gluten free, as it contains oat fiber. It is also good to use for someone who is sensitive to baking soda and baking powder.

Vegan Meringue Alternative: 6 T *aquafaba* (the liquid from ½ can of chickpeas), ¼ t cream of tartar, ½ C turbinado sugar, 1 t vanilla extract. Whip *aquafaba* and cream of tartar until foamy, slowly add sugar and continue whipping until glossy and firm peaks, at the end add vanilla extract.

Dried Herbs and Spices: The varieties of dried spices are too numerous to mention here but a few whole spices that are good to have in your pantry are: nutmeg (freshly grate on the fine side of a citrus zester), dried cinnamon bark, and of course, black pepper, ground fresh, as needed. If you use dried herbs, wake them up by rubbing them together with your hand or give them a quick pounding in a mortar and pestle. I shop at a store that sells spices in bulk so I can purchase very small quantities of a more obscure spice like celery seeds or dried sage—ones that I may use for a specific recipe. (See sidebars in this chapter, as well as the next chapter, *For Everything There is a Seasoning*.)

Garlic: Garlic is a wonderful tonic, used in many main dishes and salads; when combined with parsley, its strong aroma is tamed. Baked garlic tones down its bite and is transformed into mellow softness.

You can also make a lovely garlic oil (see page 98). I often kept a long braid of garlic dangling from a hook on my kitchen pot rack. Here's a mail order store where you can buy one (in California the season is October-November): www.bluequail.com.

Ginger: My personal favorite spice is ginger. It has remarkable digestive properties and helps to stimulate metabolism. Use it fresh, as often as possible. Ginger keeps quite well stored in a plastic bag; refrigerated it will last for about two weeks. Simply grate the end of the ginger root every time you want to add ginger to a recipe (using the finest side of a hand grater), which for me, is almost always. To peel, use the back side of a spoon or a vegetable peeler, so you don't remove too much of the skin. A lot of the nutrients are just below the surface.

WHEAT FLOUR SUBSTITUTES
CUP FOR CUP

Barley	1¼ cups
Cornmeal	1 cup
Corn	1 cup
flour	1¼ cups
Oat	3/4 cup
Potato	1¼ cups
Rice	3/4 cup
Rye	1¼ cups
Soy	1 cup
Tapioca	1¼ cups

Liquid Smoke: I like the "Wrights" brand, it's a natural product and is very powerful. Never use too much; just a drop or two will do.

Flour: Whole wheat flour is best when it's fresh and stone-ground, and should, if possible, be stored in the refrigerator. Bread baked with whole wheat flour, which isn't fresh doesn't rise as well, and sometimes not at all. Whole wheat pastry flour is finely ground and best used for quick breads, cookies and desserts. Whole-wheat pastry flour is made from a softer wheat and has less protein and gluten than regular flour, which may be taken into account for people with sensitive digestion or who are wheat sensitive. Heritage wheat, Farro, an ancient wheat flour grain that is less glutinous than wheat flour, has become popular once again.

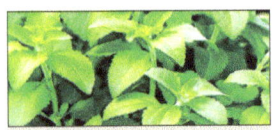

STEVIA

About 240 species of herbs and shrubs are in the sunflower stevia family (Asteraceae). Native to subtropical and tropical regions from Western North America to South America. As a sweetener and sugar substitute, it has a slower onset and longer duration than sugar, although some of its extracts may have a bitter or licorice-like aftertaste. Because it is 300 times sweeter than sugar, it is a boon for a low-carbohydrate, low-sugar food diet. To bake with stevia, follow a few basic guidelines: baking should not exceed 400 degrees, and for each cup of sugar substitute 1 teaspoon of powered or liquid stevia.

A simple solution for flour pests is adding a bay leaf to your flour container.

Gluten-Free Flours: Wheat flour contains gluten, which keep cookies, cakes and pies light and prevents them from crumbling. It does this by trapping pockets of air. In order to help retain a gluten-like structure when using non-gluten flour, binding additives like xanthan gum are needed. You can also add either potato, arrowroot, or corn starch in combination with other non-gluten flours to lighten up the mix. A great combination for baking sweets is almond and coconut flour. There are many commercial quality gluten-free flour blends available, such as: *Arrowhead Mills*, *Bob's Red Mill*, and *Barry Farm*. (See page 94 for gluten-free flour blends.)

Xanthan Gum: *Main binding agent for gluten-free baking.* Should be stored in a tight-fitting container in a cold dark place or in the freezer. (See page 288 for more information.)
 Other Alternatives are:
 Guar Gum: 1½ times the amount of xanthan gum.
 Agar Agar: 1:1 ratio the amount of xanthan gum
 Psyllium Husk Powder: 1:1 ratio with xanthan gum
 Flaxseed Meal: 1: 1 ration as xanthan gum, mixed with 2x water
 Chia Seeds: 1 T chia seeds to 2 T water for every 1 t of xanthan gum
 Egg White: one extra egg white for every teaspoon of xanthan gum
 Gelatin: 1 t xanthan gum to 2 t gelatin

Breadcrumbs: I love using Japanese Panko instead of ordinary breadcrumbs because they are crisper and lighter. Store in an airtight container as they get stale quickly. For wheat sensitivities you can make your own breadcrumbs from non-gluten bread, rice crackers, corn flakes, corn chips, or buy a commercial brand of gluten-free breadcrumbs or Panko.

Sweeteners: It's advisable to use white sugar sparingly. There are a variety of sugar choices which include: natural turbinado, Billington's muscovado sugar, and Indian jaggery. Other alternatives include date, maple and coconut sugar. They can all be used interchangeably in recipes but have a bit stronger flavor. When replacing maple syrup or honey for sugar, you might have to adjust the liquid in the recipe by decreasing it by one-fourth.

Other sugar alternatives, which can be used in certain recipes that call for corn syrup is brown rice syrup. It is also healthier than regular corn syrup. Stevia is also a good substitute; the new powdered version is not as bitter as it used to be. Monk fruit blend with xylitol is another substitute, use it cup for cup to replace sugar. One my favorite sweeteners is agave nectar or syrup. It is an all-natural plant-based sweetener derived from the agave cactus, native to Mexico, and has been used for centuries to make tequila. It's a light, golden syrup that is 1½ times sweeter than sugar.

Agave's glycemic index is 28 to 32 compared with honey which is 58. It doesn't spike blood sugar levels the way that sugar does. It's 90% fructose, which means it processes more slowly in the body than glucose. Agave is suitable for those with type 2 diabetes and is often recommended for an anti-candida diet. You can easily use it as a replacement for honey or maple syrup in any recipe but use about three quarters of the amount called for, due to its greater sweetness. When you are using it to replace one cup of sugar use ¾ cup agave and decrease the liquid by ¼ of the amount.

Salt: *Kosher Salt* dissolves fast and its flavor disperses quickly. I use a medium size grain most of the time and enjoy using my hands to feel the correct amount of salt going into the food. *Crystalline Sea Salt* adds a pungent burst of flavor to just-cooked foods, coming in both fine and coarse grades. *Fleur de Sel* can be used for special occasions; it has a delicate flavor which adds a perfect hint of saltiness to a freshly sliced tomato or cut melon. It comes from coastal salt ponds in France where conditions have to be just right (lots of sun and wind) for it to "bloom" like a flower on the surface of the water. *Himalayan Crystal Salt* includes trace minerals and elements: potassium, calcium and magnesium that help promote a healthy balance by maintaining fluids and replenishing your supply of electrolytes. *Flake Salt* sticks better, dissolves faster, and blends more evenly. Its "pinchable" texture allows you to crush it between your fingertips and deliver better seasoning control.

Chemical Removal: To remove excess chemicals from vegetables and fruit, especially tomatoes, apples, green peppers, zucchini, and eggplant, use a drop of all-natural dish soap, or any natural commercial product. You can also make your own veggie wash by combining 1 tablespoon of lemon juice to 2 tablespoons of baking soda with 1 cup of water. Put this mixture in a sprayer bottle. Spray veggies, rub slightly, let them sit for a few minutes, then rinse. Use on any vegetable except mushrooms. To clean mushrooms, simply wipe with a slightly damp kitchen towel.

FOR EVERYTHING THERE IS A SEASONING

WHAT DO YOU DO TO SPICE UP YOUR MEALS? The possibilities are endless, but where to start? Learning to cook with spices and herbs can literally change your palate and health. We all have our favorites. Most likely it's time to check out your herb and spice cabinet for a long overdue spring cleaning—anything that is aged over one or two years simply toss out and start fresh. Dried herbs lose their power and flavor with time. That's why starting with whole spices and herbs, roasting and grinding them when needed, captures the ultimate freshness and taste. You can always keep a few pots of fresh herbs on your windowsill or in a ball jar on your counter. Watching them as they grow and plucking them as you need them is a delight.

New discoveries of the remarkable properties of spices and herbs are being uncovered almost daily. The Indian healing and culinary system, known as Ayurveda, is thousands of years old, and has been on the leading edge of scientific research. Bharat Aggarwal, M.D., Ph.D., is professor at the University of Texas, Anderson Cancer Center in Houston, and author of *Healing Spices*. Dr. Aggarwal is just one physician of many who promotes the use of herbs and spices as a good dietary plan, he writes:

"When Indians eat more westernized foods, they're getting much fewer spices than their traditional diet contains, and they lose the protection those spices are conveying."

Spice Tools
You can buy a stainless-steel spice dubba and grinder or a granite mortar and pestle on:
www.Amazon.com
www.webstaurantstore.com
www.worldmarket.com

There is compelling evidence that herbs and spices are helpful for treating some chronic conditions and cooking with them enhances every dish. Because they are sensitive to light, always store your herbs and spices in sealed containers in a dark, dry place. Here are a few health benefits of some of my favorite herbs and spices along with storage and growing ideas.

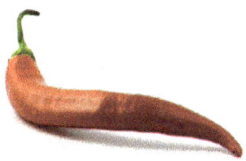

Chili Peppers
Health Benefit: *Boost metabolism*

Chili peppers obviously add a jolt of heat to our dishes. There are many varieties and heat levels to choose from. It's the capsaicin in the compound that gives chilis their kick. Studies have shown that capsaicin can increase the body's metabolic rate and stimulate brain chemicals that help us feel less hungry. Capsaicin may also lower risk of ulcers by boosting the ability of stomach cells to resist infection by ulcer-causing bacteria. It also may help the heart by keeping "bad" LDL cholesterol from turning into a more dangerous, artery-clogging substance.

> *Grow and Store:* Chili peppers are easy to grow in the summer; you can pick them fresh and dry them for use in the winter. Use them whole or de-seed for less of a punch, you can also grind dried peppers into cayenne powder. Cayenne powder can last for up to a year when stored in a tight-fitting jar.

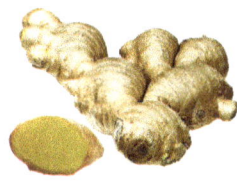

Ginger
Health Benefits: *Soothes an upset stomach and fights arthritis pain*

Ginger lends a sweet, spicy, and peppery essence to any food preparation, and it has a well-deserved reputation for relieving an unsettled stomach and aiding in digestion. Many studies show that ginger extract can help reduce nausea caused by morning sickness following surgery or chemotherapy, although it's less effective for motion sickness. Ginger, an inflammation-fighting powerhouse, has a compound known as *gingerols*, which is being investigated for fighting some cancers, reducing the aches of osteoarthritis and soothing sore muscles.

> *Storage:* Wrap fresh ginger root in a paper towel and place in a plastic bag in the refrigerator. Ground ginger should be replaced every 6 months.

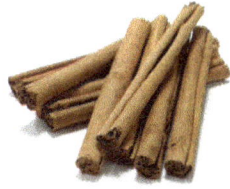

Cinnamon
Health Benefit: *Stabilizes blood sugar*

Who doesn't have cinnamon in their cupboard? It's more than just for sweets, as it works well with many savory dishes. In the Mediterranean, Africa and Northern India, cinnamon is used in many savory preparations. A few studies have found that adding cinnamon to food—up to a teaspoon a day, for people with type 2 diabetes—helps control blood sugar levels, by lowering post-meal, blood-sugar spikes.

Storage: Cinnamon needs to be fresh so don't buy too much at a time. You can store cinnamon sticks in mason jars and grind it into powder as you need it. Cinnamon powder losses its punch and health value after 6 months.

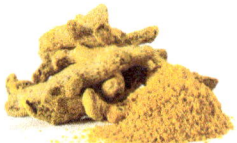

Turmeric

Health Benefits: *Quells inflammation and may inhibit tumors*

Turmeric is probably the most important spice to have on hand. This golden-colored spice is used in just about every Indian dish. It's also used in many Asian specialties to give it a warm yellow glow and is the main ingredient in the curry powder blend of spices. It's often used in India to help wounds heal (applied as a paste) and made into a tea to relieve colds and respiratory problems. The main component providing its health benefits is *curcumin*, a compound in turmeric that has potent antioxidants and anti-inflammatory properties. *Curcumin* is being studied for use in treating arthritis, heart disease, diabetes, and Alzheimer's. It may be found to inhibit tumor cell growth and suppress enzymes that activate carcinogens. These are quite impressive benefits!

Storage: In India, the root is often used fresh and ground into a paste with other spices. Here, in the West, we simply buy turmeric powder. If stored in an airtight container it could last for up to one year. Use the "smell test" to determine when it should be replaced. Fresh turmeric has a sweet and potent smell, which begins to lessen with time.

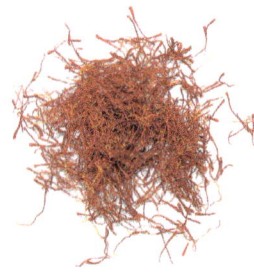

Saffron

Health Benefit: *A mood lifter*

Saffron has long been used in traditional Persian cuisine, and also as a fabric dye because of its strong, orange color. It has a sweet, grassy flavor and a little goes a long way, which is good because it's quite expensive. Saffron is used in rice preparations and other Middle Eastern dishes, and in Indian sweets. It is useful as a mood lifter and can be steeped into a medicinal tea.

Storage and Use: Saffron threads should be crushed before using them. If you need ground saffron, lightly toast and grind the threads yourself. You can also steep them in a cooking liquid before using. The longer you steep the saffron threads, the stronger the flavor and color. Store them in a tight-fitting jar and they will last for almost 6 months.

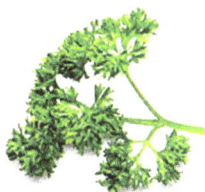

Parsley
Health Benefit: *May inhibit breast cancer cell growth*
A sprig of parsley is often a forgotten garnish on the plate, but its peppery and almost anise flavor is an important herb to use often. Further, it goes with practically any type of dish. Because of ongoing studies confirming parsley's health benefits, it's beneficial to garnish with minced fresh or dried parsley as a standard cooking practice. A study conducted by the University of Missouri scientists found that this herb can actually inhibit breast cancer cell growth, though excessive amounts are not recommended for pregnant women.

Grow and Store: Growing parsley on your windowsill or summer garden is very easy. It's like a weed; the more you pick, the more it grows. You can put fresh parsley in a mason jar filled with water and keep it on your kitchen counter, change the water every other day or wrap fresh parsley sprigs in a paper towel and place in a plastic bag in the refrigerator. Dried parsley can last up to a year, but after 6 months it begins to lose its potency.

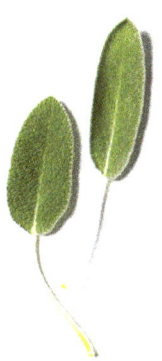

Sage
Health Benefits: *Helps to preserve memory, soothes sore throats*
This potent, earthy herb should be used sparingly, but it adds a unique touch to dishes both savory and sweet. You can sip sage tea for an upset stomach or sore throat. Preliminary research suggests it may improve some symptoms of early Alzheimer's by preventing a key enzyme from destroying acetylcholine, a brain chemical involved in memory and learning. In another study, college students who took sage extract in capsule form performed significantly better on memory tests, and their moods improved, too.

Grow and Store: Sage is a shrub that can't be cultivated in very cold climates. It loves the sun, but not a lot of wind, so keep it sheltered. You can store fresh sage leaves by wrapping them in a paper towel and then placing in a plastic bag. Ground sage will last about six months; then it loses its aroma.

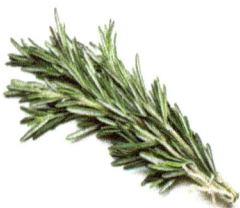

Rosemary

Health Benefits: *May enhance mental focus and fight food-borne bacteria*

Rosemary is a hardy, aromatic, evergreen shrub. With its strong, musky flavor, a little goes a long way. When the sprigs are burnt, they emit a mustard-like smell. One recent rosemary study found that people performed better on memory and alertness tests when misted with aromatic rosemary oil. In rosemary's early beginnings, it was often used in marinades, and there's scientific wisdom behind that tradition: rosmarinic acid and other antioxidant compounds in the herb fight bacteria and prevent food from spoiling.

Grow and Store: Rosemary is a hardy, beautiful ornamental plant. While often associated with the Mediterranean area, it can be grown almost anywhere. In fact, rosemary plants often suffer from too much attention, rather than too little. You can store fresh rosemary in a plastic bag or in a glass of water in the refrigerator.

RESOURCES

FOOD SUPPLIES

Here are some online food resources, sometimes the URLs may change with time, so keep that in mind.

Indian Food Company
Tel: 10877-786 to 8876 • www.ishopindian.com
One of the most extensive Indian food websites.

Organic Provisions
Thrive Market • www.thrivemarket.com
Offers boundless natural foods items from some of the industry's best-known names.

Jaffe Brothers, Inc.
105 Copperwood Way suite F, Oceanside, CA • Tel: (760) 749-1133
www.organicfruitsandnuts.com
Features an extensive line of organic dried fruits, nuts, seeds, grains, snack foods and pastas made with organically grown wheat.

International Foods
www.cmcfoodsus.com
Ingredients from African, Chinese, India, Japan, Mexico, Thailand are included on this website.

Lundberg Family Farms
Richvale, CA • Tel: 959-74-0369 • www.lundberg.com
A family-owned and operated farm that grows and produces brown rice, specialty rice varieties and brown rice products.

Cooking Apps

A number of great new apps for smart phones can help you navigate through ingredients, calories and cooking information:
- Fooducate
- Kitchen Calculator PRO
- Cook it Allergy Free
- Substitutions
- Foodily
- How to Cook Everything
- Kitchen Math
- Harvest

HERBS & SPICES

Here are few good websites to find online herbs and spices for sale:
www.myspicesage.com
www.thespicehouse.com
www.pureindianfoods.com
www.atlanticspice.com
www.penzeys.com

GLUTEN-FREE SUPPLIES

Barry Farm Enterprises
20086 Mudsock Road, Wapakoneta, Ohio 45895 • 419-228-4640
www.barryfarm.com

Gluten-free, dairy-free, vegan, sugar-free, salt-free, and wheat-free.
www.healthy-eating.com
www.glutenfreemall.com
www.glutensolutions.com
www.glutenfree.com
www.kinnikinnick.com
www.holgrain.com
www.123glutenfree.com
www.livingwithout.com

ORGANIZATIONS

The Food Allergy and Anaphylaxis Network (FAAN):
www.foodallergy.org

National Institute of Allergy and Infectious Diseases (NIAID):
www.niaid.nih.gov

The Bastyr University Natural Health Clinic:
www.bastyr.edu

Low FODMAP: Allergy Connection Information:
www.monashfodmap.com

THE ALLERGY CONNECTION

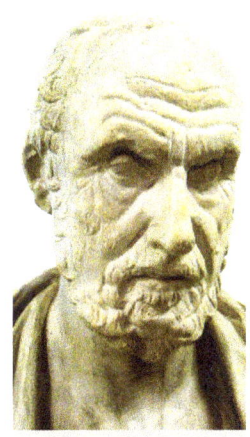

"Natural forces within us are the true healers of disease."
—Hippocrates

BECAUSE THIS BOOK FEATURES ALLERGY ALTERNATIVES, I felt it would be helpful to explore some of the more common food allergies now affecting an ever-increasing number of people.

Allergic reactions to food date back to the writings of Hippocrates in 400 BC. It wasn't until the twentieth century that findings of formal research studies on food allergies were published in respected scientific journals. The term "food allergy" is an umbrella term that describes many adverse reactions to specific foods or food groups.

According to the latest research, 1 in every 12 births of children under the age of 18 may have some form of food allergy. In fact, this malady may now affect up to 12 million people in American alone.

Dramatic findings reveal the damaging factors of gluten, casein, and sugar allergies, especially in autistic children. In fact, it is estimated that 1 in 88 children have some form of autism spectrum disorder (ASD).

Researchers have found that gluten and casein affect the developing brains of certain children, often leading to autistic behaviors. By simply eliminating one or more of these foods many of the debilitating symptoms often improve. This is a powerful example of the connection between food and its effect on the mind and body.

ALLERGIC REACTIONS

When one has a food allergy, the immune system repels the specific food item assessing its harm to the body. Once the alarm is raised, the immune system then proceeds to create specific antibodies to counteract the received threat. The next time you eat that particular food, the immune system releases large amounts of chemicals, including histamine, to protect the body. These chemicals often trigger a cascade of allergic symptoms that can affect the respiratory system, gastrointestinal tract, skin, or cardiovascular system. In general, we simply don't feel well.

There are degrees of food allergies. In some cases, hypersensitive reactions may occur within hours—or even a few minutes—after a food is eaten, causing obvious physical symptoms such as rash, hives, runny nose, or a headache. In rare cases, immediate hypersensitive reactions may cause anaphylactic shock, a life-threatening condition in which the throat swells and blocks the passage of air. Luckily, this type of hypersensitivity affects only a small percentage of people who have extreme food allergies.

One of the most common types of food allergies is lactose intolerance. As many as 30% of all adults are affected. Lactose intolerance is particularly prevalent in the African and Asian communities. People who are lactose intolerant do not produce enough of the digestive enzyme called "lactase," which breaks down the milk sugar (lactose) found in dairy products. The first sign of a problem is when we feel bloated and gassy. In a small amount of children peanut allergies are prevalent, protecting them from peanut products or additives may be challenging.

Many people are also unable to "tolerate" natural and synthetic chemicals such as sulfates, which often hide in our food supply. These sulfur-containing preservatives are often used to preserve dried fruits, wines, and many other processed foods. Another glaring food additive that can create an adverse reaction is food dye, especially yellow color No. 5 (tartrazine). One of the earliest instances of harmful food products that affected a large portion of the population is monosodium glutamate (MSG), often used to increase flavor, particularly in Asian foods.

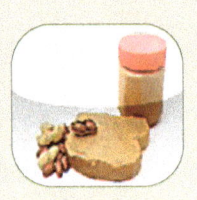

3 Allergy Apps

Am I Allergic?
An allergen thesaurus is useful when you're out shopping to ensure you avoid all the many different words used in ingredient lists for dairy (e.g., caseinate, lactose, whey, curd, etc.) It's information at your fingertips.

Allergy Guard Lite
Allergen data that this app lists is in the hundreds of food types, in alphabetical order. If you're interested in further information, click on the food type to get a more detailed list of associated foods and ingredients.

Allergy Tracker
Track of your allergies, monitor changes, add notes to each log, understand your pollen diary. Any new updates are free once you've downloaded it.

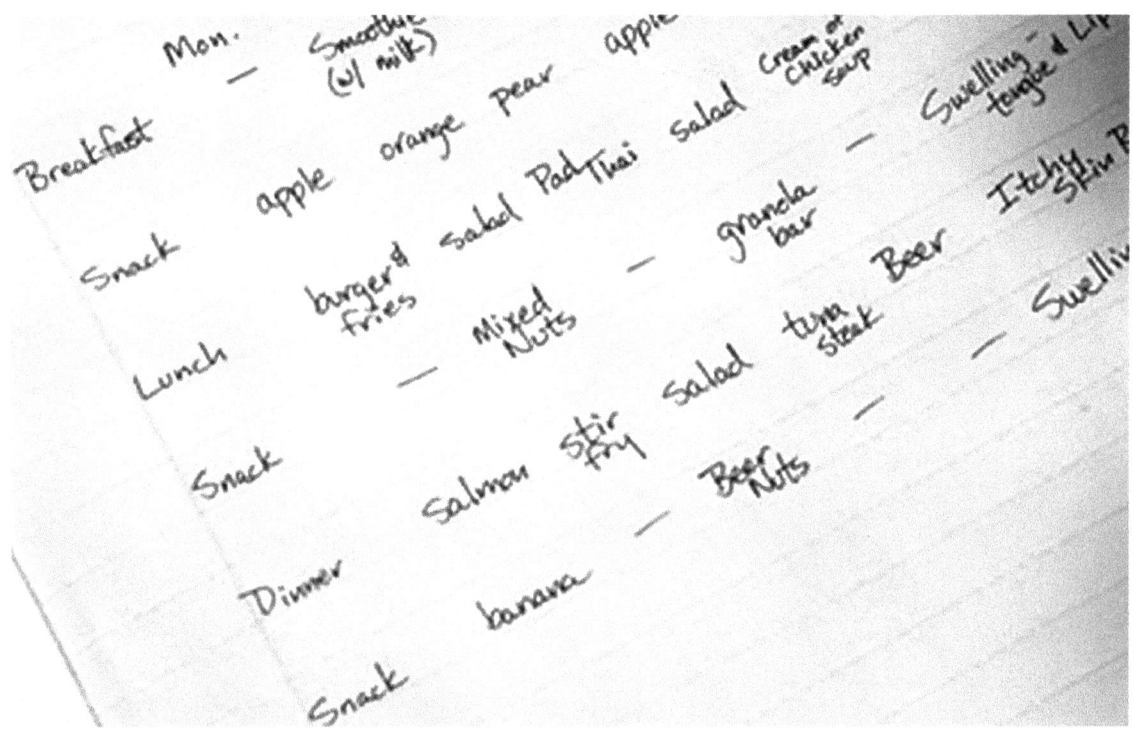

DISCOVERING ALLERGIES

Discovering foods you may be allergic to is often the first step in getting your vitality and health back on track. There are a number of tests that can be taken to confirm a food allergy: a blood test, skin (scratch) test and patch test. These tests assess the body's level of IgE antibodies to determine the immune system's response to a particular allergen. Each test method has positives and negatives. And the test results alone may not definitively diagnose allergies.

All results should be interpreted along with one's medical and family history. For example, testing for celiac disease is much more extensive, and can often run-in families. It requires a biopsy while the patient is still ingesting gluten.

Another helpful tool in the allergy arsenal is "The Elimination Diet." One needs to eliminate each suspected food for at least a month and observe whether any symptoms improve at the end of that time. Then each food can be introduced back, one at a time, to determine if that particular food causes reactions. This experiment may need to be repeated. I would suggest keeping a daily diary of meals, noting any possible symptoms that may result.

Select a Category to Eliminate Each Month: *Dairy products, Gluten-based foods, Corn, Egg, Soy, Nut, Seeds, or Yeast.*

A "rotation diet" uses the same categories as above. It's quicker, but not as extensive as the elimination diet. On this diet, potentially problematic food groups are eaten only once every four days. Again, keep a diary to record and monitor any or all symptoms.

Estimated Food Allergy Rates in North America

Prevalence	Infant/Child	Adult
Milk	2.5%	0.3%
Peanuts	1.5%	0.2%
Tree Nuts	0.5%	0.6%
Fish	0.1%	0.4%
Shellfish	0.1%	2%
Wheat, Soy	0.4%	0.3%
Sesame	0.1%	0.1%
Overall	5%	3 to 4%

REASONS FOR THE RISE IN THE NUMBER OF FOOD ALLERGIES

Repeated Foods: People tend to favor limited food groups, especially wheat and gluten products. The number one offender in this group is wheat products. Corn, milk, nuts, seeds, and eggs are also problematic. These are also common "hidden" ingredients found in many processed foods.

Digestive Tract: The digestive tract plays such a vital role in preventing illness and disease. When the intestinal barrier is compromised, partially digested dietary protein can be absorbed into the bloodstream. This causes an allergic response which produces symptoms in the intestines and often throughout the body.

Immune System on Overload: Daily stress, exposure to environmental pollution; in our air, water, and food puts a strain on our immune system. It becomes more challenging for the immune system to respond when it encounters antigens in food.

Genetics: As far as we know, food allergies and intolerances can often, but not always, be hereditary. If both parents have allergies, their children have a 67% chance of developing similar allergies—if one parent has allergies the child has about a 33% chance of developing them in their lifetime.

> **HINT**
>
> **GLUTEN-FREE ALTERNATIVES**
>
> Rice, corn, soy, potato, tapioca, sorghum, quinoa, buckwheat, bean flour, garfava, millet, arrowroot, amaranth, hemp, teff, montina, flax and nut flours.
>
> **Possible hidden gluten sources**
>
> Wheat, farro, graham, kamut, semolina, spelt, tabbouleh, bulger, rye, barley, couscous, and triticale.

Hidden Dangers

Dairy: One of the most common sources of allergies is cow's milk, which contains the protein casein. An ingredient list on a food item will indicate the presence of milk derivatives as a food source: casein, caseinate, calcium caseinate, ammonia caseinate, magnesium caseinate, potassium caseinate, and sodium caseinate. Casein is used in food processing, especially as an extender, tenderizer, and protein fortifier. It can also be found in unexpected food items like chewing gum.

Wheat and Gluten: Wheat is only one type of grain that contains gluten, but it's the most common one used in bread and pasta products. It is often hidden in products, like soy sauce. In the world of commercial baked goods, gluten is the gummy, yellow-gray material that is left over after dough (wheat flour and water) has been washed. During the washing process, many of the water-soluble substances and starches are removed, and what's left is a complicated mixture that is commonly referred to as gluten. All of wheat's components are glutinous: wheat bran, wheat germ, wheat starch, wheat nuts, and wheat berries.

Dextrin: This is an incomplete hydrolyzed starch that is often derived from the dry heating of corn, potato, rice, tapioca, arrowroot, or wheat.

Caramel: This can be made by heating several different food-grade carbohydrates, such as sugar or corn syrup.

Vanilla: This extract often uses grain alcohol during preparation and may also contain wheat protein residue.

Eggs: Baked goods and baking mixes often contain eggs. Eggs will also be in hollandaise sauce, egg-based mayonnaise, and some soups. The fat substitute *Simplesse*™ contains microparticulated egg protein. Even egg substitutes may contain egg white powder.

Soy: An ever-increasing number of products now contain soy-derivitives. These would include hydrolyzed soy protein, hydrolyzed plant protein, hydrolyzed vegetable protein, isolated vegetable protein, vegetable gum, vegetable broth, or natural flavoring. Of course, an obvious source is soy sauce as well as: *shoyu*, tamari, miso, tofu, tempeh, soy curd and soy granules.

FODMAP DIET

In 2005, researchers in the Dept. of Gastroenterology at Monash University, in Australia, identified a group of short-chain carbohydrates found in foods that are either poorly absorbed in the small intestine or difficult to digest. The Monash team named these carbohydrates FODMAPs.

The research team measured the FODMAP content of a wide range of foods. The food composition information allowed the team to develop the first low FODMAP diet.

Yeast: Small amounts of yeast are present during the drying of tea, coffee, and spices. The culturing of yeast is used as a starting point for commercial production of fermented products, like vinegars and ciders. Many milk-based products also contain yeast since yeasts thrive on milk sugar (lactose). Some of these products include sour cream, buttermilk, cream cheese, ricotta cheese, and powdered milk. Yeast extracts are sometimes hidden in canned and frozen fruit juices, and in several fruit juice concentrates.

OTHER DIGESTIVE ISSUES

It's important to figure out what type of allergies you have or if other digestive problems such as coeliac disease, ulcerative colitis, and Crohn's disease, are related to or exacerbating allergies:

Irritable Bowel Syndrome (IBS)

Recent studies have found a correlation between many patients with IBS suffering from allergies. In one of those studies, it was found that up to 80% of people with IBS, also suffer seasonal allergies, and a percentage also have an intolerance to lactose and fermentable carbohydrates.

Small Intestinal Bacterial Overgrowth (SIBO)

This is a recently researched issue that is now being explored. It occurs when there is an abnormal increase in the overall bacterial population in the small intestine—particularly types of bacteria not commonly found in that part of the digestive tract.

SIBO creates a slow passage of food and waste products in the digestive tract, creating a breeding ground for bacteria. The excess bacteria often cause many reactions such as: bloating, diarrhea, weight loss and malnutrition, which also may be caused by diet or food allergies. There is a rather complicated test you get to confirm if you have SIBO and the treatment can include antibiotics, herbs, and diet.

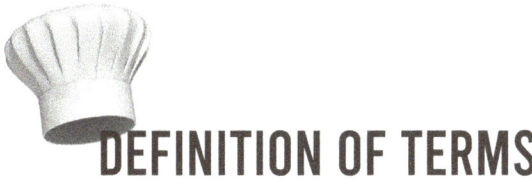
DEFINITION OF TERMS

AL DENTÉ
Cook until tender but firm to the bite.

BAKE
To cook using dry heat inside an oven.

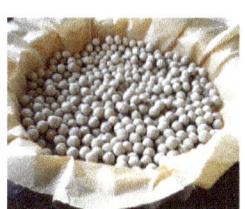

BAKE BLIND
To bake a pastry crust without a filling. To prevent shrinkage, pierce the bottom pastry with the prongs of a fork. Or put a piece of greased wax or parchment paper on the top of crust, fill with beans or dried peas kept for this purpose, before baking.

BASTE
To moisten food with fat or other liquids while cooking.

BEAT
To stir vigorously or whip briskly using a fork or whisk in order to work air into liquid or food, making it smooth and light.

BIND
Thicken liquids by the adding agents, e.g., flour or starch.

BLANCH
Plunge food into boiling water for a few seconds, followed by cold water; then drain.

BLEND
Mix ingredients so thoroughly that each loses its identity.

BOIL
Cook food in a generous amount of liquid, which should bubble continuously (boiling temperature is 225 degrees).

BOUILLON
A strained broth, homemade or dried cube.

BOUQUET GARNI
A mixture of herbs used to flavor soups, stews and sauces, etc.

BREADCRUMBS
Dried bread, made into a coarse meal to coat food.

CARAMELIZE
Gently heat foods until the sugars turn golden brown.

CHOP
Cut up in small chunks.

CLARIFY
Remove impurities from liquid or fat by heating, skimming, straining.

CREAM
Mix and beat with a spoon or fork until soft and fluffy.

CROÛTONS
Tiny cubes of bread, baked or fried until golden brown and crisp, used to garnish soups, salads, and other dishes.

CROUSTADE
A French culinary term meaning a small crust or pie-crust of any type, often made of flaky pastry or puff pastry.

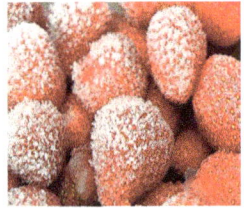

DEEP FRY
Immerse in sufficient hot fat or oil to cover food.

DREDGE
Sprinkle over food, usually with flour or sugar.

DRIZZLE
Pour liquid very slowly and gently over food.

DRY FRY
Quickly fry in pan without oil or fat.

EMULSIFY
Quickly whisk two liquids that do not easily blend (e.g., oil and vinegar in a dressing).

EXTRACT (juice)
Separate solid and liquid components of fruit or vegetables by squeezing or pressing.

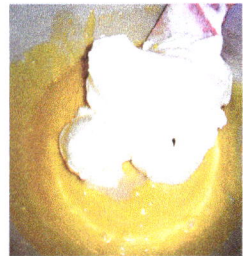

FOLD
Combine whisked mixtures by cutting and turning with a metal spoon to retain lightness.

FRY
Cook with fat in an open pan.

GARNISH
Decorate or embellish.

GLACÉ
Coat with a thin sugar or syrup.

GLAZE
Coat food to give glossy finish, usually with beaten egg, egg white, milk, syrup, sugar glaze or reduced juices.

GRATE
Reduce food to small strips by rubbing on a serrated surface.

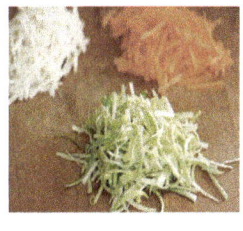

GRILL
Cook food under a heat source, with or without the addition of fat.

JULIENNE
This is a culinary knife cut in which the food item is cut into long thin strips, similar to matchsticks.

KNEAD
Work dough by folding, stretching, and pummeling with heel of hand.

MARINATE
Soak food in seasoned liquid to tenderize and flavor before cooking.

PARE
Thinly peel vegetables or fruit.

PARBOIL
Boil or simmer until partially cooked.

PICKLE
Preserve vegetables in brine, vinegar, oil, and spices.

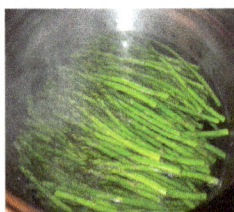

PLUNGE
Cool rapidly by immersing in cold water or crushed ice.

POACH
Cook food in liquid which must be kept just below boiling point.

PROOFING Active dry yeast
Adding a small amount of water and sweetener to yeast so that it activates and bubbles.

PURÉE
Pulp of vegetables or fruit sieved, mashed, or ground to a smooth paste.

REDUCE
Rapidly boil a liquid to reduce in volume, thereby thickening and concentrating the flavor.

ROAST
Bake with some fat in the oven.

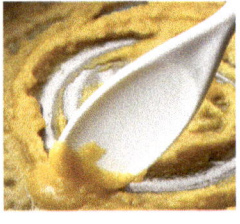

ROUX
Melted butter or fat combined with an equal amount of flour, used for thickening sauces, soups or gravies.

SAUTÉ
Cook food quickly in hot fat on a medium-hot heat, shaking or stirring pan often to prevent sticking or browning.

SCALD
Heat liquid to a temperature just below boiling point.

SCORE
To make cuts or slashes with the point of a knife.

SIEVE/SIFT
Pass dried goods through a fine mesh in order to remove lumps.

SIMMER
Cook food immersed in a liquid kept just below boiling point, similar to poaching, but for longer periods of cooking. (Soups and stews are simmered without ever being brought to the boil.)

SKIM
Remove film from surface after first boiling fruit, sugar, or stock.

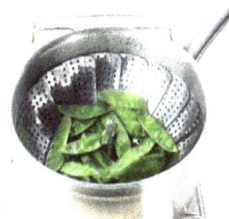

STEAM
Cook with steam. Can be done in a steamer, which is a covered sieved container placed over boiling water, or food placed in a basin which is then put into, but not covered by, boiling water in a covered container.

STEW
Cook food with liquid slowly in a covered container.

STIR FRY
Cook small pieces of vegetables, etc., rapidly by stirring them in a wok or frying pan over high heat.

TINE
Prong the bottom of dough with a fork.

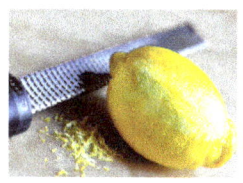

ZEST
Thinly peel or grate outer skin of citrus without getting to the inner white pith.

RECIPE INDEX BY CHAPTER

CHAPTER ONE: HEALING FOODS

Magical Greens
- Saag Paneer (or Tofu) 25
- Kale and White Bean Soup 26
- Healing Green Drinks.. 27

Healing Soups
- Chetna's Chilled Summer Soups 29
- Fire Roasted Gazpacho 30
- Chilled Mango Soup—Two Ways 31
- Grandma's Hungarian Cabbage Soup................ 32

Cooking with Flower Essences
- Tranquility Potato Salad 34
- Contented Hummus Lavash Roll 35
- Confident Lassi Drink 36
- Orange Mango Energy Punch 36

CHAPTER TWO: THE WORLDWIDE BLUE ZONES

Blue Zone Diet
- Lemony Red Lentil Stew....................................... 40
- Simple Everyday Soup 41
- Simple Spicy Tofu Stir Fry.................................... 42
- Green Pesto 43
- Black Bean Cornbread Casserole 44
- Sardinian Minestrone Stew and Lemon Couscous 45

Blue Zone Breads
- Limey Sweet Potato Cake 47
- Simple Sourdough.. 48
- Corn Tortillas.. 50
- Whole Grain Pita Bread 51
- Adventist Unleavened Communion Bread....... 52

CHAPTER THREE: VEGETABLES AND TOFU

Vegetables from the Farm
- Carrot/Sweet Potato Custard Bake 56
- Homemade Rainbow Coleslaw 57
- Crusty Homefried Potatoes & Peas with Spicy Dill Sauce... 58
- Garden Fresh-Baked Herbed Tomatoes 59
- Caramelized Double-Baked Squash 60
- Everyday Garlic Broccoli Stir Fry....................... 61
- Carrots and Pine Nut Medley 62
- A Day in the Life of Tofu...................................... 63
- Smokin' Veggie Tofu Chili.................................... 64
- Olive Tofu-Herb Salad 65
- Marinaded & Grilled Tofu with Thai Sauce 66

Veggie Burgers
- Spicy Japanese Tofu-Eggplant Burger................ 68
- Portobello Lentil Burger 69
- Madras Red Pepper-Peanut Burger.................... 70
- Zucchini-Black Bean-Chipotle Burgers 71

Saturday Market Morning
- Chopped Salad with Tempeh............................... 73
- Cranberry/Orange Relish..................................... 74
- Zesty Zucchini Stir Fry 75
- Sesame Brown Rice and Red Scallions 76

Summer Tomatoes
    Chetna's Tomato Mozzarella Salad 78
    Red Pepper-Lentil-Tomato Blended Soup 79
    Roasted Tomato Salsauce 80

CHAPTER FOUR: BREAKFAST, BREAD, AND SOUP

The Rooster's Call
    Homemade Yogurt 83
    Homemade Soy Yogurt 84
    Homemade Coconut Yogurt 84
    Nova Scotia Maple Granola 85
    Low-fat Nutty and Seedy Granola 85
    Oatmeal and Fruit 86

Bread of Life
    Whole Grain Brown Bread 88
    Coconut-Apple Braided Bread 91
    Thyme for Sweet Potato Rolls 92
    The 1 - 2 Paradox Rice Bread 93
    New York Gluten-Free Bagels 94
    Delightful Gluten-Free Sandwich Bread 95

Soup Daze
    Pea in the Bonnet Soup 97
    Roasted Garlic Carrot/Ginger Soup 98
    Ramani's Cheesy Potato Soup 99
    Madame Lepape's Leek and Potato Soup 100
    Jeanne's Kabocha Pumpkin Soup 101
    Chickpea/Sweet Potato Soup 102

CHAPTER FIVE: QUICK & SIMPLE

The Pasta & Sauce Party
    Elegant Eggplant Tomato Sauce surprise 105
    Simple Light Tomato Sauce 106
    Miso Tomato Sauce 106
    Toasted Pine-Walnut Pesto 107
    Creamy Tofu Sauce 107
    Tomato/Basil Bruschetta 108
    Simple Pasta 108

Simple Yet Elegant
    Conscious Couscous and Vegetables 110
    No-Pressure Veggie Soup 111
    A Maj Jongg Afternoon 112

    Roasted Veggie Soup 113
    Savory Potato Puffs 114
    The Easiest and Best Darn Cornbread Ever! .. 115
    Ginger/Banana/Pecan Fingers 116

CHAPTER SIX: SAUCES, SALADS, DRESSINGS, AND SPICES

Toppings that Sing
    Fresh Spicy Tofu-Peanut Sauce 119
    All Purpose Nutty Sauce 119
    Creamy Vegan Cashew Sauce 120
    Simple Miso Sauce 120
    Double Seed Dip 121
    Sweet and Sour Mango/Ginger Chutney 121
    Easy Coconut Sauce 122
    Triple-Smoked Barbecue Sauce 122
    Green Tea Dipping Sauce, Two Ways 123

Dressing the Salad
    Dad's Salad Bar 125
    Oriental Ginger Dressing 126
    Everyday Herb Dressing 126
    Miso/Carrot Dressing 127

Spice Mixtures
    Joan's Curry Powder Blend 131
    Garam Masala 132

Herbs de Provence
    Anne's Ratatouille 134
    Herbed Baked Pita Triangles 134
    Rainy Day Herbed Sesame-Rye Crackers 135
    Roasted Herbed Sweet Potatoes 136
    Savory Herb-Infused Rice 136

CHAPTER SEVEN: SEASONAL DISHES

Spring Lightness
    Tofu Non-Egg Salad Wrap 139
    Matthew's Famous Guacamole 140
    Roasted Red Pepper, Mushroom,
        Asparagus Sandwich 141
    Salsa Fresca 141
Spring Fare
    Country Kasha Varniskas: Buckwheat &
        Noodles 143

Just-Picked Steamed Asparagus
    with Dilly White Sauce 144
Rhubarb and Strawberry Crisp 145

Spring Cleansing
    Healing Juice Fast 147
    Simple Healing Soup 147
    Edamame Salad with Gomasio 148
    Curry Tempeh Stir Fry 149
    Grape and Dried Fig Cobbler 150

New Year's Feast: 2001: Year of the Snake
    Simple and Traditional Lotus-Root Salad 153
    Delightful Tofu-Spinach Salad 153
    Sweet & Sour So Simple Black Beans 154
    Chestnut Mount Fuji Dessert 154
    Traditional Soba Noodle New Year's Dinner .. 155

Coming Together: 2003: Year of the Sheep
    Herb-Crusted Roasted Veggies 157
    Saffron/Cardamom Thai Rice 158
    Savory Spinach Pockets 159
    Maple/Lemony Tarts 160

CHAPTER EIGHT: INTERNATIONAL CUISINE

Grandma's Specialties
    Grandma's Everyday Eggplant Spread 163
    Two Unique Spreads 164
    Kasha Knish Appetizer 165
    Kasha Knish Appetizer (cont'd) 166
    Grandma's Rugelach 167
    Grandma Pauline's Thumbprint Cookies 168

Stuffing the Pita
    Homemade Falafel 170
    Punchy Baba Ghanouj 171
    Authentic Pita Bread 172

A Japanese Meal
    Broccoli & Carrot Salad with
        Sesame-Ginger Dressing 175
    Traditional Udon Noodle Soup 176
    Broiled Tofu Steak 177
    Miso 178
    Tomiko's Miso Show 179
    Orange Almond Miso Vinaigrette 180
    Miso Sauce & Spread 181
    Classic Miso Stir Fry 182

CHAPTER NINE: GUEST RECIPES

Ki's
    Grilled Tempeh Marinade 186
    Avocado Salsa 187
    Ki's Roasted Vegetables 188
    Roasted Tofu 188

Garden Taste
    Sheila's Famous Garden Taste Roll 190
    Classic Lentil Soup 191
    Garden Taste Salad with Sesame Dressing 192

Kitchen Consciousness
    Red Lentil Dahl 196
    Whole Wheat Chapatis 197
    Tomato Vegetable Sauce 198
    Pumpkin Pasta Salad 199
    French Bread 200

Baking at the Edge of the Universe
    Country Pear Cake 203
    Spicy Persimmon Jam 204
    Russian River Sourdough Rye Bread 205

Dasaprakash
    Sambar (Lentil Soup) 209
    Mixed Vegetable Kurma 210

CHAPTER TEN: COOKING FOR KIDS

Fun Projects in the Kitchen
    Three Kid Friendly Activities 213
    Kids Mealtime 214

School Ideas
    Corny Cornbread 215
    Lentil Balls 216
    Simple Zucchini Patties 217
    Super Creamy Rainbow Spaghetti
        and Spirals 218
Snacks and Healthy Desserts
    Crunchy Trail Mix 220

Gaga Muffins..221
Kid friendly Cookies 222
Fresh Berry Cake or Cupcakes 223
Mini Banana Bread 224

CHAPTER ELEVEN: EAST INDIAN COOKING

A Day in the Indian Kitchen: Indian Vegetables
Pan-Fried Green Beans..................................227
Eggplant Curry..228
Tofu or Paneer and Zucchini Red Curry 229
Coconut Cauliflower and Potato Curry 230

An Indian Meal
Upma 233
Potato and Green Pepper Vegetables.............234
Vegetable Yogurt Sauce—Raita.....................235
Fried Okra 236

South Indian Specialties
Dosa 238
Idli 240
Tiffin..241
Dahi Vada..242
Pakora: Vegetable Fritters.............................243
Chana Dhokla 244
Crispy Chickpea Cookie Bread 245

Chutney
Coconut Chutney 247
Mint or Coriander Chutney............................248
Tomato Chutney...249

Rice
Fragrant Vegetable Rice................................254
Soothing Yogurt Rice 255
Lemon Rice 256

Dhal Day
Savory Split Mung Dhal with Spinach..........259
Split Pea Dhal..260
Hearty Chickpea Curry..................................261

Mumbai Kitchen
Stir-Fried Gourd or Zucchini 263
Ujju's Heavenly Tomato Soup 264
Bombay Baigan Bharta (Eggplant Curry)........265
Eggplant Masala (Spice) Rice Balls 266

CHAPTER TWELVE: TIMELESS SWEETS

Pies
Traditional Pie Crusts....................................269
Wheat-Free Crusts 270
More Wheat-Free Crusts 271
Blueberry Crumble Pie 272
Mom's Apple Pie 273
Creamy Pecan Pie 274
Holiday Pumpkin Pie 275
Intense Chocolate Tart...................................276

Cakes, Cookies, and Bars
Organic Pineapple-Carrot
    Celebration Cake 278
Holiday Biscotti 279
Rhubarb-Raspberry Cobbler 280
Raspberry-Pecan Bars 281
Oatmeal-Date Squares...................................282
Healthy Dark Chocolate Mocha Brownies 283
Aunt Bea's Poppy Seed Moon Cookies...........284
Peanut Butter/Nut Chip Cookie.....................285
Mini Chocolate Chip Coconut Cookies..........286
Oatmeal/Walnut-Raisin Cookies 287
Vegan Mango/Sorbet Gluten-Free Sandwich .288
Gluten-Free Cardamom Rose Cupcakes.........289
Gluten-Free Chip Blondies 290

Creamy Creations
Cashew Cheese 291
Spicy Pumpkin Custard..................................292
Fruity Yogurt Tart 293
Easy Loganberry Light Ice Cream 294
Strawberry or Raspberry Ice Cream...............295

Indian Desserts
Halva Pudding...297
Mataji's Carrot Burfi (Fudge)............................298
Rice Pudding...299
Tropical Fruit Salad.......................................300
Refreshing Indian Mango Sorbet...................301
Traditional Almond Milk (Badam Kheer)......302
Chai Tea..302

RECIPE INDEX BY TITLE

ADVENTIST UNLEAVENED COMMUNION BREAD 52
ALL PURPOSE NUTTY SAUCE 119
ANNE'S RATATOUILLE 134
AUNT BEA'S POPPY SEED MOON COOKIES 284
AUTHENTIC PITA BREAD 172
AVOCADO SALSA 187
BLACK BEAN CORNBREAD CASSEROLE 44
BLUEBERRY CRUMBLE PIE 272
BOMBAY BAIGAN BHARTA (EGGPLANT CURRY) 265
BROCCOLI & CARROT SALAD WITH SESAME-GINGER DRESSING 175
BROILED TOFU STEAK 177
CARAMELIZED DOUBLE-BAKED SQUASH 60
CARROT/SWEET POTATO CUSTARD BAKE 56
CARROTS AND PINE NUT MEDLEY 62
CASHEW CHEESE 291
CHAI TEA 302
CHANA DHOKLA 244
CHESTNUT MOUNT FUJI DESSERT 154
CHETNA'S CHILLED SUMMER SOUPS 29
CHETNA'S TOMATO MOZZARELLA SALAD 78
CHICKPEA/SWEET POTATO SOUP 102
CHILLED MANGO SOUP—TWO WAYS 31
CHOPPED SALAD WITH TEMPEH 73
CLASSIC LENTIL SOUP 191
CLASSIC MISO STIR FRY 182
COCONUT-APPLE BRAIDED BREAD 91
COCONUT CAULIFLOWER AND POTATO CURRY 230
COCONUT CHUTNEY 247
CONFIDENT LASSI DRINK 36
CONSCIOUS COUSCOUS AND VEGETABLES 110
CONTENTED HUMMUS LAVASH ROLL 35
CORN TORTILLAS 50
CORNY CORNBREAD 215
COUNTRY KASHA VARNISKAS: BUCKWHEAT & NOODLES 143
COUNTRY PEAR CAKE 203
CRANBERRY/ORANGE RELISH 74
CRCREAMY PECAN PIE 274
CREAMY TOFU SAUCE 107
CREAMY VEGAN CASHEW SAUCE 120
CRISPY CHICKPEA COOKIE BREAD 245
CRUNCHY TRAIL MIX 220
CRUSTY HOMEFRIED POTATOES &
    PEAS WITH SPICY DILL SAUCE 58
CURRY TEMPEH STIR FRY 149
DAD'S SALAD BAR 125
DAHI VADA 242
DELIGHTFUL GLUTEN-FREE SANDWICH BREAD 95
DELIGHTFUL TOFU-SPINACH SALAD 153
DOSA 238
DOUBLE SEED DIP 121
EASY COCONUT SAUCE 122
EASY LOGANBERRY LIGHT ICE CREAM 294
EDAMAME SALAD WITH GOMASIO 148
EGGPLANT CURRY 228
EGGPLANT MASALA (SPICE) RICE BALLS 266
ELEGANT EGGPLANT TOMATO SAUCE SURPRISE 105
EVERYDAY HERB DRESSING 126
EVERYDAY GARLIC BROCCOLI STIR FRY 61
FIRE ROASTED GAZPACHO 30
FRAGRANT VEGETABLE RICE 254
FRENCH BREAD 200
FRESH SPICY TOFU-PEANUT SAUCE 119
FRESH BERRY CAKE OR CUPCAKES 223
FRIED OKRA 236
FRUITY YOGURT TART 293
GAGA MUFFINS 221

GARAM MASALA	132
GARDEN FRESH-BAKED HERBED TOMATOES	59
GARDEN TASTE SALAD WITH SESAME DRESSING	192
GINGER/BANANA/PECAN FINGERS	116
GLUTEN-FREE CARDAMOM ROSE CUPCAKES	289
GLUTEN-FREE CHIP BLONDIES	290
GRANDMA PAULINE'S THUMBPRINT COOKIES	168
GRANDMA'S EVERYDAY EGGPLANT SPREAD	163
GRANDMA'S HUNGARIAN CABBAGE SOUP	32
GRANDMA'S RUGELACH	167
GRAPE AND DRIED FIG COBBLER	150
GREEN PESTO	43
GREEN TEA DIPPING SAUCE, TWO WAYS	123
GRILLED TEMPEH MARINADE	186
HALVA PUDDING	297
HEALING GREEN DRINKS	27
HEALING JUICE FAST	147
HEALTHY DARK CHOCOLATE MOCHA BROWNIES	283
HEARTY CHICKPEA CURRY	261
HERB-CRUSTED ROASTED VEGGIES	157
HERBED BAKED PITA TRIANGLES	134
HOLIDAY BISCOTTI	279
HOLIDAY PUMPKIN PIE	275
HOMEMADE COCONUT YOGURT	84
HOMEMADE FALAFEL	170
HOMEMADE RAINBOW COLESLAW	57
HOMEMADE SOY YOGURT	84
HOMEMADE YOGURT	83
IDLI	240
INTENSE CHOCOLATE TART	276
JEANNE'S KABOCHA PUMPKIN SOUP	101
JOAN'S CURRY POWDER BLEND	131
JUST-PICKED STEAMED ASPARAGUS WITH DILLY WHITE SAUCE	144
KALE AND WHITE BEAN SOUP	26
KASHA KNISH APPETIZER (CONT'D)	166
KASHA KNISH APPETIZER	165
KI'S ROASTED VEGETABLES	188
KID FRIENDLY COOKIES	222
LEMON RICE	256
LEMONY RED LENTIL STEW	40
LENTIL BALLS	216
LIMEY SWEET POTATO CAKE	47
LOW-FAT NUTTY AND SEEDY GRANOLA	85
MADAME LEPAPE'S LEEK AND POTATO SOUP	100
MADRAS RED PEPPER-PEANUT BURGER	70
MAPLE/LEMONY TARTS	160
MARINADED & GRILLED TOFU WITH THAI SAUCE	66
MATAJI'S CARROT BURFI (FUDGE)	298
MATTHEW'S FAMOUS GUACAMOLE	140
MINI BANANA BREAD	224
MINI CHOCOLATE CHIP COCONUT COOKIES	286
MINT OR CORIANDER CHUTNEY	248
MISO SAUCE & SPREAD	181
MISO TOMATO SAUCE	106
MISO/CARROT DRESSING	127
MIXED VEGETABLE KURMA	210
MOM'S APPLE PIE	273
MORE WHEAT-FREE CRUSTS	271
NEW YORK GLUTEN-FREE BAGELS	94
NO-PRESSURE VEGGIE SOUP	111
NOVA SCOTIA MAPLE GRANOLA	85
OATMEAL AND FRUIT	86
OATMEAL/WALNUT-RAISIN COOKIES	287
OATMEAL-DATE SQUARES	282
OLIVE TOFU-HERB SALAD	65
ORANGE ALMOND MISO VINAIGRETTE	180
ORANGE MANGO ENERGY PUNCH	36
ORGANIC PINEAPPLE-CARROT CELEBRATION CAKE	278
ORIENTAL GINGER DRESSING	126
PAKORA: VEGETABLE FRITTERS	243
PAN-FRIED GREEN BEANS	227
PEA IN THE BONNET SOUP	97
PEANUT BUTTER/NUT CHIP COOKIE	285
PORTOBELLO LENTIL BURGER	69
POTATO AND GREEN PEPPER VEGETABLES	234
PUMPKIN PASTA SALAD	199
PUNCHY BABA GHANOUJ	171
RAINY DAY HERBED SESAME-RYE CRACKERS	135
RAMANI'S CHEESY POTATO SOUP	99
RASPBERRY-PECAN BARS	281
RED LENTIL DAHL	196
RED PEPPER-LENTIL-TOMATO BLENDED SOUP	79
REFRESHING INDIAN MANGO SORBET	301
RHUBARB AND STRAWBERRY CRISP	145
RHUBARB-RASPBERRY COBBLER	280
RICE PUDDING	299
ROASTED GARLIC CARROT/GINGER SOUP	98
ROASTED HERBED SWEET POTATOES	136
ROASTED RED PEPPER, MUSHROOM ASPARAGUS SANDWICH	141
ROASTED TOFU	188
ROASTED TOMATO SALSAUCE	80
ROASTED VEGGIE SOUP	113
RUSSIAN RIVER SOURDOUGH RYE BREAD	205
SAAG PANEER (OR TOFU)	25

SAFFRON/CARDAMOM THAI RICE	158
SALSA FRESCA	141
SAMBAR (LENTIL SOUP)	209
SARDINIAN MINESTRONE STEW AND LEMON COUSCOUS	45
SAVORY HERB-INFUSED RICE	136
SAVORY POTATO PUFFS	114
SAVORY SPINACH POCKETS	159
SAVORY SPLIT MUNG DHAL WITH SPINACH	259
SCHOOL IDEAS	215
SESAME BROWN RICE AND RED SCALLIONS	76
SHEILA'S FAMOUS GARDEN TASTE ROLL	190
SIMPLE AND TRADITIONAL LOTUS-ROOT SALAD	153
SIMPLE EVERYDAY SOUP	41
SIMPLE HEALING SOUP	147
SIMPLE LIGHT TOMATO SAUCE	106
SIMPLE MISO SAUCE	120
SIMPLE PASTA	108
SIMPLE SOURDOUGH	48
SIMPLE SPICY TOFU STIR FRY	42
SIMPLE ZUCCHINI PATTIES	217
SPICY MAYO	141
SMOKIN' VEGGIE TOFU CHILI	64
SOOTHING YOGURT RICE	255
SPICY JAPANESE TOFU-EGGPLANT BURGER	68
SPICY PERSIMMON JAM	204
SPICY PUMPKIN CUSTARD	292
SPLIT PEA DHAL	260
STIR-FRIED GOURD OR ZUCCHINI	263
STRAWBERRY OR RASPBERRY ICE CREAM	295
SUPER CREAMY RAINBOW SPAGHETTI AND SPIRALS	218
SWEET & SOUR SO SIMPLE BLACK BEANS	154
SWEET AND SOUR MANGO/GINGER CHUTNEY	121
THE 1 - 2 PARADOX RICE BREAD	93
THE EASIEST AND BEST DARN CORNBREAD EVER!	115
THREE KID FRIENDLY ACTIVITIES	213
THYME FOR SWEET POTATO ROLLS	92
TOASTED PINE-WALNUT PESTO	107
TOFU NON-EGG SALAD WRAP	139
TOFU OR PANEER AND ZUCCHINI RED CURRY	229
TOMATO CHUTNEY	249
TOMATO VEGETABLE SAUCE	198
TOMATO/BASIL BRUSCHETTA	108
TOMIKO'S MISO SHOW	179
TRADITIONAL ALMOND MILK (BADAM KHEER)	302
TRADITIONAL PIE CRUSTS	269
TRADITIONAL SOBA NOODLE NEW YEAR'S DINNER	155
TRADITIONAL UDON NOODLE SOUP	176
TRANQUILITY POTATO SALAD	34
TRIPLE-SMOKED BARBECUE SAUCE	122
TROPICAL FRUIT SALAD	300
TWO UNIQUE SPREADS	164
UJJU'S HEAVENLY TOMATO SOUP	264
UPMA	233
VEGAN FETA	73
VEGAN MANGO/SORBET GLUTEN-FREE SANDWICH	288
VEGAN RICOTTA	58
VEGETABLE YOGURT SAUCE - RAITA	235
WHEAT-FREE CRUSTS	270
WHOLE GRAIN BROWN BREAD	88
WHOLE GRAIN PITA BREAD	51
WHOLE WHEAT CHAPATIS	197
ZESTY ZUCCHINI STIR FRY	75
ZUCCHINI-BLACK BEAN-CHIPOTLE BURGERS	71

GENERAL INDEX

A
Acknowledgments 7
　A Day in the Indian
　　Kitchen 226
　　Coconut Cauliflower and
　　　Potato Curry 230
　　Eggplant Curry 228
　　Pan-Fried Green Beans 227
　　Tofu or Paneer and Zucchini
　　　Red Curry 229
A Day in the Life of Tofu 63
　Marinated & Grilled Tofu with
　　Thai Sauce 66
　Olive Tofu-Herb Salad 65
　Smokin' Veggie Tofu Chili 64
Adventist Unleavened
　Communion Bread 52
A Japanese Meal 173
　Broccoli & Carrot Salad with
　　Sesame-Ginger
　　Dressing 175
　Broiled Tofu Steak 177
　Growing Ginger in Your Home
　　Garden 174
　Traditional Udon Noodle
　　Soup 176
Allergic Reactions 319
All Purpose Nutty Sauce 119
A Mah Jongg Afternoon 112
　Ginger/Banana/Pecan
　　Fingers 116
　Roasted Veggie Soup 113
　Savory Potato Puffs 114
　The Easiest and Best Darn
　　Cornbread Ever 115
An Indian Meal 231
　Fried Okra 236
　Potato and Green Pepper
　　Vegetables 234
　Upma 233
　Vegetable Yogurt Sauce -
　　Raita 235
Anne's Ratatouille 134
Aunt Bea's Poppy Seed Moon
　Cookies 284
Authentic Pita Bread 172
Avocado Salsa 187

B
Baking at the Edge of the
　Universe 201
　Country Pear Cake 203
　Russian River Sourdough Rye
　　Bread 205
　Spicy Persimmon Jam 204
Baking Supplies 306
Berry Frosting 273
Blueberry Crumble Pie 272
Black Bean Cornbread
　Casserole 44
Blooming Active Dry Yeast 88
Blue Zone Diet 38
　Lemony Red Lentil
　　Stew 40
　Simple Everyday Soup 41
　Simple Spicy Tofu Stir fry 42
　Green Pesto 43
　Black Bean Cornbread
　　Casserole 44
　Sardinian Minestrone Stew and
　　Lemon Couscous 45
Blanching Almonds 29
Blue Zone Breads 46
　Limey Sweet Potato Cake 47
　Simple Sourdough 48
　Corn Tortillas 50
　Whole Grain Pita Bread 51
　Adventist Unleavened
　　Communion Bread 52
Bombay Baigan Bharta
　(Eggplant Curry) 265
Bread of Life 87
　Coconut-Apple Braided
　　Bread 91
　New York Gluten-Free
　　Bagels 94
　The 1 - 2 Paradox Rice
　　Bread 93
　Thyme for Sweet Potato
　　Rolls 92
　Whole Grain Brown Bread 88
Broccoli & Carrot Salad with
　Sesame-Ginger Dressing 175
Broiled Tofu Steak 177

C
Cakes, Cookies, and Bars 277
　Aunt Bea's Poppy Seed Moon
　　Cookies 284

Gluten-Free Cardamom Rose Cupcakes 289
Gluten-Free Chip Blondies 290
Healthy Dark Chocolate Mocha Brownies 283
Mini Chocolate Chip Coconut Cookies 286
Oatmeal-Date Squares 282
Oatmeal/Walnut-Raisin Cookies 287
Organic Pineapple-Carrot Celebration Cake 278
Peanut Butter/Nut Chip Cookie 285
Raspberry-Pecan Bars 281
Vegan Mango/Sorbet Gluten-Free Sandwich 288
Caramelized Double-Baked Squash 60
Carrots and Pine Nut Medley 62
Carrot/Sweet Potato Custard Bake 38
Cashew Cheese 291
Chai Tea 302
Chestnut Mount Fuji Dessert 154
Chetna's Chilled Summer Soups 29
Chetna's Tomato Mozzarella Salad 78
Chickpea/Sweet Potato Soup 102
Chilled Mango Soup: Two Ways 31
Chopped Salad with Tempeh 73
Chutney 246
    Coconut Chutney 247
    Mint or Coriander Chutney 248
    Tomato Chutney 249
    Classic Lentil Soup 191
    Classic Miso Stir Fry 182
    Coconut Chutney 247
Coconut-Apple Braided Bread 91
Coming Together: New Year 2003 156
Corny Cornbread 215
Cream Cheese Icing 278

Curry Leaf Powder 249
Herb-Crusted Roasted Veggies 157
Maple/Lemony Tarts 160
Saffron/Cardamom Thai Rice 158
Savory Spinach Pockets 159
Complementary Herbs and Spices 130
Confident Lassi Drink 36
Conscious Couscous and Vegetables 110
Contented Hummus Lavash Roll 35
Cooking with Flower Essences 33
    Confident Lassi Drink 36
    Contented Hummus Lavash Roll 35
    Orange Mango Energy Punch 36
    Tranquility Potato Salad 34
Corn Tortillas 50
Country Kasha Varniskas: Buckwheat & Noodles 143
Country Pear Cake 203
Cranberry/Orange Relish 74
Creamy Creations 291
    Easy Loganberry Light Ice Cream 294
    Fruity Yogurt Tart 293
    Spicy Pumpkin Custard 292
Creamy Pecan Pie 274
Creamy Tofu Sauce 107
Creamy Vegan Cashew Sauce 120
Crunchy Trail Mix 220
Crusty Homefried Potatoes & Peas with Spicy Dill Sauce 58
Curry Tempeh Stir Fry 149

D
Dahi Vada 242
Dad's Salad Bar 125
Dasaprakash 207
    Mixed Vegetable Kurma 210
    Sambar (Lentil Soup) 209
Dashi Japanese stock base 155
Definition of Terms 325

Delightful Gluten-Free Sandwich Bread 95
Delightful Tofu-Spinach Salad 153
Dhal Day 257
Dilly Sauce 58
Dressing for Roasted Veggies 157
Hearty Chickpea Curry 261
Savory Split Mung Dhal with Spinach 259
Split Pea Dhal 260
Discovering Allergies 321
Dosa 238
Double Seed Dip 121
Dressing the Salad 124

E
Easy Baked Applesauce 217
Easy Coconut Sauce 122
Easy Lemon Pickle 258
Easy Low-Sugar Strawberry Jam 215
Edamame Salad with Gomasio 148
Eggplant Curry 228
Eggplant Masala (Spice) Rice Balls 266
Elegant Eggplant Tomato Sauce Surprise 105
Everyday Garlic Broccoli Stir fry 61
Everyday Herb Dressing 126
Exploring Herbs, Spices and Healing Foods 17
    The Color of Healing Foods 19

F
Festive Flavored Butter 92
Fire Roasted Gazpacho 30
For Everything There is a Seasoning 312
Fragrant Vegetable Rice 254
French Bread 200
Fresh Spicy Tofu-Peanut Sauce 119
Fresh Berry Cake or Cupcakes 223
Fried Okra 236

Fruity Yogurt Tart 293
Fun Projects in the Kitchen 212
   Three Kid Friendly Activities 213

G
Gaga Muffins 221
Garam Masala 132
Garnish Seasoning 248
Garden Fresh-Baked Herbed Tomatoes 59
Garden Taste 189
   Classic Lentil Soup 191
   Garden Taste Salad with Sesame Dressing 192
   Sheila's Famous Garden Taste Roll 190
   Garden Taste Salad with Sesame Dressing 192
Ginger/Banana/Pecan Fingers 116
Ginger/Chili Paste 263
Gluten-Free Cardamom Rose Cupcakes 289
Gluten-Free Flour Blends 94
Gluten-Free Chip Blondies 290
Gomasio 148
Grandma Pauline's Thumbprint Cookies 168
Grandma's Hungarian Cabbage Soup 32
Grandma's Everyday Eggplant Spread 163
Grandma's Rugelach 167
Grandma's Specialties 162
   Grandma Pauline's Thumbprint Cookies 148
   Grandma's Everyday Eggplant Spread 163
   Grandma's Rugelach 167
   Kasha Knish Appetizer 165
   Two Unique Spreads 164
Grape and Dried Fig Cobbler 150
Green Beans with Cashews 164
Green Pesto 43
Green Tea Dipping Sauce, Two Ways 123
Grilled Tempeh Marinade 186

Growing Ginger in Your Home Garden 174

H
Halva Pudding 297
Healing Green Drinks 27
Healing Juice Fast 147
Healing Soups 28
   Chetna's Chilled Summer Soups 29
   Chilled Mango Soup—Two Ways 31
   Fire Roasted Gazpacho 30
   Grandma's Hungarian Cabbage Soup 32
Healthy Dark Chocolate Mocha Brownie 283
Hearty Chickpea Curry 261
Herb and Spice Combinations 109
Herb-Crusted Roasted Veggies 157
Herbed Baked Pita Triangles 134
Herbs de Provence 133
   Anne's Ratatouille 134
   Herbed Baked Pita Triangles 134
   Rainy Day Herbed Sesame-Rye Crackers 135
   Roasted Herbed Sweet Potatoes 136
   Savory Herb-Infused Rice 136
Herby Vegetable Peel Stock 41
Holiday Pumpkin Pie 275
Homemade Coconut Yogurt 84
Homemade Falafel 170
Homemade Rainbow Coleslaw 57
Homemade Soy Yogurt 84
Homemade Yogurt 83
How to Make Your Own Pomegranate Juice 69

I
Idli 240
Indian Desserts 296
   Chai Tea 302

   Halva Pudding 297
   Mataji's Carrot Burfi (Fudge) 298
   Refreshing Indian Mango Sorbet 301
   Rice Pudding 299
   Traditional Almond Milk (Badam Kheer) 302
   Tropical Fruit Salad 300
Intense Chocolate Tart 276

J
Jeanne's Kabocha Pumpkin Soup 101
Joan's Curry Powder Blend 131

K
Kale and White Bean Soup 26
Kasha Knish Appetizer 166
Kid Friendly Cookies 222
Kids Mealtime 214
   School Ideas 215
   Lentil Balls 216
   Simple Zucchini Patties 217
   Super Creamy Rainbow Spaghetti and Spirals 218
Ki's 184
   Avocado Salsa 187
   Grilled Tempeh Marinade 186
   Ki's Roasted Vegetables 188
   Roasted Tofu 188
Ki's Roasted Vegetables 188
Kitchen Consciousness 193
   French Bread 200
   Pumpkin Pasta Salad 199
   Red Lentil Dahl 196
   Tomato Vegetable Sauce 198
   Whole Wheat Chapatis 197

L
Lemon Couscous 45
Lemon Juice Extraction 61
Lemon Rice 256
Lemony Red Lentil Stew 40
Lentil Balls 216
Lentil Spread 164
Limey Sweet Potato Cake 47

Living in Harmony 22
Low-fat Nutty and Seedy Granola 85
Low Sugar Strawberry or Raspberry freezer Jam 289

M
Madame Lepape's Leek and Potato Soup 100
Madras Red Pepper-Peanut Burger 70
Magical Greens 24
    Healing Green Drinks 27
    Kale and White Bean Soup 26
    Saag Paneer (or Tofu) 25
Making Paneer (Indian Cheese) 229
Making Your Own Sprouts 42
Maple Glaze for Cookies 168
Maple/Lemony Tarts 160
Marinated & Grilled Tofu with Thai Sauce 66
Mataji's Carrot Burfi (Fudge) 298
Matthew's Famous Guacamole 140
Mini Banana Bread 224
Mini Chocolate Chip Coconut Cookies 286
Mint or Coriander Chutney 248
Miso 178
    Classic Miso Stir Fry 182
    Miso Sauce & Spread 181
    Orange Almond Miso Vinaigrette 180
Miso Topping 47
Tomiko's Miso Show 179
Miso Sauce & Spread 181
Miso Tomato Sauce 106
Miso/Carrot Dressing 127
Mixed Vegetable Kurma 210
Mom's Apple Pie 278
More Wheat-Free Crusts 271
Mumbai Kitchen 262
    Bombay Baigan Bharta (Eggplant Curry) 265
    Eggplant Masala (Spice) Rice Balls 266
    Stir-Fried Gourd or Zucchini 263
    Ujju's Heavenly Tomato Soup 264
My Culinary Journey 16

N
New Year's Feast: 2001 151
    Chestnut Mount Fuji Dessert 154
    Delightful Tofu-Spinach Salad 153
    Ringing of the Bells 152
    Simple and Traditional Lotus-Root Salad 153
    Sweet & Sour So Simple Black Beans 154
    Traditional Soba Noodle New Year's Dinner 155
New York Gluten-Free Bagels 94
No-Pressure Veggie Soup 111
Nova Scotia Maple Granola 85

O
Oatmeal and Fruit 86
Oatmeal-Date Squares 282
Oatmeal/Walnut-Raisin Cookies 287
Olive Tofu-Herb Salad 65
Orange Almond Miso Vinaigrette 180
Orange Mango Energy Punch 36
Organic Pineapple-Carrot Celebration Cake 278

P
Pan-Fried Green Beans 227
Pantry Items and Alternatives 306
Pea in the Bonnet Soup 97
Peanut Butter Chip Cookie 285
Pies 268
    Blueberry Crumble Pie 272
    Creamy Pecan Pie 274
    Holiday Pumpkin Pie 275
    Intense Chocolate Tart 276
    Mom's Apple Pie 273
    More Wheat-Free Crusts 271
    Traditional Pie Crusts 269
Portobello Lentil Burger 69
Potato and Green Pepper Vegetables 234
Potato Package Surprise 55
Pots and Pans 267
Pumpkin Pasta Salad 199
Punchy Baba Ghanouj 171

R
Rainy Day Herbed Sesame-Rye Crackers 135
Ramani's Cheesy Potato Soup 99
Raspberry-Pecan Bars 281
Reasons for the Rise in the Number of Food Allergies 322
Red Lentil Dahl 196
Red Pepper-Lentil-Tomato Blended Soup 79
Refreshing Indian Mango Sorbet 301
Resources 317
Rhubarb and Strawberry Crisp 145
Rhubarb-Raspberry Cobbler 280
Rice 250
    Fragrant Vegetable Rice 254
    Lemon Rice 256
    Soothing Yogurt Rice 255
Rice Pudding 299
Ringing of the Bells 132
Roasted Garlic Carrot/Ginger Soup 98
Roasted Red Pepper, Mushroom, Asparagus Sandwich 141
Roasted Sesame Tofu Soup Garnish 96
Roasted Tofu 188
Roasted Veggie Soup 113
Russian River Sourdough Rye Bread 205

S
Saag Paneer (or Tofu) 25
Saffron/Cardamom Thai Rice 158
Shaken Light Dressing 73
Salsa Fresca 141

Salt and Yeast 91
Sambar (Lentil Soup) 209
Sardinian Minestrone Stew and Lemon Couscous 45
Saturday Market Morning 72
   Chopped Salad with Tempeh 73
   Cranberry/Orange Relish 74
   Sesame Brown Rice and Red Scallions 76
   Zesty Zucchini Stir Fry 75
Savory Herb-Infused Rice 136
Savory Potato Puffs 114
Savory Spinach Pockets 159
Savory Split Mung Dhal with Spinach 259
Sesame Brown Rice and Red Scallions 76
Sheila's Famous Garden Taste Roll 190
Simple and Traditional Lotus-Root Salad 153
Super Creamy Rainbow Spaghetti and Spirals 218
Simple Everyday Soup 41
Simple Healing Soup 147
Simple Light Tomato Sauce 106
Simple Miso Sauce 120
Simple Pasta 108
Simple Miso Sauce 120
Simple Sourdough 48
Simple Spicy Tofu Stir fry 42
Simple Zucchini Patties 217
Simple Yet Elegant 109
   Conscious Couscous and Vegetables 110
   No-Pressure Veggie Soup 111
Smokin' Veggie Tofu Chili 64
Smoky Roasted Garlic Oil 98
Snacks and Healthy Desserts 219
   Crunchy Trail Mix 220
   Fresh Strawberry Cake or Cupcakes 223
   Gaga Muffins 221
   Kid friendly Cookies 222
   Mini Banana Bread 224
Soothing Yogurt Rice 255

Soup Daze 96
   Chickpea/Sweet Potato Soup 102
   Elegant Eggplant Tomato Sauce Surprise 105
   Jeanne's Kabocha Pumpkin Soup 101
   Madame Lepape's Leek and Potato Soup 100
   Pea in the Bonnet Soup 97
   Ramani's Cheesy Potato Soup 99
   Roasted Garlic Carrot/Ginger Soup 98
Soup Base 176
South Indian Specialties 237
   Dosa 238
   Idli 240
Sourdough Starter 48
Spice Mixtures 128
   Complementary Herbs and Spices 130
   Garam Masala 132
   Herb and Spice Combinations 129
   Joan's Curry Powder Blend 131
Spicy Japanese Tofu-Eggplant Burger 68
Spicy Mayo 141
Spicy Pumpkin Custard 292
Spicy Persimmon Jam 204
Spicy-Sweet Dill Pickles 67
Split Pea Dhal 260
Spring Cleansing 146
   Curry Tempeh Stir Fry 149
   Edamame Salad with Gomasio 148
   Grape and Dried Fig Cobbler 150
   Healing Juice Fast 147
   Simple Healing Soup 147
Spring Fare 142
   Country Kasha Varniskas: Buckwheat & Noodles 143
   Just-Picked Steamed Asparagus with Dilly White Sauce 144

   Rhubarb and Strawberry Crisp 145
Spring Lightness 138
   Matthew's Famous Guacamole 140
   Roasted Red Pepper, Mushroom, Asparagus Sandwich 141
   Salsa Fresca 141
   Tofu Non-Egg Salad Wrap 139
Stir-Fried Gourd or Zucchini 263
Stocking the Pantry 304
   Baking Supplies 306
   Pantry Items and Alternatives 306
   Pots and Pans 305
Strawberry or Raspberry Ice Cream 295
Stuffing the Pita 169
   Authentic Pita Bread 172
   Homemade Falafel 170
   Punchy Baba Ghanouj 171
Summer Tomatoes 77
   Chetna's Tomato Mozzarella Salad 78
   Red Pepper-Lentil-Tomato Blended Soup 79
   Roasted Tomato Salsauce 80
Super Creamy Rainbow Spaghetti and Spirals 218
Sweet and Sour Mango/Ginger Chutney 121

T
Tahini Sauce 170
The 1 - 2 Paradox Rice Bread 93
The Allergy Connection 319
   Allergic Reactions 320
   Discovering Allergies 312
   Hidden Dangers 323
   Reasons for the Rise in the Number of Food Allergies 322
The Cold Chaser 192
The Color of Healing Foods 19
The Easiest and Best Darn Cornbread Ever 115

The Genesis of a Manuscript 20
   Living in Harmony 22
The Interdependent Circle 15
   My Culinary Journey 16
The Pasta & Sauce Party 104
   Creamy Tofu Sauce 107
   Elegant Eggplant Tomato Sauce Surprise 105
   Miso Tomato Sauce 106
   Simple Light Tomato Sauce 106
   Simple Pasta 108
   Toasted Pine-Walnut Pesto 107
   Tomato/Basil Bruschetta 108
The Rooster's Call 82
   Homemade Coconut Yogurt 84
   Homemade Soy Yogurt 84
   Homemade Yogurt 83
   Low-fat Nutty and Seedy Granola 85
   Nova Scotia Maple Granola 85
   Oatmeal and Fruit 86
Thyme for Sweet Potato Rolls 92
Tiffin 241
   Chana Dhokla 244
   Crispy Chickpea Cookie Bread 245
   Dahi Vada 242
   Pakora: Vegetable Fritters 243
Toasted Pine-Walnut Pesto 107
Tofu Cream 154
Tofu Non-Egg Salad Wrap 139
Tomato/Basil Bruschetta 108
Tomato Chutney 249
Tomato Vegetable Sauce 198
Tomiko's Miso Show 179

Toppings that Sing 118
   All Purpose Nutty Sauce 119
   Creamy Vegan Cashew Sauce 120
   Double Seed Dip 121
   Easy Coconut Sauce 122
   Fresh Spicy Tofu-Peanut Sauce 119
   Green Tea Dipping Sauce, Two Ways 123
   Simple Miso Sauce 120
   Sweet and Sour Mango/Ginger Chutney 121
   Triple-Smoked Barbecue Sauce 122
Traditional Almond Milk (Badam Kheer) 302
Traditional Pie Crusts 269
Traditional Soba Noodle New Year's Dinner 155
Traditional Udon Noodle Soup 176
Tranquility Potato Salad 34
Triple-Smoked Barbecue Sauce 122
Tropical Fruit Salad 300
Two Unique Spreads 164
Tzatziki Sauce 169

U
Ujju's Heavenly Tomato Soup 264
Upma 233
Upma Cutlets 233

V
Vegetables from the Farm 54
   Caramelized Double-Baked Squash 60
   Carrots and Pine Nut Medley 62
   Carrot/Sweet Potato Custard Bake 56
   Crusty Homefried Potatoes & Peas with Spicy Dill Sauce 58
   Everyday Garlic Broccoli Stir Fry 61
   Garden Fresh-Baked Herbed Tomatoes 59
   Homemade Rainbow Coleslaw 57
Vegan Feta 73
Vegan Mango/Sorbet Gluten-Free Sandwich 288
Vegan Ricotta Cheese 58
Vegetable Yogurt Sauce - Raita 235
Veggie Burgers 49
   Madras Red Pepper-Peanut Burger 70
   Portobello Lentil Burger 69
   Spicy Japanese Tofu-Eggplant Burger 68
   Zucchini-Black Bean-Chipotle Burgers 71

W
Wheat-Free Crusts 270
Whole Grain Brown Bread 88
Whole Grain Pita Bread 51

Z
Zesty Zucchini Stir Fry 75
Zucchini-Black Bean-Chipotle Burgers 71

ABOUT THE AUTHOR

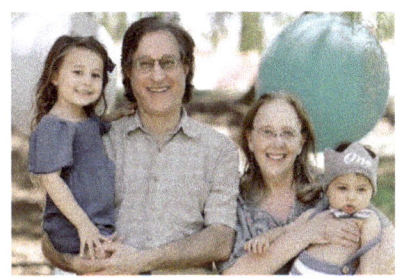 Joan Greenblatt is a magazine columnist, a graphic designer, and a certified flower essence practitioner. She is also a gourmet vegetarian cook. Through her travels and interaction with the cooking styles of diverse cultures, Joan has skillfully captured their essence and fundamental cuisines, which she regularly shared through her cooking column in the award-winning *Inner Directions Journal*. A considerable number of those columns appear throughout this book, along with her culinary reminiscences, which explore the basis of many of the recipes.

Joan, along with her husband Matthew, are co-founders of the INNER DIRECTIONS FOUNDATION. She is also the author of *Healing with Flower Essences: How to Use Natural Botanicals for Spiritual and Emotional Well-Being*. They currently reside in Ventura County, California where they work in the print and online publishing fields. They can often be found taking an evening walk along the beach.

NOTES

USE THIS SPACE FOR TAKING CULINARY NOTES, AS YOU GO THROUGH THE BOOK.

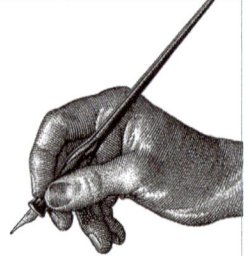

www.ingramcontent.com/pod-product-compliance
Lightning Source LLC
Chambersburg PA
CBHW061809290426
44110CB00026B/2838